Facial Palsy: Diagnostic and Therapeutic Management

Editors

TERESA M. O
NATE JOWETT
TESSA A. HADLOCK

OTOLARYNGOLOGIC CLINICS OF NORTH AMERICA

www.oto.theclinics.com

Consulting Editor
SUJANA S. CHANDRASEKHAR

December 2018 • Volume 51 • Number 6

ELSEVIER

1600 John F. Kennedy Boulevard • Suite 1800 • Philadelphia, Pennsylvania, 19103-2899

http://www.oto.theclinics.com

OTOLARYNGOLOGIC CLINICS OF NORTH AMERICA Volume 51, Number 6
December 2018 ISSN 0030-6665, ISBN-13: 978-0-323-64215-6

Editor: Jessica McCool
Developmental Editor: Sara Watkins

Otolaryngologic Clinics of North America (ISSN 0030-6665) is published bimonthly by Elsevier, Inc., 360 Park Avenue South, New York, NY 10010-1710. Months of issue are February, April, June, August, October, and December. Business and Editorial Offices: 1600 John F. Kennedy Blvd., Suite 1800, Philadelphia, PA 19103-2899. Customer Service Office: 6277 Sea Harbor Drive, Orlando, FL 32887-4800. Periodicals postage paid at New York, NY and additional mailing offices. Subscription prices are $396.00 per year (US individuals), $835.00 per year (US institutions), $100.00 per year (US student/resident), $519.00 per year (Canadian individuals), $1058.00 per year (Canadian institutions), $556.00 per year (international individuals), $1058.00 per year (international institutions), $270.00 per year (international & Canadian student/resident). Foreign air speed delivery is included in all *Clinics'* subscription prices. All prices are subject to change without notice. **POSTMASTER:** Send address changes to *Otolaryngologic Clinics of North America*, Elsevier Health Sciences Division, Subscription Customer Service, 3251 Riverport Lane, Maryland Heights, MO 63043. **Telephone: 1-800-654-2452 (U.S. and Canada); 314-447-8871 (outside U.S. and Canada). Fax: 314-447-8029. E-mail: journalscustomerservice-usa@elsevier.com (for print support); journalsonlinesupport-usa@elsevier.com (for online support).**

Reprints. For copies of 100 or more of articles in this publication, please contact the Commercial Reprints Department, Elsevier Inc., 360 Park Avenue South, New York, NY 10010-1710. Tel.: 212-633-3874; Fax: 212-633-3820; E-mail: reprints@elsevier.com.

Otolaryngologic Clinics of North America is also published in Spanish by McGraw-Hill Interamericana Editores S.A., P.O. Box 5-237, 06500 Mexico D.F., Mexico.

Otolaryngologic Clinics of North America is covered in *MEDLINE/PubMed (Index Medicus), Current Contents/Clinical Medicine, Excerpta Medica, BIOSIS, Science Citation Index,* and *ISI/BIOMED.*

PROGRAM OBJECTIVE

The goal of the *Otolaryngologic Clinics of North America* is to provide information on the latest trends in patient management, the newest advances; and provide a sound basis for choosing treatment options in the field of otolaryngology.

LEARNING OBJECTIVES

Upon completion of this activity, participants will be able to:

1. Review the multimodal approach to outcome tracking for facial palsy.
2. Discuss diagnostic and therapeutic interventions in the management of facial palsy.
3. Recognize the importance of facial expression in social interactions.

ACCREDITATION

The Elsevier Office of Continuing Medical Education (EOCME) is accredited by the Accreditation Council for Continuing Medical Education (ACCME) to provide continuing medical education for physicians.

The EOCME designates this enduring material for a maximum of 15 *AMA PRA Category 1 Credit*(s)™. Physicians should claim only the credit commensurate with the extent of their participation in the activity.

All other health care professionals requesting continuing education credit for this enduring material will be issued a certificate of participation.

DISCLOSURE OF CONFLICTS OF INTEREST

The EOCME assesses conflict of interest with its instructors, faculty, planners, and other individuals who are in a position to control the content of CME activities. All relevant conflicts of interest that are identified are thoroughly vetted by EOCME for fair balance, scientific objectivity, and patient care recommendations. EOCME is committed to providing its learners with CME activities that promote improvements or quality in healthcare and not a specific proprietary business or a commercial interest.

The planning committee, staff, authors and editors listed below have identified no financial relationships or relationships to products or devices they or their spouse/life partner have with commercial interest related to the content of this CME activity:
Nicholas S. Andresen, MD; Jennifer Baiungo, PT, MS; Kofi Derek Boahene, MD; Gregory Borschel, MD, FACS, FAAP; Patrick Byrne, MD; Sujana S. Chandrasekhar, MD; Maura K. Cosetti, MD; Leahthan F. Domeshek, MD; Joseph R. Dusseldorp, MBBS, MS, FRACS; Aaron Fay, MD; Julia L. Frisenda, MD; Bruce J. Gantz, MD; Tessa A. Hadlock, MD; Natalie Homer, MD; Lisa E. Ishii, MD, MHS; Masaru Ishii, MD, PhD; Andrew William Joseph, MD, MPH; Nate Jowett, MD; Vivian Kaul, MD; Alison Kemp; Jennifer C. Kim, MD; Marissa Purcelli Lafer, MD; Jessica McCool; Suresh Mohan, MD; Jason C. Nellis, MD; Teresa M. O, MD, MArch, FACS; James A. Owusu, MD; Alicia M. Quesnel, MD; Mara Wernick Robinson, PT, MS, NCS; Felipe Santos, MD; Daniel Q. Sun, MD; Subhalakshmi Vaidyanathan; Martinus M. van Veen, MD; Sara Watkins; Ronald Zuker, MD, FRCS, FACS, FAAP.

The planning committee, staff, authors and editors listed below have identified financial relationships or relationships to products or devices they or their spouse/life partner have with commercial interest related to the content of this CME activity:
Babak Azizzadeh, MD, FACS: receives royalties from John Wiley & Sons, Inc., Thieme Medical Publishers, Inc., Elsevier, and Springer Nature Switzerland AG.

UNAPPROVED/OFF-LABEL USE DISCLOSURE

The EOCME requires CME faculty to disclose to the participants:

1. When products or procedures being discussed are off-label, unlabelled, experimental, and/or investigational (not US Food and Drug Administration [FDA] approved); and
2. Any limitations on the information presented, such as data that are preliminary or that represent ongoing research, interim analyses, and/or unsupported opinions. Faculty may discuss information about pharmaceutical agents that is outside of FDA-approved labelling. This information is intended solely for CME and is not intended to promote off-label use of these medications. If you have any questions, contact the medical affairs department of the manufacturer for the most recent prescribing information.

TO ENROLL

To enroll in the *Otolaryngologic Clinics of North America* Continuing Medical Education program, call customer service at 1-800-654-2452 or sign up online at http://www.theclinics.com/home/cme. The CME program is available to subscribers for an additional annual fee of USD 260.

METHOD OF PARTICIPATION

In order to claim credit, participants must complete the following:

1. Complete enrolment as indicated above.
2. Read the activity.
3. Complete the CME Test and Evaluation. Participants must achieve a score of 70% on the test. All CME Tests and Evaluations must be completed online.

CME INQUIRIES/SPECIAL NEEDS

For all CME inquiries or special needs, please contact elsevierCME@elsevier.com.

Contributors

CONSULTING EDITOR

SUJANA S. CHANDRASEKHAR, MD, FACS, FAAOHNS
Past President, American Academy of Otolaryngology–Head and Neck Surgery, Partner, ENT & Allergy Associates, LLP, Clinical Professor, Department of Otolaryngology–Head and Neck Surgery, Zucker School of Medicine at Hofstra-Northwell, Hempstead, New York, USA; Clinical Associate Professor, Department of Otolaryngology–Head and Neck Surgery, Icahn School of Medicine at Mount Sinai, New York, New York, USA

EDITORS

TERESA M. O, MD, MArch, FACS
Director, Facial Nerve Center, Vascular Birthmark Institute of New York, Department of Otolaryngology–Head and Neck Surgery, Manhattan Eye, Ear, and Throat Hospital, Lenox Hill Hospital, New York, New York, USA

NATE JOWETT, MD
Assistant Professor, Department of Otolaryngology, Division of Facial Plastic and Reconstructive Surgery, Massachusetts Eye and Ear, Harvard Medical School, Boston, Massachusetts, USA

TESSA A. HADLOCK, MD
Chief, Division of Facial Plastic and Reconstructive Surgery, Professor, Department of Otolaryngology–Head and Neck Surgery, Massachusetts Eye and Ear, Harvard Medical School, Boston, Massachusetts, USA

AUTHORS

NICHOLAS S. ANDRESEN, MD
Department of Otolaryngology–Head and Neck Surgery, Johns Hopkins School of Medicine, Baltimore, Maryland, USA

BABAK AZIZZADEH, MD, FACS
Associate Clinical Professor, Division of Head and Neck Surgery, David Geffen School of Medicine at UCLA, Los Angeles, California, USA; Center for Advanced Facial Plastic Surgery, Beverly Hills, California, USA

JENNIFER BAIUNGO, PT, MS
Physical Therapist, Facial Plastic and Reconstructive Surgery Department, Facial Nerve Center, Massachusetts Eye and Ear, Facial Nerve Center, Boston, Massachusetts, USA

KOFI DEREK BOAHENE, MD
Professor, Otolaryngology–Head and Neck Surgery, Johns Hopkins School of Medicine, Department of Otorhinolaryngology, The Johns Hopkins Hospital, Baltimore, Maryland, USA

GREGORY H. BORSCHEL, MD, FACS, FAAP
Division of Plastic and Reconstructive Surgery, The Hospital for Sick Children, Toronto, Ontario, Canada

PATRICK BYRNE, MD
Professor, Otolaryngology–Head and Neck Surgery, Johns Hopkins School of Medicine, Baltimore, Maryland, USA

MAURA K. COSETTI, MD
Department of Otolaryngology–Head and Neck Surgery, Icahn School of Medicine at Mount Sinai, New York Eye and Ear Infirmary of Mount Sinai, New York, New York, USA

LEAHTHAN F. DOMESHEK, MD
Division of Plastic and Reconstructive Surgery, The Hospital for Sick Children, Toronto, Ontario, Canada

JOSEPH R. DUSSELDORP, MBBS, MS, FRACS
Senior Lecturer, Department of Otolaryngology–Head and Neck Surgery, Massachusetts Eye and Ear, Harvard Medical School, Boston, Massachusetts, USA; Department of Plastic and Reconstructive Surgery, Royal Australasian College of Surgeons, University of Sydney, Sydney, Australia

AARON FAY, MD
Massachusetts Eye and Ear, Boston, Massachusetts, USA

JULIA L. FRISENDA, MD
Center for Advanced Facial Plastic Surgery, Beverly Hills, California, USA

BRUCE J. GANTZ, MD
Professor and Chair, Department of Otolaryngology–Head and Neck Surgery, University of Iowa Hospitals & Clinics, Iowa City, Iowa, USA

TESSA A. HADLOCK, MD
Chief, Division of Facial Plastic and Reconstructive Surgery, Professor, Department of Otolaryngology–Head and Neck Surgery, Massachusetts Eye and Ear, Harvard Medical School, Boston, Massachusetts, USA

NATALIE HOMER, MD
Department of Ophthalmology, Massachusetts Eye and Ear, Harvard Medical School, Boston, Massachusetts, USA

LISA E. ISHII, MD, MHS
Professor, Otolaryngology–Head and Neck Surgery, Johns Hopkins School of Medicine, Baltimore, Maryland, USA

MASARU ISHII, MD, PhD
Associate Professor, Otolaryngology–Head and Neck Surgery, Johns Hopkins School of Medicine, Baltimore, Maryland, USA

ANDREW WILLIAM JOSEPH, MD, MPH
Clinical Lecturer, Department of Otorhinolaryngology–Head and Neck Surgery, Division of Facial Plastic and Reconstructive Surgery, University of Michigan Medical School, Ann Arbor, Michigan, USA

NATE JOWETT, MD
Assistant Professor, Department of Otolaryngology, Division of Facial Plastic and Reconstructive Surgery, Massachusetts Eye and Ear, Harvard Medical School, Boston, Massachusetts, USA

VIVIAN KAUL, MD
Department of Otolaryngology–Head and Neck Surgery, Icahn School of Medicine at Mount Sinai, New York Eye and Ear Infirmary of Mount Sinai, New York, New York, USA

JENNIFER C. KIM, MD
Associate Professor, Department of Otorhinolaryngology–Head and Neck Surgery, Division of Facial Plastic and Reconstructive Surgery, University of Michigan Medical School, Ann Arbor, Michigan, USA

MARISSA PURCELLI LAFER, MD
Resident, Department of Otolaryngology–Head and Neck Surgery, New York University, New York, New York, USA

SURESH MOHAN, MD
Department of Otolaryngology–Head and Neck Surgery, Massachusetts Eye and Ear, Harvard Medical School, Boston, Massachusetts, USA

JASON C. NELLIS, MD
Resident, Otolaryngology–Head and Neck Surgery, Johns Hopkins School of Medicine, Baltimore, Maryland, USA

TERESA M. O, MD, MArch, FACS
Director, Facial Nerve Center, Vascular Birthmark Institute of New York, Department of Otolaryngology–Head and Neck Surgery, Manhattan Eye, Ear, and Throat Hospital, Lenox Hill Hospital, New York, New York, USA

JAMES A. OWUSU, MD
Department of Head and Neck Surgery, Mid-Atlanatic Permanente Medical Group, McLean, Virginia, USA

ALICIA M. QUESNEL, MD
Assistant Professor, Department of Otolaryngology, Otology, Neurotology, and Skull Base Surgery, Massachusetts Eye and Ear, Harvard Medical School, Boston, Massachusetts, USA

MARA WERNICK ROBINSON, PT, MS, NCS
Physical Therapist, Facial Plastic and Reconstructive Surgery Department, Facial Nerve Center, Massachusetts Eye and Ear, Boston, Massachusetts, USA

FELIPE SANTOS, MD
Assistant Professor, Department of Otolaryngology, Otology, Neurotology, and Skull Base Surgery, Massachusetts Eye and Ear, Harvard Medical School, Boston, Massachusetts, USA

DANIEL Q. SUN, MD
Assistant Professor, Department of Otolaryngology–Head and Neck Surgery, Johns Hopkins University School of Medicine, Baltimore, Maryland, USA

MARTINUS M. VAN VEEN, MD
Department of Otolaryngology–Head and Neck Surgery, Massachusetts Eye and Ear, Harvard Medical School, Boston, Massachusetts, USA; Department of Plastic Surgery, University Medical Center Groningen, University of Groningen, Groningen, The Netherlands

RONALD M. ZUKER, MD, FRCS, FACS, FAAP
Division of Plastic and Reconstructive Surgery, The Hospital for Sick Children, Toronto, Ontario, Canada

Contents

occurs within a few hours to days. The differential diagnosis is broad; however, the most common cause is viral-associated Bell Palsy. A comprehensive history and physical examination are essential in arriving at a diagnosis. Medical treatment for acute FP depends on the specific diagnosis; however, corticosteroids and antiviral medications are the cornerstone of therapy. Lack of recovery after 4 months should prompt further diagnostic workup.

Bell palsy and traumatic facial nerve injury are two common causes of acute facial palsy. Most patients with Bell palsy recover favorably with medical therapy alone. However, those with complete paralysis (House-Brackmann 6/6), greater than 90% degeneration on electroneurography, and absent electromyography activity may benefit from surgical decompression via a middle cranial fossa (MCF) approach. Patients with acute facial palsy from traumatic temporal bone fracture who meet these same criteria may be candidates for decompression via an MCF or translabyrinthine approach based on hearing status.

Flaccid facial paralysis results in disfiguring facial changes. The treatment of flaccid facial paralysis is complex and treatment approaches should be determined based on duration and the causes of paralysis, status and accessibility of the affected facial nerve, medical comorbidities, and patient-specific goals. Although primary nerve repair is the preferred treatment strategy when possible, nerve substitution procedures are the mainstay of treatment for patients with flaccid facial paralysis of less than 2 years duration.

Ineffective eyelid closure can pose a serious risk of injury to the ocular surface and eye. In cases of eyelid paresis, systematic examination of the eye and ocular adnexa will direct appropriate interventions. Specifically, 4 distinct periorbital regions should be independently assessed: eyebrow, upper eyelid, ocular surface, and lower eyelid. Corneal exposure can lead to dehydration, thinning, scarring, infection, perforation, and blindness. Long-term sequelae following facial nerve palsy may also include epiphora, gustatory lacrimation, and synkinesis.

Masseter and temporalis muscle transfer is an effective technique for restoring facial symmetry and commissure excursion in flaccid facial paralysis. Adherence to the principles and biomechanics of muscle transfer is essential for achieving optimal results. Muscle transfer has the advantage of being single staged with fast recovery of function. It is particularly useful in patients with low life expectancy or multiple comorbidities where a more complex, multiple stage procedure may be detrimental.

 Video content accompanies this article at https://www.oto.theclinics.com/.

This article presents an approach to reanimation of the midface in long-standing flaccid facial palsy by means of functional free gracilis transfer and static facial suspension.

Chronic flaccid facial paralysis (FFP>2 years) may be approached with static and dynamic techniques. A horizontal zonal assessment evaluates the upper, middle, and lower thirds of the face. Surgery is tailored to an individual's deficits, goals, and health status. While dynamic reanimation is the gold standard for rehabilitation, there are cases in which static approaches are more appropriate or may be used as an adjunct to dynamic techniques. This article focuses on the surgical management of FFP primarily using static approaches to the individual zones of the face to create resting symmetry.

 Video content accompanies this article at http://oto.theclinics.com/.

This article describes the most widely used clinician-graded and patient-reported outcome measures, and describes facial rehabilitation strategies for acute and chronic facial palsy, and rehabilitation following dynamic facial reanimation surgery. The multimodality rehabilitation of the facial palsy patient is determined by the extent of facial nerve injury, specific functional deficits, the presence of synkinesis, and the patient's individual goals. Appropriate intervention, including patient education, soft tissue mobilization, neuromuscular reeducation, and chemodenervation, decreases facial tension and improves facial muscle motor control, physical function, facial expression, and quality of life.

 Video content accompanies this article at http://www.oto.theclinics.com/.

Modified selective neurectomy of the distal branches of the buccal, zygomatic, and cervical branches of the facial nerve in addition to platysmal myotomy is an effective surgical procedure for the treatment of postfacial paralysis synkinesis. Success of this procedure depends on identification of the peripheral facial nerve branches, preservation of zygomatic and marginal mandibular branches that innervate key smile muscles, and ablation of buccal and cervical branches that cause lateral and/or inferior excursion of the oral commissure. Results are long-lasting; objective improvements in electronic clinician-graded facial function scale score, House-Brackmann score, and decreased botulinum toxin-A requirements have been observed.

Facial nerve schwannomas are benign peripheral nerve sheath tumors that arise from Schwann cells, and most commonly present with facial paresis and/or hearing loss. Computed tomography and MRI are critical to diagnosis. Management decisions are based on tumor size, facial function, and hearing status. Observation is usually the best option in patients with good facial function. For patients with poor facial function, the authors favor surgical resection with facial reanimation. There is growing evidence to support radiation treatment in patients with progressively worsening moderate facial paresis and growing tumors.

Current consensus on optimal treatment of vestibular schwannoma remains poorly established; treatment options include observation, stereotactic radiosurgery, microsurgical resection, medical therapy, or a combination of these. Treatment should be individualized and incorporate the multitude of patient- and tumor-specific characteristics known to affect outcome. Treatment paradigms for sporadic and neurofibromatosis type 2–related tumors are distinct and decision-making in neurofibromatosis type 2 is uniquely challenging. In all cases, treatment should maximize tumor control and minimize functional deficit.

Bilateral facial paralysis is a rare entity that occurs in both pediatric and adult patients and can have congenital or acquired causes. When paralysis does not resolve with conservative or medical management, surgical intervention may be indicated. This article presents the authors' preferred technique for facial reanimation in patients with bilateral congenital facial paralysis. Specifically, a staged bilateral segmental gracilis transfer to ipsilateral nerve to masseter is discussed.

OTOLARYNGOLOGIC CLINICS
OF NORTH AMERICA

SERIES OF RELATED INTEREST

Facial Plastic Surgery Clinics November 2017 (Vol. 25, No. 4)
Trauma in Facial Plastic Surgery
Kris S. Moe, *Editor*
Available at: https://www.facialplastic.theclinics.com/

THE CLINICS ARE AVAILABLE ONLINE!
Access your subscription at:
www.theclinics.com

Foreword

You're Never Fully Dressed Without a Smile

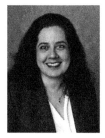

Sujana S. Chandrasekhar, MD, FACS, FAAOHNS
Consulting Editor

Whether we like it or not, judgments based on facial appearance play a powerful role in how we treat others and how we ourselves are treated. Psychologists have long known that attractive people achieve better outcomes in practically all walks of life. We have all heard, "You never get a second chance to make a first impression." What is striking is that the judgment during the first impression is made within 1/10th of one second.[1]

It is obvious, therefore, that people with acute facial palsy or paralysis are immediately aware of their deformity and are extremely frightened that it will be permanent. Individuals with residual facial palsy have higher rates of depression and social withdrawal.[2]

The parents of a child born with unilateral or bilateral facial palsy seek help and need qualified counseling and intervention quickly. Acquired isolated facial palsy affects 25 to 120 per 100,000, and is idiopathic, which is called Bell palsy, in 70% of cases. However, because it can be mistaken for a stroke (cerebrovascular accident), these patients are evaluated on an emergent basis. Moreover, whether it is idiopathic, viral, related to tumor, infection, trauma, or iatrogenic, this likewise demands comprehensive and timely intervention.

Drs O, Jowett, and Hadlock have compiled this issue of *Otolaryngologic Clinics of North America* addressing all the issues that arise when managing these patients and helping to restore their quality of life, starting with an article devoted to the psychology of facial expression. Having an outline of the approach to facial palsy aids the clinician when they are confronted with a scared and worried patient and family. Knowing how to track outcomes allows us to be honest and ethical in our estimations of our own work and to communicate with other clinicians accurately.

Because of the emotional response to acute facial paralysis, patients seek, and physicians provide, all sorts of medical interventions. The article on medical management cuts through the haze to offer evidence-based options. Surgery for acute facial palsy,

Otolaryngol Clin N Am 51 (2018) xv–xvi
https://doi.org/10.1016/j.otc.2018.08.019
0030-6665/18/© 2018 Published by Elsevier Inc.

discussed in detail, is challenging, due to potential delays in presentation, difficulty pinpointing the site of the injury, and, in some cases, surgical team discomfort with the middle cranial fossa approach needed to decompress the 3-mm labyrinthine segment of the nerve.

Flaccid facial paralysis is divided into that of less than 2 years' duration, and that of more. Different approaches are needed for each, and for the various muscle groups supplied by each branch of the facial nerve. These considerations, and the medical and surgical treatment options for them, are explored in each of the corresponding articles. Just as with all other facets of medicine and surgery, physicians cannot work in isolation if the patient is to have the best outcome. The article on facial rehabilitation illustrates what can be done to achieve success. Synkinesis is a very troubling consequence of facial paralysis, and that article highlights methods to address this.

Rare disorders affect facial nerve function and are addressed in the last three articles. Benign tumors affecting the facial nerve have consequences that are not benign at all. The articles on facial nerve schwannoma and on management of the facial nerve in both sporadic and neurofibromatosis-2–related vestibular schwannomas are helpful guides on how to assess, plan, counsel, and act. Bilateral facial nerve palsy, which accounts for less than 2% of all facial palsy, demands a comprehensive workup to look for the underlying cause, and then creative interventions.

The line, "You're never fully dressed without a smile," was written by Martin Charnin for the Broadway musical *Annie*.[3,4] In the show, a beaming smile transforms surly New Yorkers into happy, friendly people, illustrating the potent power of facial expression. I again congratulate Drs Teresa O, Nate Jowett, and Tessa Hadlock on putting together this thorough issue of *Otolaryngologic Clinics of North America* with such excellent authors and articles. I hope you enjoy reading all of it, as I have.

Sujana S. Chandrasekhar, MD, FACS, FAAOHNS
ENT & Allergy Associates, LLP
18 East 48th Street, 2nd Floor
New York, NY 10017, USA

Zucker School of Medicine at Hofstra-Northwell
Hempstead, NY 11549, USA

Icahn School of Medicine at Mount Sinai
New York, NY 10029, USA

E-mail address:
ssc@nyotology.com

REFERENCES

1. Willis J, Todorov A. First impressions: making up your mind after a 100-ms exposure to a face. Psychol Sci 2006;17(7):592–8.
2. Chang Y-S, Choi JE, Kim SW, et al. Prevalence and associated factors of facial palsy and lifestyle characteristics: data from the Korean National Health and Nutrition Examination Survey 2010–2012. BMJ Open 2016;6(11):e012628.
3. Erlewine S. "Annie [Original Broadway Cast] [Remastered]". AllMusic.com. All Media Network.
4. "Charnin overview". Allmusic.com.

Preface

Facial Palsy: Diagnostic and Therapeutic Management

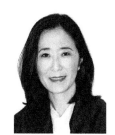
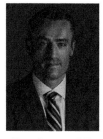
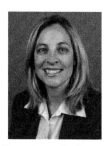

Teresa M. O, MD, MArch   Nate Jowett, MD   Tessa A. Hadlock, MD
Editors

Facial expression is an evolutionary adaption facilitating successful social interaction. Muscles of facial expression are pivotal to nonverbal communication, articulation, and corneal protection. Facial palsy results in functional, communicative, and social impairment with profound negative impact on quality of life and emotional well-being. Congenital absence or acute facial nerve insult results in flaccid paralysis. Ultimate recovery following facial nerve insult lies on a spectrum from persistence of dense paralysis to return of normal function; in between zonal permutations of varying degrees of static and kinetic hypoactivity and hyperactivity and synkinesis exist. Owing to the tireless efforts of innovators in the field, such as Korte, Gillies, Smith, House, Fisch, Harii, and O'Brien among others, manifold therapeutic options to reduce long-term sequelae and restore facial balance and function to patients stricken with this devastating condition exist.

Management of facial palsy can be daunting. This issue of *Otolaryngologic Clinics of North America* provides a framework for classification and state-of-the-art management of facial palsy deficits by zone and duration of palsy, with articles authored by leading experts in the field. We hope it becomes a valuable addition to the libraries

Otolaryngol Clin N Am 51 (2018) xvii–xviii
https://doi.org/10.1016/j.otc.2018.08.018
0030-6665/18/© 2018 Published by Elsevier Inc.

of facial nerve clinicians across the globe and serves as inspiration to future generations to advance the field.

Teresa M. O, MD, MArch
Facial Nerve Center, Department of Otolaryngology–
Head and Neck Surgery
Manhattan Eye, Ear, and Throat Hospital
210 East 64th Street
New York, NY 10065, USA

Nate Jowett, MD
Division of Facial Plastic &
Reconstructive Surgery
Massachusetts Eye & Ear
Harvard Medical School
243 Charles Street
Boston, MA 02114, USA

Tessa A. Hadlock, MD
Division of Facial Plastic &
Reconstructive Surgery
Massachusetts Eye & Ear
Harvard Medical School
243 Charles Street
Boston, MA 02114, USA

E-mail addresses:
to@vbiny.org (T.M. O)
nate_jowett@meei.harvard.edu (N. Jowett)
tessa_hadlock@meei.harvard.edu (T.A. Hadlock)

The Importance and Psychology of Facial Expression

Lisa E. Ishii, MD, MHS*, Jason C. Nellis, MD,
Kofi Derek Boahene, MD, Patrick Byrne, MD, Masaru Ishii, MD, PhD

KEYWORDS

- Facial paralysis • Smile • Psychology • Facial expression • Quality of life
- Psychosocial heath • Social perceptions • Psychological distress

KEY POINTS

- Facial expression is critical in successful social engagement.
- Individuals with impaired facial expression from facial paralysis experience impaired social engagement.
- Reconstructive surgery to restore facial expression in patients with facial paralysis normalizes their social perception.

INTRODUCTION

The human face is critical in social interactions, providing nonverbal cues regarding a person's identity, race, sexual dimorphism, emotion, and overall health.[1] In the normal state, emotional contagion and mimicry occur through the exchange of facial expressions and subconscious mimicry.[2] Thus, when facial appearance is disrupted, as occurs when a person has a facial deformity, this may lead to significant psychosocial distress. The specific facial deformity of facial paralysis where facial movement impairment occurs thus has the potential to substantially impact social interaction.

The psychological distress associated with facial deformity has been well characterized.[3] Several studies have evaluated the relationship between societal perceptions, patient perceptions, and the penalty on social interactions caused by limited facial expression. Herein, the authors describe the relevant literature and discuss the penalties of limited facial expression associated with facial paralysis.

Disclosure Statement: Nothing to disclose.
Otolaryngology–Head and Neck Surgery, Johns Hopkins School of Medicine, 601 North Caroline Street, Baltimore, MD 21287, USA
* Corresponding author.
E-mail address: learnes2@jhmi.edu

Impact of Limited Facial Expression on Observer Perceptions

To investigate social perceptions of facial paralysis and limited facial expression, various approaches have been used to compare how casual observers gaze on faces with facial paralysis and impaired facial expression as compared with those who have normal facial function. A series of studies have been performed to measure the impact of impaired facial expression on casual observer gaze. In a randomized controlled experiment including 60 casual observers, Ishii and colleagues[4] used infrared eye-gaze tracker technology to record observers gazing on paralyzed and normal faces. The study found that casual observers gaze on a paralyzed face differently, with greater attention to the mouth, compared with a normal face, especially when smiling. In addition, when Su and colleagues[5] showed a large group of close to 400 casual observers images of paralyzed faces, the casual observers were remarkably good at identifying that facial paralysis was present. Furthermore, the accuracy of detection increased when they were shown faces smiling as compared with faces in repose.

Other studies have used wisdom-of-the-crowds methodology, where random observers were surveyed to rate patients with facial paralysis across various domains. To understand the effect of facial paralysis on affect display, Ishii and colleagues[6] showed 40 random naïve observers pictures of paralyzed faces and normal faces, capturing observer-perceived emotion, including happiness, disgust, anger, sadness, or fear, and whether patients appeared trustworthy, friendly, tired, hostile, energetic, or neutral. In this study, observers perceived paralyzed faces as having a negative affect most of the time compared with normal faces. In a similar study investigating layperson perception of emotions, Bogart and colleagues[7] showed 121 undergraduate students short videos of patients with facial paralysis across a range of severity. The observers were asked to rate the faces on intensity of happiness or sadness. In this study, participants rated individuals with severe facial paralysis as much less happy than those with mild facial paralysis.

Other studies have shown that facial paralysis and loss of facial expression result in other negative perceptions. Ishii and colleagues[8] asked 40 casual observers to identify a paralyzed face and rate the attractiveness of paralyzed faces as compared with normal faces. Observers accurately identified facial paralysis and rated paralyzed faces as significantly less attractive compared with normal faces. Furthermore, Li and colleagues[9] demonstrated that casual observers perceive patients with facial paralysis as less normal, more distressed, less trustworthy, and less intelligent. A supplementary investigation of isolated facial palsies revealed that isolated upper zygomatic branch palsy (ie, impaired eye closure) results in the highest social penalty, whereas frontal palsy results in the lowest social penalty.

With casual observer perception as a backdrop, additional studies examined the relationship between patient and observer perceptions. In a prospective study by Goines and colleagues[10] investigating quality of life and disability, 84 naïve observers rated perceived quality of life and facial paralysis–related disability in patients with facial paralysis and control patients while simultaneously capturing patient-reported quality of life. They found that observers rated quality of life lower than the patients rated themselves. Furthermore, Dey and colleagues[11] found that clinicians also perceive patients with facial paralysis more negatively than patients perceive themselves with regards to attractiveness, severity of facial dysfunction, and quality of life.

Does Facial Reanimation Surgery Restore Normalcy?

Clearly, impaired facial expression results in significant social penalty that increases with the severity of facial paralysis and subsequent impairment in facial expression.

Numerous facial reanimation procedures exist, with many of them having the primary goal of restoring facial expression. A series of studies have been carried out to measure the impact of various facial reanimation procedures on restoring normalcy of facial expression. Dey and colleagues[12] investigated the impact of facial reanimation surgery on affect display. In this study, 90 naïve observers rated affect display for 20 patients with severe facial paralysis (ie, HB [House Brackmann] IV or greater) before and after facial reanimation surgery. Casual observers viewed photographs of patients who underwent both dynamic and static procedures as well as control patients. It was shown that facial reanimation significantly improved affect display, especially when smiling. There was no significant difference between postoperative and control ratings when in repose.

In a different study investigating attractiveness, Dey and colleagues[13] noted that casual observers rated patients significantly more attractive after surgery. However, patients were not completely normalized when compared with controls. To further understand the impact of surgery on social perceptions, Su and colleagues[14] measured observer-graded health state utilities, quality of life, and willingness to pay for surgery for patients before and after facial reanimation surgery. In this study, casual observers viewed images of patients with facial paralysis. Observers rated facial reanimation surgery as highly valuable with a mean willingness to pay per quality-adjusted life-year of $10,167 for low-grade facial paralysis, and $17,008 for high-grade facial paralysis.

Next, researchers investigated the ability of facial reanimation surgery to normalize the way that casual observers gaze on faces with impaired facial expression from facial paralysis. An eye-tracker was used to measure the gaze patterns of casual observers gazing on paralyzed faces before and after facial reanimation surgery.[15] Analysis of the eye-gaze patterns showed that surgery normalized many of the hemifacial gaze asymmetries resulting from facial paralysis. This objective evidence provided additional support for the effectiveness of facial reanimation surgery to restore facial expression and normalcy.

IMPACT OF FACIAL PARALYSIS FROM PATIENT PERSPECTIVE
Quality of Life

In addition to investigating the impact of facial paralysis and impaired facial expression on societal perceptions, multiple studies have also investigated the psychosocial effect that patients with impaired facial expression from facial paralysis experience. In fact, multiple validated quality-of-life metrics exist, including the Facial Clinimetric Evaluation Scale (FaCE) and the Facial Disability Index (FDI).[16,17] In a cross-sectional survey mailed to approximately 1600 patients following extirpation of vestibular schwannoma, Ryzenman and colleagues[18] found that approximately one-third of patients were significantly distressed by their facial paralysis even though most of them had some form of treatment to address the facial paralysis.

Studying patients with facial nerve weakness after parotidectomy, Prats-Golczer and colleagues[19] found a significant decrease in FDI scores in the first 3 months after surgery. Most of the patients included in this study had isolated marginal mandibular nerve weakness, and all had total recovery of facial nerve function at 12 months. In fact, their FDI scores improved after 12 months. In a retrospective cohort of patients with facial paralysis, Kleiss and colleagues[20] showed that facial paralysis severity and female gender were inversely correlated with FaCE scores. However, Volk and colleagues[21] were not able to demonstrate that changes in psychosocial patient-reported scores correlate with facial paralysis severity. Furthermore, Leong and

Lesser[22] demonstrated a correlation between younger age and worse social function among patients who developed facial paralysis following vestibular schwannoma surgery. In contrast, Strobel and Renner[23] did not find significantly reduced quality of life in children with Moebius syndrome compared with normative data. Several prospective observational studies have measured FaCE, FDI, and validated health status instruments in patients with facial paralysis from various causes, finding increased facial impairment leads to worse physical and social function.[24–26] A few studies have investigated the effect of facial reanimation on quality of life. In a cohort of 127 patients with flaccid facial paralysis, Lindsay and colleagues[27] demonstrated that patients had significantly improved quality of life after free gracilis muscle transfer. In addition, studies have found that botulinum toxin treatment of facial hyperkinesis can significantly improve patient quality of life.[28,29]

Depression

The distress experienced by patients with diminished capacity for facial expression may increase their risk for depression. Investigators have attempted to understand the prevalence of depression and anxiety in patients with facial paralysis. In a cross-sectional survey of 103 patients with facial paralysis, Fu and colleagues[30] found that approximately 31% of patients had significant levels of anxiety and depression as measured on the Hospital Anxiety and Depression Scale. In a similar study, Bradbury and colleagues[31] found that 11.4% of patients had depression and 35% of patients had anxiety. Furthermore, in their studies, patients with depression were more likely to be dissatisfied with reconstructive procedures. At a tertiary referral center for facial paralysis, Walker and colleagues[32] found the prevalence of depression or anxiety as high as 60%, with similar prevalence noted in other studies. However, these studies were limited by the absence of a comparison group. In a prospective observational study, Nellis and colleagues[26] found that patients with facial paralysis, and particularly those with higher grades of facial dysfunction, had significantly higher depression scores, lower self-reported attractiveness, lower mood scores, and lower quality-of-life scores compared with control patients without facial paralysis. Furthermore, female gender was associated with increased depression.

Impaired Facial Expression Leads to Other Psychosocial Distress

In addition to the anxiety and depression experienced by patients with facial paralysis and impaired facial expression, a host of other studies have demonstrated additional psychosocial penalties, including impaired nonverbal communication. One study demonstrated that patients with Moebius syndrome had significant impairment in facial expression and facial identity recognition when compared with controls.[23] When appearance-related psychological distress was measured in patients with facial palsy following vestibular schwannoma extirpation, Cross and colleagues[33] found variable levels of distress that were greatest among patients with low self-esteem using the Derriford appearance scale. Bogart and colleagues[34] demonstrated that patients with acquired facial paralysis had reduced compensatory expressive behavior as compared with patients with congenital facial paralysis, suggesting that developmental stage at onset of facial paralysis impacts long-term expressiveness.

SUMMARY

Impaired facial expression from facial paralysis results in multiple psychosocial penalties from the perspective of both the casual observer and the patient. Thus, facial paralysis and impaired facial expression dramatically influence the way patients engage with society. As described herein, multiple studies demonstrated that casual observers perceive patients with facial paralysis as less attractive, more distressed, less trustworthy, less intelligent, and more negative. Furthermore, it has been shown that casual observers gaze on paralyzed faces differently than those without. It follows that casual observers may be less inclined to engage with those patients based on those perceptions. Moreover, when casual observers do interact with individuals with facial paralysis, they may misinterpret the facial expressions leading to a negative experience for both. As was noted in the Su and colleagues study, the paralysis was more conspicuous to casual observers when patients were smiling. Thus, a patient attempting to express a positive emotion may instead be perceived negatively in society by the casual observer. Fortunately, facial reanimation surgery leads to improved perception as rated by the casual observer.

There are limitations to the current literature that must be taken into consideration. Many of the findings were from proof-of-concept studies that included as subjects patients with the highest severity levels of facial paralysis. Additional studies that include a spectrum of severity of facial paralysis and limited facial expression will be needed to fully understand the penalties. Furthermore, although a wisdom-of-the-crowds approach was used in many of the studies described herein, based on the demographics, they are not necessarily generalizable to the entire population. Additional studies exploring the full spectrum of the impaired facial expression deformity will be needed to fully characterize the impact of limited facial expression.

Nonetheless, the aggregate data clearly suggest that impaired facial expression from facial paralysis leads to psychosocial penalties. Providers should consider specific education about this for patients and their family members so that they will anticipate and cope with these social situations accordingly. Furthermore, providers should remain finely attuned for evidence of depression, anxiety, and other psychological distress in their patients with impaired facial expression from facial paralysis.

REFERENCES

1. Frith C. Role of facial expressions in social interactions. Philos Trans R Soc Lond B Biol Sci 2009;364(1535):3453–8.
2. Baaren RBV, Holland RW, Kawakami K, et al. Mimicry and prosocial behavior. Psychol Sci 2004;15(1):71–4.
3. Macgregor FC. Facial disfigurement: problems and management of social interaction and implications for mental health. Aesthetic Plast Surg 1990;14(4):249–57.
4. Ishii L, Dey J, Boahene KD, et al. The social distraction of facial paralysis: Objective measurement of social attention using eye-tracking. Laryngoscope 2016;126(2):334–9.
5. Su P, Ishii LE, Nellis J, et al. Societal identification of facial paralysis and paralysis location. JAMA Facial Plast Surg 2018;20(4):272–6.
6. Ishii LE, Godoy A, Encarnacion CO, et al. What faces reveal: impaired affect display in facial paralysis. Laryngoscope 2011;121(6):1138–43.
7. Bogart K, Tickle-Degnen L, Ambady N. Communicating without the face: holistic perception of emotions of people with facial paralysis. Basic Appl Soc Psych 2014;36(4):309–20.
8. Ishii L, Godoy A, Encarnacion CO, et al. Not just another face in the crowd: society's perceptions of facial paralysis. Laryngoscope 2012;122(3):533–8.
9. Li MK, Niles N, Gore S, et al. Social perception of morbidity in facial nerve paralysis. Head Neck 2016;38(8):1158–63.

10. Goines JB, Ishii LE, Dey JK, et al. Association of facial paralysis-related disability with patient- and observer-perceived quality of life. JAMA Facial Plast Surg 2016; 18(5):363–9.

11. Dey JK, Ishii LE, Nellis JC, et al. Comparing patient, casual observer, and expert perception of permanent unilateral facial paralysis. JAMA Facial Plast Surg 2017; 19(6):476–83.

12. Dey JK, Ishii M, Boahene KD, et al. Facial reanimation surgery restores affect display. Otol Neurotol 2014;35(1):182–7.

13. Dey JK, Ishii M, Boahene KD, et al. Changing perception: facial reanimation surgery improves attractiveness and decreases negative facial perception. Laryngoscope 2014;124(1):84–90.

14. Su P, Ishii LE, Joseph A, et al. Societal value of surgery for facial reanimation. JAMA Facial Plast Surg 2017;19(2):139–46.

15. Dey JK, Ishii LE, Byrne PJ, et al. Seeing is believing: objectively evaluating the impact of facial reanimation surgery on social perception. Laryngoscope 2014; 124(11):2489–97.

16. Ho AL, Scott AM, Klassen AF, et al. Measuring quality of life and patient satisfaction in facial paralysis patients: a systematic review of patient-reported outcome measures. Plast Reconstr Surg 2012;130(1):91–9.

17. Pavese C, Cecini M, Camerino N, et al. Functional and social limitations after facial palsy: expanded and independent validation of the Italian version of the facial disability index. Phys Ther 2014;94(9):1327–36.

18. Ryzenman JM, Pensak ML, Tew JM Jr. Facial paralysis and surgical rehabilitation: a quality of life analysis in a cohort of 1,595 patients after acoustic neuroma surgery. Otol Neurotol 2005;26(3):516–21 [discussion: 521].

19. Prats-Golczer VE, Gonzalez-Cardero E, Exposito-Tirado JA, et al. Impact of dysfunction of the facial nerve after superficial parotidectomy: a prospective study. Br J Oral Maxillofac Surg 2017;55(8):798–802.

20. Kleiss IJ, Hohman MH, Susarla SM, et al. Health-related quality of life in 794 patients with a peripheral facial palsy using the FaCE Scale: a retrospective cohort study. Clin Otolaryngol 2015;40(6):651–6.

21. Volk GF, Granitzka T, Kreysa H, et al. Nonmotor disabilities in patients with facial palsy measured by patient-reported outcome measures. Laryngoscope 2016; 126(7):1516–23.

22. Leong SC, Lesser TH. A national survey of facial paralysis on the quality of life of patients with acoustic neuroma. Otol Neurotol 2015;36(3):503–9.

23. Strobel L, Renner G. Quality of life and adjustment in children and adolescents with Moebius syndrome: Evidence for specific impairments in social functioning. Res Dev Disabil 2016;53-54:178–88.

24. VanSwearingen JM, Cohn JF, Turnbull J, et al. Psychological distress: linking impairment with disability in facial neuromotor disorders. Otolaryngol Head Neck Surg 1998;118(6):790–6.

25. Volk GF, Granitzka T, Kreysa H, et al. Initial severity of motor and non-motor disabilities in patients with facial palsy: an assessment using patient-reported outcome measures. Eur Arch Otorhinolaryngol 2017;274(1):45–52.

26. Nellis JC, Ishii M, Byrne PJ, et al. Association among facial paralysis, depression, and quality of life in facial plastic surgery patients. JAMA Facial Plast Surg 2017; 19(3):190–6.

27. Lindsay RW, Bhama P, Hadlock TA. Quality-of-life improvement after free gracilis muscle transfer for smile restoration in patients with facial paralysis. JAMA Facial Plast Surg 2014;16(6):419–24.

28. Mehta RP, Hadlock TA. Botulinum toxin and quality of life in patients with facial paralysis. Arch Facial Plast Surg 2008;10(2):84–7.
29. Streitova H, Bares M. Long-term therapy of benign essential blepharospasm and facial hemispasm with botulinum toxin A: retrospective assessment of the clinical and quality of life impact in patients treated for more than 15 years. Acta Neurol Belg 2014;114(4):285–91.
30. Fu L, Bundy C, Sadiq SA. Psychological distress in people with disfigurement from facial palsy. Eye (Lond) 2011;25(10):1322–6.
31. Bradbury ET, Simons W, Sanders R. Psychological and social factors in reconstructive surgery for hemi-facial palsy. J Plast Reconstr Aesthet Surg 2006; 59(3):272–8.
32. Walker DT, Hallam MJ, Ni Mhurchadha S, et al. The psychosocial impact of facial palsy: our experience in one hundred and twenty six patients. Clin Otolaryngol 2012;37(6):474–7.
33. Cross T, Sheard CE, Garrud P, et al. Impact of facial paralysis on patients with acoustic neuroma. Laryngoscope 2000;110(9):1539–42.
34. Bogart KR, Tickle-Degnen L, Ambady N. Compensatory expressive behavior for facial paralysis: adaptation to congenital or acquired disability. Rehabil Psychol 2012;57(1):43–51.

A General Approach to Facial Palsy

Nate Jowett, MD

KEYWORDS

- Facial palsy • Facial reanimation • Facial nerve • Synkinesis

KEY POINTS

- Facial palsy is a devastating condition encompassing a spectrum of movement disorders that range from flaccid paralysis to postparalytic facial hyperactivity.
- Timing and selection of diagnostic and therapeutic interventions in facial palsy are critical.
- Therapeutic management may comprise medical therapy, surgical decompression, physical therapy, injectable fillers, and surgical reanimation procedures.

INTRODUCTION

Facial palsy (FP) is a devastating condition with functional and esthetic sequelae resulting in profound quality-of-life (QOL) impairment.[1,2] When acquired, the inciting insult typically results in acute flaccid facial palsy (FFP). Depending on the degree of neural injury, ultimate outcomes range from persistent and complete FFP to full return of normal function. In between these extremes exist zonal permutations of hypoactivity and hyperactivity and synkinesis, often with symptomatic gustatory epiphora and facial discomfort, a condition known as postparalytic facial nerve syndrome[3,4] which arises from aberrant regeneration of the facial nerve.[5,6] For clarity, a summary of pertinent definitions is provided in **Table 1**. This article provides a diagnostic and therapeutic management approach to FP.

HISTORY AND PHYSICAL EXAMINATION

It is incumbent upon the treating clinician to establish a diagnosis for the underlying cause of the facial movement disorder. Causes of acute FP include Bell palsy, Ramsay-Hunt syndrome (varicella zoster virus), Lyme disease, otic infections and cholesteatomas, postsurgical insult (eg, following vestibular schwannoma extirpation), benign tumors (eg, facial nerve schwannomas or venous vascular malformations of

Disclosure Statement: The author has nothing to disclose.
Division of Facial Plastic and Reconstructive Surgery, Department of Otolaryngology, Massachusetts Eye and Ear Infirmary, Harvard Medical School, 243 Charles Street, Boston, MA 02114, USA
E-mail address: nate_jowett@meei.harvard.edu

Otolaryngol Clin N Am 51 (2018) 1019–1031
https://doi.org/10.1016/j.otc.2018.07.002
oto.theclinics.com

Table 1
Relevant definitions

Term	Definition
Facial palsy	Term encompassing entire spectrum of facial movement disorders, including flaccid facial palsy, facial paresis, and postparalytic facial palsy
Flaccid facial palsy	Complete or near-complete absence of facial movement and tone, without synkinesis or hyperactivity
Facial synkinesis	Involuntary and abnormal facial muscle activation accompanying volitional or spontaneous expression
Postparalytic facial nerve syndrome	Syndrome comprising facial synkinesis, facial muscle rigidity, spasm, contracture, or pain. Gustatory epiphora (also known as Bogorad syndrome or crocodile tears) is often present. The syndrome is thought to result from aberrant axonal regeneration or ephaptic transmission following facial nerve insult
Postparalytic facial palsy	Facial movement disorder of postparalyic facial nerve syndrome, comprising varying degrees of zonal synkinesis, hypoactivity, and hyperactivity

the facial nerve), or malignant tumors (eg, parotid or hematogenous primaries, regional spread of cutaneous malignancies, or solid tumor metastases), congenital malformations, systemic infections (eg, human immunodeficiency virus, syphillis), autoimmune conditions (eg, antiphospholid antibody syndrome, sarcoidosis, systemic lupus erythematosus, Sjogen's), granulomatous diseases (eg, Melkersson-Rosenthal syndrome, sarcoidosis), and trauma.[7] Although rare, pontine infarcts or hemorrhages may present with isolated FP.[8]

The time course of palsy onset, progression, prior therapies, resultant symptoms, and their impact on facial function and QOL are documented. A thorough history is invaluable in establishing the diagnosis; the clinician may inquire as to the presence of otovestibular symptoms (hearing loss, hyperacusis, vertigo, imbalance, otorrhea, otalgia), other focal neurologic deficits (eg, diplopia, facial anesthesia), constitutional symptoms (fever, chills, fatigue, malaise, sweats, weight loss), meningitic (headache, nuchal rigidity), and Lyme-specific symptoms (recent tick bite or exposure, erythema migrans rash, arthralgias, myalgias, low back pain), and inflammatory symptoms (eg, orofacial swelling or parotitis, uveitis) or known autoimmune conditions. In the setting of acute idiopathic FP, red flags suggesting a diagnosis other than Bell palsy include bilateral paralysis, slow onset of facial weakness (weakness in Bell palsy fully evolves over 24–72 hours), asymmetric weakness across facial zones at onset, constitutional symptoms (fever, lethargy, malaise, myalgias), headache (other than retroauricular pain and otalgia, which occur frequently in Bell palsy), presence of other focal neurologic deficits (diplopia, hearing loss, vertigo), and absence of recovery of facial tone within 4 months of palsy onset. Facial symptoms vary according to the timing of presentation and degree of recovery. FFP results in paralytic lagophthalmos and ocular irritation, loss of facial symmetry at rest, collapse of the external nasal valve, and oral incompetence. Postparalytic facial palsy (PFP) presents with facial synkinesis, muscle hyperactivity, contracture, and epiphora. Platysmal synkinesis results in neck discomfort and facial fatigue. Periocular synkinesis results in a narrowed palpebral fissure width. Lack of meaningful smile occurs in severe cases.

A thorough head and neck examination, including otoscopy and detailed cranial nerve examination, is performed. Zonal assessment of facial function at rest and with movement is crucial (**Fig. 1**). The brow position together with its effect on the

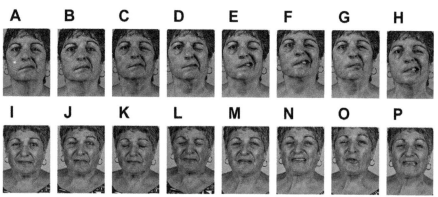

Fig. 1. Acute FFP (*top*) and subsequent PFP (*bottom*) in Ramsay-Hunt syndrome (varicella-zoster viral FP). Complete flaccid paralysis on the affected side (*asterisk*) is demonstrated at rest (*A*), and with brow elevation (*B*), gentle eye closure (*C*), full-effort eye closure (*D*), gentle smile (*E*), full-effort smile (*F*), lip pucker (*G*), and lower lip depression (*H*). The patient lacks Bell phenomenon (*C, D*). At 1 year following symptom onset, the affected brow remains depressed, while hyperactivity has developed in the orbicularis oculi, mentalis, and platysma muscles at rest (*I*). Volitional brow elevation remains impaired (*J*), while marked brow synkinesis is present with eye closure (*K, L*). As is usual in PFP, eye closure is adequate (*K, L*). Smile symmetry is improved with light effort (*M*); commissure restriction is noted with full-effort smile (*N*). Near normal return to function of the orbicularis oris muscle is noted (*O*). Lip depressor function remains weak on the affected side (*P*). Periocular, mentalis, and platysmal synkinesis is worsened by smile, pucker, and lip depression (*N–P*).

periocular complex is noted. The degree of paralytic lagophthalmos, presence or absence of Bell phenomenon, width of the palpebral fissure, and position of the lower lid are noted; laxity is assessed using distraction and snap-back tests. The depth and orientation of the nasolabial fold (NLF), position of the oral commissure, and presence and degree of brow, ocular, midfacial, depressor, mentalis, and platysmal synkinesis are evaluated. Attention is paid to the contralateral hemi-face with regard to whether weakening of a given paired muscle group, such as the hemi-brow or depressor labii inferioris, is likely to result in improved symmetry. Photography and videography to document appearance of face at rest and with 7 volitional facial movements (brow elevation, light- and full-effort eye closure, and smile, lip pucker, lower lip depression) on presentation and follow-up are essential (see **Fig. 1**). Spontaneous smile may be assessed by elicitation using humorous video clips.[9]

INVESTIGATIONS

When the history and physical examination are consistent with Bell palsy, further investigation is not required except in Lyme endemic areas, where serology is always prudent.[10–12] Imaging studies (such as a fine-cut computed tomography of the temporal bone without contrast, and/or gadolinium-enhanced MRI of the temporal bones and parotid gland) are indicated to rule out benign or malignant tumors affecting the facial nerve and should be ordered in the setting of abnormal otoscopy or tuning fork findings, palpable parotid or neck mass, slow- or asymmetric-onset or FP, slowly progressive FP, unilateral recurrent FP, or recent FP demonstrating absent recovery at 4 months. Blood work (such as complete blood count, erythrocyte sedimentation rate, C-reactive protein, rheumatoid factor, antinuclear antibody, antineutrophil cytoplasmic antibody, antiphospholipid antibodies, angiotensin converting enzyme) is indicated in recurrent cases, or where autoimmune conditions are suspected. Electroneuronography (ENoG) is indicated between 3 and 14 days of symptom onset in patients who present with delayed traumatic or idiopathic FFP who demonstrate complete absence of hemi-facial movement on examination, to assess candidacy for acute facial nerve decompression.

THERAPEUTIC MANAGEMENT

Given the breadth of therapeutic options, management of FP can be daunting. It is useful to classify patients with FP into 1 of 5 management domains, based on timing of presentation, and status of the facial nerve and facial musculature (**Fig. 2**): acute FFP, FFP with potential for spontaneous recovery, FFP with viable facial musculature with low potential for spontaneous recovery, FFP without viable facial musculature, and PFP. Therapeutic strategies may include pharmaceutical agents, corneal protective measures, physical therapy (PT), chemodenervation agents, fillers, and a myriad of surgical procedures. Organization of potential interventions by type and side of FP and facial zone is valuable for developing a therapeutic plan (**Fig. 3, Table 2**).

Acute Flaccid Facial Palsy (Intact Facial Nerve)

This domain encompasses the first 72 hours to 2 weeks following onset of acute facial nerve injury. The role of the clinician is to establish a diagnosis, initiate appropriate medical therapy (such as immunosuppressant, antiviral, or antibiotic), manage exposure keratopathy risk, and determine candidacy for acute surgical intervention. In the setting of Bell palsy, administration of high-dose corticosteroids within 72 hours of symptom onset shortens recovery time.[13] Combined use of antivirals and corticosteroids in Bell palsy may be of additional clinical benefit, especially for those with severe to complete paralysis,[14,15] and good evidence supports combination therapy in VZV.[16] Delayed onset or incomplete FP following trauma or iatrogenic insult warrants corticosteroids and observation. Iatrogenic injury resulting in immediate and complete paralysis of one or more FN branches warrants urgent surgical exploration. Patients with complete idiopathic or posttraumatic paralysis with an ENoG response demonstrating greater than 90% degeneration, and absent voluntary motor units on electromyography (EMG) are referred for neurotology consultation for consideration of surgical decompression within 14 days of symptom onset.[14,17] Lyme disease–associated FP is treated with a prolonged course of oral doxycycline or intravenous ceftriaxone.[18] Although adjuvant corticosteroid therapy is commonly prescribed, its role in Lyme is unclear.[12,19,20] Otitis media–associated FP is treated with wide myringotomy with or without mastoidectomy, corticosteroids, topical and parenteral antibiotics.[21] Eye lubrication with nighttime taping of the eye closed is typically indicated to prevent exposure keratopathy. PT for education and instruction on upper eyelid stretching to aid passive closure may be of benefit. Correction of paralytic lagophthalmos may be achieved by temporary tarsorrhaphy or upper eyelid weighting; indications include poor prognosis for rapid recovery, inability to work due to ocular symptoms, inadequate Bell phenomenon, and absent recovery at 4 months.[22]

Flaccid Facial Palsy with Potential for Spontaneous Recovery

Where nerve continuity is thought intact in the setting of FFP, for example, following resection of a vestibular schwannoma where FN stimulation was noted before closure, a potential for spontaneous recovery exists, whereby return of facial tone and movement are expected within 6 to 12 months. Patients may benefit from PT, corneal protective measures, static periocular reanimation, and temporary chemodenervation of

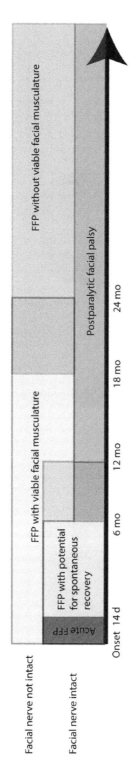

Fig. 2. FP management domains. Patients may be categorized according to timing of presentation from palsy onset, and status of the facial nerve and facial musculature. This conceptual framework is helpful in selecting appropriate therapeutic interventions. Medical therapy is often indicated in acute FFP. Close observation is indicated for a period of several months in FFP whereby there exists potential for spontaneous recovery (for example, following extirpation of a vestibular schwannoma with facial nerve preservation). Where the facial nerve is discontinuous, nerve repair or transfers (such as hypoglossal-to-facial and/or nerve-to-masseter to branches controlling smile) are immediately indicated; such transfers are also indicated in the case of persistent FFP following 6 to 12 months of observation because native facial musculature remains viable (ie, receptive to reinnervation) for a period of approximately 2 years. Where facial musculature is no longer viable (ie, absent or unreceptive to reinnervation), muscle transfers are indicated for smile reanimation. Patients with PFP (comprising synkinesis and varying degrees of zonal hypoactivity and hyperactivity) are typically managed with PT and chemodenervation; surgical reanimation is appropriate in severe cases.

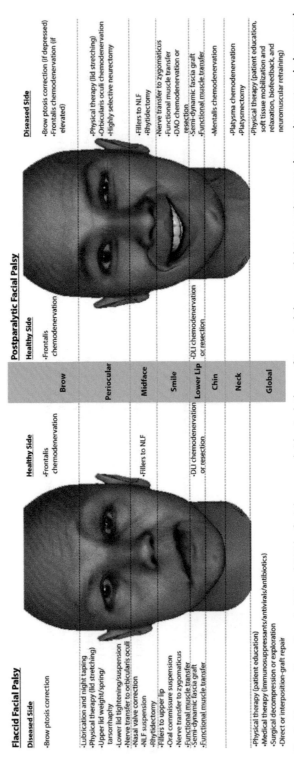

Fig. 3. Therapeutic options in FFP and PFP, by facial zone and side. A plethora of targeted therapeutic interventions may be used to restore balance and symmetry in hemi-FP.

Flaccid Facial Palsy

Diseased Side

- Brow ptosis correction

- Lubrication and night taping
- Physical therapy (lid stretching)
- Upper lid weight/spring/ tarsorrhaphy
- Lower lid tightening/suspension
- Nerve transfer to orbicularis oculi
- Nasal valve correction
- NLF suspension
- Rhytidectomy
- Fillers to upper lip
- Oral commissure suspension
- Nerve transfer to zygomaticus
- Functional muscle transfer
- Semi-dynamic fascia graft
- Functional muscle transfer.

- Physical therapy (patient education)
- Medical therapy (immunosuppressants/antivirals/antibiotics)
- Surgical decompression or exploration
- Direct or interposition-graft repair

Healthy Side

- Frontalis chemodenervation

- Fillers to NLF

- DLI chemodenervation or resection.

Postparalytic Facial Palsy

Healthy Side

- Frontalis chemodenervation

- DLI chemodenervation or resection.

Brow	
Periocular	
Midface	
Smile	
Lower Lip	
Chin	
Neck	
Global	

Diseased Side

- Brow ptosis correction (if depressed)
- Frontalis chemodenervation (if elevated)

- Physical therapy (lid stretching)
- Orbicularis oculi chemodenervation
- Highly selective neurectomy

- Fillers to NLF
- Rhytidectomy

- Nerve transfer to zygomaticus
- Functional muscle transfer
- DAO chemodenervation or resection
- Semi-dynamic fascia graft
- Functional muscle transfer

- Mentalis chemodenervation

- Platysma chemodenervation
- Platysmectomy

- Physical therapy (patient education, soft tissue mobilization and relaxation, biofeedback, and neuromuscular retraining)

Table 2
Therapeutic options in flaccid facial palsy and postparalytic facial palsy

Setting	Medical Management	PT	Injections	Surgical Management

Acute FFP (intact facial nerve)	• Corticosteroids: idiopathic (Bell), varicella zoster (VZV/Ramsay-Hunt), acute otitis associated, delayed traumatic, delayed iatrogenic
	• Antivirals: VZV, consider for idiopathic
	• Antibiotics (targeted): indicated for Lyme disease or acute otitis
	• Eye protection is always indicated
	  ○ Daytime lubricating eye drops
	  ○ Night time lubricating ointment, eyelid taping
		• Patient education
		• Eyelid stretching
			• None indicated	Adjunctive
				• Facial nerve decompression: indicated for idiopathic and posttraumatic complete FFP with ENoG response <90% and absent voluntary motor units on EMG between 3 and 14 d of symptom onset
				• Wide myringotomy ± tube placement ± mastoidectomy: indicated for acute otitis
				Static reanimation
				• Eyelid weight (reversible if recovery ensues)

FFP with potential for spontaneous recovery	• Corneal protection is always indicated
	  ○ Daytime lubricating eye drops
	  ○ Night time lubricating ointment, eyelid taping
		• Patient education
		• Eyelid stretching
			• Botulinum toxin
			  ○ Contralateral brow
			  ○ Contralateral depressor labii inferioris (DLI)
				Static reanimation
				• Eyelid weight
				• Consider lower lid tightening in elderly patients

FFP with viable facial musculature and low potential for spontaneous recovery	• Corneal protection is always indicated
	  ○ Daytime lubricating eye drops
	  ○ Night time lubricating ointment, eyelid taping
		• Patient education
		• Eyelid stretching
		• Targeted PT following dynamic reanimation
			• Botulinum toxin
			  ○ Contralateral brow
			  ○ Contralateral DLI
			• Volumizing fillers
			  ○ Contralateral NLF
			  ○ Ipsilateral lips
				Static reanimation
				• Brow ptosis correction
				• Eyelid weight
				• Lower lid tightening
				• External nasal valve correction
				• NLF suspension
				• Oral commissure suspension
				Dynamic reanimation
				• Direct end-to-end repair or interposition grafting (for facial nerve transections/resections)
				• XII–VII for facial tone
				• Cross-facial nerve grafting or V–VII for targeted reanimation of expression (blink, smile)

(continued on next page)

Table 2
(continued)

Setting	Medical Management	PT	Injections	Surgical Management

FFP without viable facial musculature	• Corneal protection is always indicated
	  ○ Daytime lubricating eye drops
	  ○ Night time lubricating ointment, eyelid taping
		• Patient education
		• Eyelid stretching
			• Botulinum toxin
			  ○ Contralateral brow
			  ○ Contralateral DLI
			• Volumizing fillers
			  ○ Contralateral NLF
			  ○ Ipsilateral lips
				Static reanimation
				• Brow ptosis correction
				• Eyelid weighting and lower lid tightening
				• Static facial sling: external nasal valve, NLF, oral commissure
				• Rhytidectomy
				• Contralateral DLI resection
				Dynamic reanimation
				• Smile reanimation
				  ○ Temporalis or free muscle transfer

PFP	• Corneal protection if blink inadequate (rare)
	  ○ Daytime lubricating eye drops
	  ○ Night time lubricating ointment, eyelid taping
		• Patient education
		• Eyelid stretching
		• Biofeedback
		• Neuromuscular retraining
		• Targeted PT following dynamic reanimation
			• Botulinum toxin
			  ○ Contralateral or bilateral brow
			  ○ Ipsilateral orbicularis oculi
			  ○ Contralateral DLI
			  ○ Ipsilateral depressor anguli oris (DAO)
			  ○ Ipsilateral mentalis
			  ○ Ipsilateral platysma
			• Volumizing fillers
			  ○ Ipsilateral or contralateral NLF
			  ○ Ipsilateral lips
				Static reanimation
				• Brow ptosis correction
				• Highly selective neurectomy
				• Ipsilateral rhytidectomy
				• Contralateral DLI resection
				• Ipsilateral DAO resection
				• Platysmectomy
				Dynamic reanimation
				• Smile reanimation
				  ○ Temporalis transfer or free muscle transfer

the healthy-side depressor labii inferioris muscle to improve oral competence and articulation during this period. Close follow-up (every 3 months) is warranted to ensure recovery of function.

Flaccid Facial Palsy with Viable Facial Musculature and Low Potential for Spontaneous Recovery

In this clinical scenario, there exists discontinuity of the facial nerve or absent recovery of facial function noted within 6 to 12 months of FP onset. Native facial musculature is intact and likely receptive to reinnervation. Common clinical scenarios involve patients presenting with dense FFP resulting from temporal bone tumors (such as facial nerve schwannomas, venous vascular malformations, or cholesteatomas), cerebellopontine angle tumor extirpations, or pontine hemorrhage. Although no definitive criteria exist, evidence from case series suggests that facial musculature remains receptive to reinnervation for periods up to 24 months following denervation in adults,[23–26] and possibly longer periods in children. Within this period, nerve repair and transfers are indicated. Interposition graft repair should be contemplated in the setting of neural discontinuity; split-hypoglossal nerve transfer to the main trunk of the facial nerve is an alternative option where interposition graft repair is unfeasible or where no recovery is noted within 12 months. The goal of main trunk repairs and transfers is to restore facial tone and some form of blink; meaningful reanimation of expression is rarely achieved. Volitional expressions may be restored through targeted nerve transfers during this period, such as nerve-to-masseter transfer to lower zygomatic branches of the facial nerve for smile reanimation, or cross-face nerve grafting to upper zygomatic branches for blink restoration. Targeted nerve transfers should be considered in patients demonstrating minimal to no improvement in facial function 7 months following vestibular schwannoma resection with facial nerve preservation, as the probability of ultimate recovery of meaningful expression is less than 10%.[27] Static periocular reanimation (such as upper lid weighting and lateral tarsal strip procedure) is offered early in the course of palsy onset where recovery is likely to take several months.

Flaccid Facial Palsy Without Viable Facial Musculature

Where native facial musculature is absent (eg, following resection or congenital absence) or unlikely to be receptive to reinnervation (eg, long denervation period or marked distal perineural spread of a malignant tumor), nerve repair or transfers are no longer indicated. In addition to PT and targeted chemodenervation of healthy side lip depression and brow elevation, surgical interventions include static facial suspensions, static periocular reanimation, and muscle transfers. Targeted suspensions of the brow, lower eyelid, and midface, nasal valve, NLF, and oral commissure may be achieved using sutures, fascia lata, or bioabsorbable or permanent implants. Tightening of the lower lid may be achieved by the lateral tarsal strip procedure[28] with or without medical canthal tendon plication. Dynamic smile reanimation may be achieved through antidromic[29] or orthodromic[30] temporalis muscle transfer, or free muscle transfer[31,32] with motor innervation provided through cranial nerve transfer. Options for dynamic reanimation of the lower lip include anterior digastric muscle transfer[33] or inlay of a T-shaped fascia graft.[34]

Postparalytic Facial Palsy

PFP develops 6 to 18 months following severe facial nerve insult with spontaneous, yet aberrant, regeneration or following main trunk nerve grafting. Once present, it is permanent. Lagophthalmos is rare. PT is first-line treatment; a comprehensive program includes patient education, soft tissue mobilization, mirror and EMG biofeed-back, and neuromuscular retraining.[35] Blunting of hyperactivity through filler injection and weakening of hyperactive muscles through targeted chemodenervation, neurec-tomy, or resection in advanced disease is indicated in conjunction with PT. For many patients, targeted chemodenervation of diseased side orbicularis oculi, mentalis, and platysma offers significant improvements. Weakening of the diseased side depressor anguli oris muscle through chemodenervation or resection can result in dramatic improvement in smile dynamics in select cases.[36,37] In cases with severe restriction of oral commissure excursion, regional (eg, temporalis) or free (eg, gracilis) muscle transfer may be considered for dynamic smile reanimation. Targeted nerve transfers, such as nerve-to-masseter transfer to diseased-side zygomatic branches for smile reanimation, are largely ineffective in the setting of PFP.

CLINICAL OUTCOMES

Systematic tracking of therapeutic outcomes is a prerequisite to clinical excellence. Outcomes tracking in FP may entail patient-reported QOL measures, clinician-assessed grading of facial function, and objective measurement of facial displace-ments. QOL impact may be assessed using generalized patient-graded scales such as the SF-36.[38] The Facial Disability Index,[39] the Facial Clinimetric Evaluation,[1] and the Synkinesis Assessment Questionnaire[40] are patient-graded scales specifically designed and validated for use in FP to concurrently assess symptom severity and impact on QOL. Although global 5- or 6-point facial function scales exist (such as the House-Brackmann,[41,42] Fisch,[43] and others[44,45]), such scales lack the resolution necessary to capture meaningful changes in zonal function over time. The Yanagihara scale[46] provides Likert scale resolution of zonal appearance with movement, but not at rest, and lacks separate grading of synkinesis. The Sunnybrook Facial Grading Sys-tem[47] provides weighted scores of zonal symmetry at rest and with motion in addition to synkinesis. A recently validated electronic facial paralysis assessment tool provides even higher resolution zonal data through use of continuous visual analogue scales to assess 5 static, 7 dynamic, and 4 synkinesis zonal parameters.[48,49] A computer vision-based facial landmark recognition algorithm has recently been used within a novel freeware application (Emotrics, Mass Eye and Ear Infirmary) for objective measure-ment of various facial displacements (eg, smile excursion) from clinical photographs.[50]

SUMMARY

Management of FP necessitates establishing a diagnosis and formulating a therapeu-tic plan according to the timing of presentation in flaccid cases, and specific pattern of facial dysfunction in patients presenting with aberrant neural regeneration. Therapeu-tic interventions include PT, injectables, and a plethora of surgical reanimation procedures.

REFERENCES

1. Kahn JB, Gliklich RE, Boyev KP, et al. Validation of a patient-graded instrument for facial nerve paralysis: the FaCE scale. Laryngoscope 2001;111(3):387–98.
2. Ishii LE, Godoy A, Encarnacion CO, et al. What faces reveal: impaired affect display in facial paralysis. Laryngoscope 2011;121(6):1138–43.
3. Valls-Sole J, Tolosa ES, Pujol M. Myokymic discharges and enhanced facial nerve reflex responses after recovery from idiopathic facial palsy. Muscle Nerve 1992; 15(1):37–42.

4. Montserrat L, Benito M. Facial synkinesis and aberrant regeneration of facial nerve. Adv Neurol 1988;49:211–24.
5. Kimura J, Rodnitzky RL, Okawara SH. Electrophysiologic analysis of aberrant regeneration after facial nerve paralysis. Neurology 1975;25(10):989–93.
6. Wetzig P. Aberrant regeneration of oculomotor and facial nerves. Rocky Mt Med J 1957;54(4):347–8.
7. Hohman MH, Hadlock TA. Etiology, diagnosis, and management of facial palsy: 2000 patients at a facial nerve center. Laryngoscope 2014;124(7):E283–93.
8. Agarwal R, Manandhar L, Saluja P, et al. Pontine stroke presenting as isolated facial nerve palsy mimicking Bell's palsy: a case report. J Med Case Rep 2011; 5(1):287.
9. Iacolucci C, Banks CA, Jowett N, et al. Development and validation of a spontaneous smile assay. JAMA Facial Plast Surg 2015;17(3):191–6.
10. Ho K, Melanson M, Desai JA. Bell palsy in lyme disease-endemic regions of canada: a cautionary case of occult bilateral peripheral facial nerve palsy due to Lyme disease. CJEM 2012;14(5):321–4.
11. Smouha EE, Coyle PK, Shukri S. Facial nerve palsy in Lyme disease: evaluation of clinical diagnostic criteria. Am J Otol 1997;18(2):257–61.
12. Jowett N, Gaudin RA, Banks CA, et al. Steroid use in Lyme disease-associated facial palsy is associated with worse long-term outcomes. Laryngoscope 2017; 127(6):1451–8.
13. Engstrom M, Berg T, Stjernquist-Desatnik A, et al. Prednisolone and valaciclovir in Bell's palsy: a randomised, double-blind, placebo-controlled, multicentre trial. Lancet Neurol 2008;7(11):993–1000.
14. McAllister K, Walker D, Donnan PT, et al. Surgical interventions for the early management of Bell's palsy. Cochrane Database Syst Rev 2013;(10):CD007468.
15. de Almeida JR, Al Khabori M, Guyatt GH, et al. Combined corticosteroid and antiviral treatment for Bell palsy: a systematic review and meta-analysis. JAMA 2009; 302(9):985–93.
16. Murakami S, Hato N, Horiuchi J, et al. Treatment of Ramsay Hunt syndrome with acyclovir-prednisone: significance of early diagnosis and treatment. Ann Neurol 1997;41(3):353–7.
17. Gantz BJ, Rubinstein JT, Gidley P, et al. Surgical management of Bell's palsy. Laryngoscope 1999;109(8):1177–88.
18. Wormser GP, Dattwyler RJ, Shapiro ED, et al. The clinical assessment, treatment, and prevention of lyme disease, human granulocytic anaplasmosis, and babesiosis: clinical practice guidelines by the Infectious Diseases Society of America. Clin Infect Dis 2006;43(9):1089–134.
19. Clark JR, Carlson RD, Sasaki CT, et al. Facial paralysis in Lyme disease. Laryngoscope 1985;95(11):1341–5.
20. Halperin JJ, Shapiro ED, Logigian E, et al. Practice parameter: treatment of nervous system Lyme disease (an evidence-based review): report of the Quality Standards Subcommittee of the American Academy of Neurology. Neurology 2007;69(1):91–102.
21. Redaelli de Zinis LO, Gamba P, Balzanelli C. Acute otitis media and facial nerve paralysis in adults. Otol Neurotol 2003;24(1):113–7.
22. Jowett N, Hadlock TA. Contemporary management of Bell palsy. Facial Plast Surg 2015;31(2):93–102.
23. Wu P, Chawla A, Spinner RJ, et al. Key changes in denervated muscles and their impact on regeneration and reinnervation. Neural Regen Res 2014;9(20): 1796–809.

24. Conley J. Hypoglossal crossover–122 cases. Trans Sect Otolaryngol Am Acad Ophthalmol Otolaryngol 1977;84(4 Pt 1). Orl-763–8.

25. Gavron JP, Clemis JD. Hypoglossal-facial nerve anastomosis: a review of forty cases caused by facial nerve injuries in the posterior fossa. Laryngoscope 1984;94(11 Pt 1):1447–50.

26. Kunihiro T, Kanzaki J, Yoshihara S, et al. Hypoglossal-facial nerve anastomosis after acoustic neuroma resection: influence of the time anastomosis on recovery of facial movement. ORL J Otorhinolaryngol Relat Spec 1996;58(1):32–5.

27. Rivas A, Boahene KD, Bravo HC, et al. A model for early prediction of facial nerve recovery after vestibular schwannoma surgery. Otol Neurotol 2011;32(5):826–33.

28. Anderson RL, Gordy DD. The tarsal strip procedure. Arch Ophthalmol 1979; 97(11):2192–6.

29. Gillies H. Experiences with fascia lata grafts in the operative treatment of facial paralysis: (section of otology and section of laryngology). Proc R Soc Med 1934;27(10):1372–82.

30. McLaughlin CR. Permanent facial paralysis; the role of surgical support. Lancet 1952;2(6736):647–51.

31. Harii K, Ohmori K, Torii S. Free gracilis muscle transplantation, with microneurovascular anastomoses for the treatment of facial paralysis. A preliminary report. Plast Reconstr Surg 1976;57(2):133–43.

32. Harii K, Asato H, Yoshimura K, et al. One-stage transfer of the latissimus dorsi muscle for reanimation of a paralyzed face: a new alternative. Plast Reconstr Surg 1998;102(4):941–51.

33. Edgerton MT. Surgical correction of facial paralysis: a plea for better reconstructions. Ann Surg 1967;165(6):985–98.

34. Watanabe Y, Sasaki R, Agawa K, et al. Bidirectional/double fascia grafting for simple and semi-dynamic reconstruction of lower lip deformity in facial paralysis. J Plast Reconstr Aesthet Surg 2015;68(3):321–8.

35. Wernick Robinson M, Baiungo J, Hohman M, et al. Facial rehabilitation. Oper Tech Otolaryngol Head Neck Surg 2012;23(4):288–96.

36. Jowett N, Malka R, Hadlock TA. Effect of weakening of ipsilateral depressor anguli oris on smile symmetry in postparalysis facial palsy. JAMA Facial Plast Surg 2016;19(1):29–33.

37. Labbe D, Benichou L, Iodice A, et al. Depressor anguli oris sign (DAO) in facial paresis. How to search it and release the smile (technical note). Ann Chir Plast Esthet 2012;57(3):281–5 [in French].

38. Ware JE Jr, Sherbourne CD. The MOS 36-item short-form health survey (SF-36). I. Conceptual framework and item selection. Med Care 1992;30(6):473–83.

39. VanSwearingen JM, Brach JS. The Facial Disability Index: reliability and validity of a disability assessment instrument for disorders of the facial neuromuscular system. Phys Ther 1996;76(12):1288–98 [discussion: 1298–300].

40. Mehta RP, WernickRobinson M, Hadlock TA. Validation of the synkinesis assessment questionnaire. Laryngoscope 2007;117(5):923–6.

41. House JW. Facial nerve grading systems. Laryngoscope 1983;93(8):1056–69.

42. House JW, Brackmann DE. Facial nerve grading system. Otolaryngol Head Neck Surg 1985;93(2):146–7.

43. Fisch U. Surgery for Bell's palsy. Arch Otolaryngol 1981;107(1):1–11.

44. Botman JW, Jongkees LB. The result of intratemporal treatment of facial palsy. Pract Otorhinolaryngol (Basel) 1955;17(2):80–100.

45. May M, Blumenthal F, Taylor FH. Bell's palsy: surgery based upon prognostic indicators and results. Laryngoscope 1981;91(12):2092–103.

46. Yanagihara N. On standardised documentation of facial palsy (author's transl). Nihon Jibiinkoka Gakkai Kaiho 1977;80(8):799–805 [in Japanese].
47. Ross BG, Fradet G, Nedzelski JM. Development of a sensitive clinical facial grading system. Otolaryngol Head Neck Surg 1996;114(3):380–6.
48. Banks CA, Hadlock TA. Pediatric facial nerve rehabilitation. Facial Plast Surg Clin North Am 2014;22(4):487–502.
49. Banks CA, Bhama PK, Park J, et al. Clinician-graded electronic facial paralysis assessment: the eFACE. Plast Reconstr Surg 2015;136(2):223e–30e.
50. Guarin DL, Dusseldorp JR, Hadlock TA, et al. A machine learning approach for automated facial measurements in facial palsy. JAMA Facial Plast Surg 2018; 20(4):335–7.

Outcome Tracking in Facial Palsy

Joseph R. Dusseldorp, MBBS, MS, FRACS[a,b,*], Martinus M. van Veen, MD[a,c],
Suresh Mohan, MD[a], Tessa A. Hadlock, MD[a]

KEYWORDS

- Facial palsy • eFACE • Emotrics • Emotionality quotient • Spontaneous smile
- Machine learning • Layperson

KEY POINTS

- Outcome tracking in facial palsy is multimodal, consisting of patient-reported outcome measures, clinician-graded scoring systems, objective assessment tools, and novel tools for layperson and spontaneity assessment.
- Patient-reported outcome measures are critical to understanding burden of disease in facial palsy and effects of interventions from the patient perspective.
- Clinician-graded scoring systems have been the focus of intensive study for more than half a century. No 1 system is perfect for all needs and many systems have been described and validated.
- Objective assessment tools quantify facial movements for both research and clinical purposes. Recent advances in facial recognition technology have enabled automated facial measurements.
- Novel assessment tools have been developed to analyze more complex facial attributes, such as spontaneous smile, emotional expressivity, disfigurement, and attractiveness, as determined by laypersons.

INTRODUCTION

Current outcome tracking in facial palsy is multimodal, consisting of patient-reported outcome measures, clinician-graded scoring systems, objective assessment tools, and novel tools for layperson and spontaneity assessment.

Patient-reported outcome measures (PROMs) are critical to understanding the burden of disease in facial palsy and effects of interventions from the patient

Disclosure: The authors have nothing to disclose. No funding was received for this article.
[a] Department of Otolaryngology/Head and Neck Surgery, Massachusetts Eye and Ear Infirmary, Harvard Medical School, 243 Charles Street, Boston, MA 02114, USA; [b] Department of Plastic and Reconstructive Surgery, Royal Australasian College of Surgeons, University of Sydney, City Road, Camperdown, Sydney, NSW, Australia 2006; [c] Department of Plastic Surgery, University Medical Center Groningen, University of Groningen, Hanzeplein 1, 9713 GZ Groningen, Netherlands
* Corresponding author. Massachusetts Eye and Ear Infirmary, 243 Charles Street, Boston, MA.
E-mail address: joeduss@gmail.com

perspective. Such measures should be sensitive to change and targeted to patients with facial palsy. As interventions are modified over time, outcome measures must also be updated to capture the full range of patient experience following any procedure.

Clinician-graded scoring systems have been the focus of intensive study for more than half a century.[1] Many systems have been described and validated, but no 1 system has gained universal acceptance. House-Brackmann was the first widely accepted outcome measure in facial palsy. It continues to be used because of its familiarity with clinicians from multiple disciplines even though it is unable to quantify the full spectrum of facial palsy management. As automated facial grading systems become common, outdated systems should be replaced.

Many objective assessment tools have been developed to quantify facial movements for both research and clinical purposes. Most systems are time consuming, require expensive and complicated hardware, and can be difficult to implement in clinical practice. Recent advances in machine learning technology have enabled automated facial measurements to be made, dramatically improving the efficiency and objectivity of making automated facial measurements.[2]

Novel assessment tools have been developed to analyze more complex facial attributes such as emotional expressivity, disfigurement, and attractiveness as defined by both clinician and layperson. Technological advances in facial recognition have already led to multiple insights. Eye tracking, which analyses the gaze pattern of laypersons, has been used to understand the differences in the observer's experience when confronted with an image of someone with facial palsy.[3,4] These insights have helped clinicians to understand why laypersons score facial palsy lower in attractiveness, and give an overall negative facial impression. However, routine use of layperson assessments to measure outcomes is not practical.

Machine learning has made inroads into decoding the emotional content of facial expressions. Commercially available software trained from millions of encounters with normal facial expressions has been applied to patients with facial palsy, showing the profound impact of facial palsy on not only the ability to express joy when smiling but also the inadvertent expression of negative emotions, such as contempt. Findings such as this will allow clinicians to educate patients, tailor treatments, and quantify the improvements following procedures. Increased negative emotion expression when patients with facial palsy try to smile has been consistently found in layperson assessments and quantified by machine learning algorithms.[4–7] Machine learning algorithms may eventually be validated as layperson equivalents.

No current methodology exists for quantifying the presence or absence of a spontaneous smile other than the impression of the treating surgeon. Given the importance that both surgeons and patients place on a spontaneous smile, a standardized approach is required. Machine learning technology may hold the key to future analysis of this elusive attribute.

The Ideal Outcome Measure Panel in Facial Palsy

No single outcome measure can capture all of the complex domains of facial palsy. An optimal panel of outcome measures is required, with measures that are objective, sensitive to change, and easy to implement.[8] It is only by agreeing on a common, data-driven language that clinicians will be able to compare outcomes for the benefit of patients with facial palsy. An optimal outcome measure panel in facial palsy should include:

1. PROMs
2. Automated and clinician-graded facial palsy grading systems

3. Layperson assessment equivalent
4. Spontaneous smile analysis

   Tools in all 4 of these categories are currently being developed. This article outlines the background of outcome tracking in facial palsy and highlights recent advances.

PATIENT-REPORTED OUTCOME MEASURES

Facial palsy has a profound psychosocial impact and negatively affects quality of life.[9-11] Thus, PROMs should be an integral part of routine assessment and outcome measurement in facial palsy. According to a recent survey of the Sir Charles Bell Society, most facial nerve clinicians do not use a PROM in routine assessment of facial palsy, and, among those who do, there are a multitude of different surveys in use.[12] Two validated, facial palsy–specific quality-of-life questionnaires are the Facial Disability Index (FDI) and the Facial Clinimetric Evaluation (FaCE) scale.[13] Neither the FDI nor the FaCE scale incorporates questions specifically assessing the effect of synkinesis on quality of life. The Synkinesis Assessment Questionnaire (SAQ) was developed to address this problem.[14] The SAQ can be used as a standalone tool in established synkinesis or as an adjunct to other quality-of-life questionnaires to obtain specific information relevant to synkinetic patients.

Facial Disability Index (1996)

The first facial palsy–specific quality-of-life questionnaire was the FDI, published in 1996.[15] The FDI consists of 10 questions, each with 6 answer options. Five questions relate to physical function of the face, 5 to psychosocial wellbeing. Scores in each of these domains are calculated, ranging from 0 (worst) to 100 (best). The FDI is available in German,[16] Italian,[17] Spanish,[18] and Swedish.[19]

Facial Clinimetric Evaluation Scale (2001)

The FaCE scale was developed in 2001 and since then has become the most widely used quality-of-life questionnaire in facial palsy.[12,20,21] The FaCE scale is composed of 15 questions with 5-point Likert scale responses ranging from 1 (worst) to 5 (best). Based on these 15 questions, 6 domain subscores are calculated for facial movement, facial comfort, oral function, eye comfort, lacrimal control, and social function. The subscores are collated to yield a FaCE scale total score ranging from 0 (worst) to 100 (best). The FaCE scale is available in Chinese,[22] Dutch,[10] German,[16] and Swedish.[19] The FaCE scale is thought to assess psychometric parameters more accurately than FDI, although both scales have advantages and disadvantages.[13]

Synkinesis Assessment Questionnaire (2007)

The SAQ was developed in 2007 in response to the lack of synkinesis-specific items in earlier PROMs for facial palsy.[14] A computerized facial synkinesis assessment tool had been published but was more suited to research purposes.[23] The SAQ is a 9-item questionnaire with 5-point Likert scale responses. The raw score is converted to a total score, ranging from 20 (worst) to 100 (best). Note that SAQ is not a quality-of-life questionnaire but rather a questionnaire regarding patient perception of facial synkinesis. SAQ can easily be combined with a facial palsy–specific quality-of-life questionnaire (ie, FDI or FaCE scale).

CLINICIAN-GRADED SCORING SYSTEMS

Numerous clinician-graded facial nerve scales have been introduced into the literature over the past 50 years. Although each tool has attempted to improve the resolution of facial grading, limitations persist and an optimal tool remains elusive.

Yanagihara (1977)

The Yanagihara method, introduced at the Third International Symposium on Facial Nerve Surgery in 1976, is one of the earliest widely accepted facial grading scales.[24] Ten facial movements are each graded on a 4-point scale, and facial function is measured by the sum of scores. The summed score represents the spectrum from no movement to normal facial movement (0–40, respectively). Recovery from facial palsy has been defined as a score higher than 36 points without accompanying facial contracture or synkinesis.[25,26] Although the variety of expressions evaluated provides regional information and the scale correlates well with patient self-evaluation,[27] limitations include that the scale is unweighted, leading to an inability to differentially emphasize the various facial movements[28]; there is a low intraobserver reliability; and it captures only ocular synkinesis.

House-Brackmann (1985)

The most popular and widely used tool for facial grading in the United States remains the House-Brackmann scale,[29] a 6-point scale intended for categorizing overall facial nerve function from normal to complete paralysis (grades 1–6). It has good intraobserver[29–32] and interobserver reliability,[24,28,29,31–36] accounts for synkinesis (albeit nonspecifically), and can measure gross changes over time.[28,37] However, such widespread usage has led to multiple iterations[35,38] and interpretations of the original scale, obscuring analyses attempting to clarify its true efficacy. In addition, it has been extensively criticized for its subjective and gross nature resulting in an inability to measure nuanced regional changes after interventions.[39–42] Nevertheless, its ease of use as a communication tool has perpetuated its widespread adoption.

Sunnybrook Facial Grading Scale (1996)

The Sunnybrook scale was introduced in 1996 by Ross and colleagues[41] and addresses many of the weaknesses of the House-Brackmann scale. The system is divided into three sections: resting symmetry, symmetry of voluntary movement, and synkinesis, with score weighting and regionality incorporated. Higher sensitivity to change and a wider response range of the composite score (0–100) provide greater resolution of grading as opposed to the ordinal categorization of the House-Brackmann scale.[43] Further, correlation with the House-Brackmann scale has been well shown.[28,43] High intraobserver and interobserver reliability have also been shown in both expert and nonexpert raters.[34,39,44–47] Areas of improvement remain. Synkinesis is adequately incorporated into the composite score, although, like most other clinician-graded tools, scoring remains subjective.

Terzis and Noah (1997)

Terzis and Noah's[48] classification system uses a 5-tier scale (poor to excellent) to rate the aesthetic and functional outcomes of facial reanimation using the parameters of symmetry and contraction. It offers dynamic movement assessment and has been used for assessment of changes over time through preoperative and postoperative evaluations by experts.[49,50] However, it does not provide regional scoring or synkinesis analysis and has not undergone validated reliability studies. It has been used in numerous studies primarily because of a lack of any other outcome measure and its ease of use.[51–56]

Sydney (2005)

The Sydney facial grading system, used since 1988 in Australia, assesses function of facial movements associated with the five facial nerve zones and their corresponding muscle groups.[34] Each movement is given a rating from 0 to 3, as is overall synkinesis. Although the Sydney system provides regionality and accounts for synkinesis, it is nonspecific and has limited comparison with other scales, such as the Sunnybrook. In addition, it does not provide static assessment, has not been validated for changes over time, and has not been evaluated for intraobserver reliability, leaving room for further study.

Facial Nerve Grading System 2.0 (2009)

To combat the limitations of the original House-Brackmann scale, nearly 15 years later, the revised Facial Nerve Grading Scale 2.0 (FNGS2.0) was introduced with directed improvements.[57] Four separate regions are scored from 1 to 6, based on degree of movement, and synkinesis is scored on a scale of 0 to 3. In addition, the total summed score of 4 to 24 is converted to a House-Brackmann scale grade. Interobserver reliability using expert raters has been shown to be consistently high,[1,36,42,58] with Vrabec and colleagues[57] reporting a mean Pearson correlation coefficient with the House-Brackmann scale of 0.91. Lee and colleagues[36] also found a moderate agreement between the scales with regard to change over time but showed FNGS2.0 to be a better measure of synkinesis.

eFACE (2015)

The electronic facial paralysis assessment tool (eFACE), described by Banks and colleagues[59] in 2015, combines many of the strengths of earlier clinician-graded tools into a digital interface. Each item is scored using a visual analog scale in 3 sections (static, dynamic, and synkinesis). Most subscores range from 0 to 100, with 100 representing normal facial function. The 0 to 100 scale is easy to understand, compared with the scales that run from 0 to 6, 0 to 20, or 0 to 40. Certain parameters range from 0 to 200, where 100 is balanced, 0 represents a flaccid state, and 200 represents a synkinetic state. Static and dynamic assessment, subregional scoring, high-resolution synkinesis scoring, sensitivity to change, convenience of digital data, high intraobserver and interobserver reliability, and high test-retest reliability have all been shown.[60] The eFACE has been compared with overall disfigurement by experts,[61] been assessed in person and from video recordings,[60] and has been examined by international facial nerve experts showing high interrater reliability in early use.[62] Despite its many merits, like all other clinician-graded tools, this measure is subject to bias and human error (**Fig. 1**).

OBJECTIVE ASSESSMENT TOOLS
Photographic

Documentation of facial palsy has focused more on clinician-graded scales than on objective outcome measures. However, in order to evaluate treatment options, clinicians need to compare outcomes, and so the need for standard objective outcome measures has been consistently recognized.[1,8] Clinical photography in repose and with staged facial movements is a simple measure that is commonly used in clinical practice, although rarely in exactly the same manner. A systematic review from 2015 described 13 different photographic assessment methods.[63]

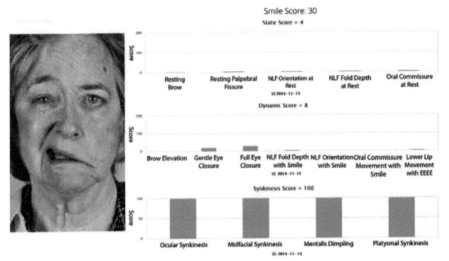

Fig. 1. Example of an eFACE assessment of the flaccid face. (*Left*) A patient at rest, showing total flaccidity. (*Right*) Each item in bar chart formats, generated by the eFACE software. NLF, nasolabial fold. (*From* Banks CA, Bhama PK, Park J, et. al. Clinician-graded electronic facial paralysis assessment. Plast Reconstr Surg 2015;136(2):225e; with permission.)

Photographic analysis tools related to Photoshop (Adobe Systems, San Jose, CA) are among the most widely used. Advantages are the low cost and no need for specialized equipment. Manual systems may or may not require placement of reflective dots on the patient's face, which can limit use in clinical practice. Two semi-automated tools that do not require dot placement have been published and are freely available: the MEEI Facegram[8] and the Emotrics software.[2]

MEEI Facegram (2012)

The Facial Assessment by Computer Evaluation software was developed by Hadlock and colleagues[8] in 2012 and was made freely available on the Sir Charles Bell Society Web site, where it has become known as the MEEI Facegram. No markers need to be placed and the system can analyze any frontal-view photograph. Measurements are scaled using average iris diameter of 11.8 mm in humans. Measurements of smile excursion, brow height, palpebral fissure width, nasal and philtral deviation, and lip measurements can be obtained and exported. Although this tool significantly reduced the time and effort of analyzing facial photographs, each measurement was individually calculated and there was no automation of landmark placement.[8]

Emotrics (2018)

Recent advances in machine learning technology have enabled development of an objective tool for facial analysis in facial palsy, known as Emotrics.[2] The tool automatically places dots on key facial landmarks of standard frontal photographs and, once verified by the clinician, automatically calculates a full set of measurements relevant to facial palsy. In addition, multiple photographs can be analyzed simultaneously, allowing an automated calculation of smile excursion, among many other features. This tool is freely available for download from the Sir Charles Bell Society Web site (**Figs. 2–4**).

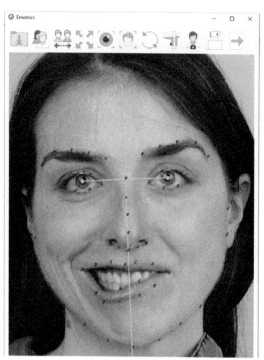

Fig. 2. Graphical user interface of Emotrics. Icon bar displays the different functionalities, including load patient, compare 2 images, find iris diameter, find facial midline, reposition landmarks, show facial measurements. Emotrics automatically displays the facial image with 68 facial landmark dots (*red dots*) and bilateral iris positions (*green circles*). The facial midline (*green line*) can be displayed as a reference. (*From* Guarin D, Dusseldrop J, Hadlock T, et. al. A machine learning approach for automated facial measurements in facial palsy. JAMA Facial Plast Surg 2018;e1. https://doi.org/10.1001/jamafacial.2018.0030; with permission.)

Videographic

Facial palsy vastly affects the kinetics of facial movement, but a gold standard videography assessment tool has not been developed. Several techniques have been published, but none of them has been universally adopted because they are mostly complex, time consuming, and expensive. Four methods that have been well studied are from Frey and colleagues,[64,65] the FACIAL CLIMA,[66] and Sforza and colleagues.[67,68] Whether in 2 or 3 dimensions, objective video analysis remains a research tool, not yet integrated into clinical practice.

Frey and colleagues (1994; 1999)

In 1994, Frey and colleagues[64] published an innovative method for quantifying facial movements, involving placement of reflective markers on the face and an installation of 4 video cameras allowing three-dimensional (3D) dynamic analysis. Although this was the first system to offer both dynamic and 3D analysis in facial palsy, the extensive setup, need to place markers, and time-consuming analysis were inhibitory to its widespread use.

In 1999, Frey and colleagues[65] published a novel 3D method of facial palsy documentation. This method used a single camera combined with 2 mirrors placed at a

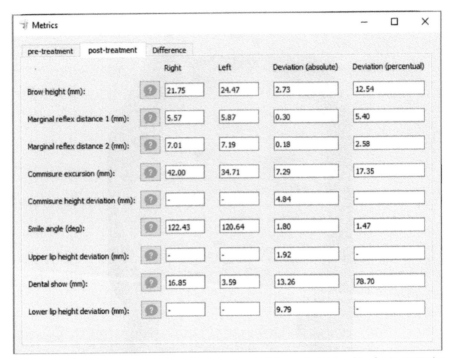

Fig. 3. Facial measurements automatically computed from facial landmarks in Emotrics. Pixel width is automatically normalized using a mean iris diameter of 11.77 mm. (*From* Guarin D, Dusseldrop J, Hadlock T, et. al. A machine learning approach for automated facial measurements in facial palsy. JAMA Facial Plast Surg 2018;e1. https://doi.org/10.1001/jamafacial.2018.0030; with permission.)

fixed angle behind the patient. Using complex computer software, 3D measurements could be obtained from a single video recording. This system had many advantages, but complexity of software analysis precluded further use.

FACIAL CLIMA (2008)

In 2008, Hontanilla and Aubá[66] published their 3D videography assessment method. The system used reflective markers and 3 infrared cameras to track facial movements. 3D displacement and facial movement velocity were calculated. Similarly, the disadvantages were the requirement for specialized equipment, the placing of markers on the face, and the time-consuming nature of the analysis.

Sforza and colleagues (2010)

Sforza and colleagues[67] described the use of an optoelectronic 3D motion analyzer in 2010. The system consisted of 6 infrared cameras and 21 reflective markers. Although highly accurate, this tool is not routinely used in clinical practice.

Three-dimensional versus Two-dimensional

The ongoing development of 3D stereophotogrammetry methods will continue to be of interest to facial nerve clinicians. Systems that rely on surface-based assessment of the face rather than landmark-based assessment have been shown to be more sensitive.[69] In addition, such systems are becoming less complex and less expensive

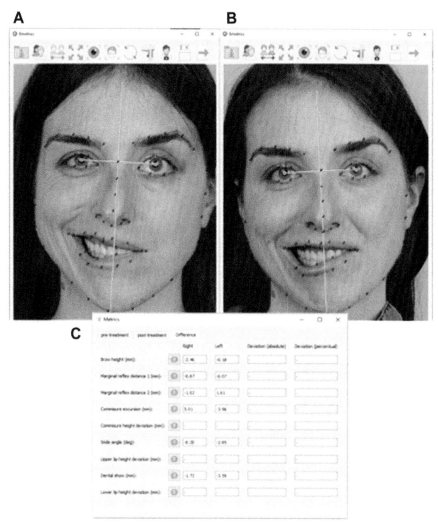

Fig. 4. Case example of a partially recovered left-sided Bell palsy showing comparison between prerecovery (*A*) and postrecovery (*B*). The facial midline is shown in both images computed as a perpendicular line to the interpupillary plane at the midpupillary point. (*C*) The difference in facial measurements between photographs. (*From* Guarin D, Dusseldrop J, Hadlock T, et. al. A machine learning approach for automated facial measurements in facial palsy. JAMA Facial Plast Surg 2018;e2. https://doi.org/10.1001/jamafacial. 2018.0030; with permission.)

over time. Some systems have been used in facial palsy for research purposes and may become more integrated with clinical practice.[70]

Although 3D analysis of facial motion is promising, two-dimensional (2D) videographic analysis may still have a role to play. 2D videography is exceedingly simple to record and software analysis tools are intuitive to use. In addition, machine learning models have been trained on large volumes of data using 2D photographs.[71] Machine learning approaches using 2D videography are currently being developed to aid assessment of spontaneous smile videos with good success.

NOVEL OUTCOME MEASURES

The face acts as a platform for social integration and nonverbal communication.[9,72] Although it is clear that patients with facial palsy have marked difficulties in these domains, few studies have sought to quantify this deficit or to show improvement following various interventions.[5,9,13,73]

Layperson Assessment

Naive observers may be best suited to determine whether patients with facial palsy are able to communicate effectively and integrate socially. Laypersons have been considered the ideal outcome measurement tool to determine the effectiveness of facial palsy treatment.[74] However, patient confidentiality makes routine use of layperson assessments impractical.

Attractiveness (2012; 2014)

Two studies recently performed by Ishii and colleagues[5] have determined the aesthetic penalty paid for unilateral facial palsy. Forty laypersons were asked to analyze normal and affected faces in a randomized sequence by rating their attractiveness. Significantly lower attractiveness was found in patients with facial palsy. In 2014, layperson assessments were used to test the difference in preoperative and postoperative attractiveness. Ninety laypersons analyzed a random sequence of paralyzed faces before and after reanimation surgery, as well as normal faces. Facial paralysis yielded an attractiveness penalty of 2.51 out of 10 at rest and 3.38 with smiling.[73] Reanimation surgery improved attractiveness at rest by 0.84 and with smiling by 1.24 points. They reported that laypersons had an overall negative facial perception of the facial palsy group, indicating the potential protective effect of smile reanimation surgery on social reintegration.

Eye tracking (2014; 2016)

In 2014, eye-tracking technology was used to analyze the scan paths of 86 laypersons while gazing on the faces of a random sequence of patients with facial palsy, both before and after smile reanimation surgery, and normal subjects, at rest and with smiling. In patients with facial palsy, fixation of gaze was directed to different points within the central triangle region. Although in normal subjects the nose held most fixation, this was directed toward the mouth in patients with facial palsy. Smile reanimation surgery was able to normalize the gaze asymmetries. In 2016, attention pattern of 60 laypersons was found to be significantly different when gazing on paralyzed faces compared with normal faces, a finding exacerbated by smiling (**Fig. 5**).

Disfigurement (2018)

In 2017, more than 500 laypersons assessed disfigurement in videos of smiles in patients with facial palsy over a broad spectrum of severity.[6] A significant correlation with degree of facial palsy (lower eFACE score) and disfigurement was discovered. Furthermore, laypersons considered patients with worse dynamic subscores to be more disfigured.

Emotional Expressivity of Voluntary Smile

Nonverbal communication from facial expressions is critical to normal social functioning and is dramatically reduced in patients with facial palsy.[9,75,76] These differences in facial expression can be detected by laypersons. Automated facial expression analysis using machine learning tools trained on millions of normal facial

A

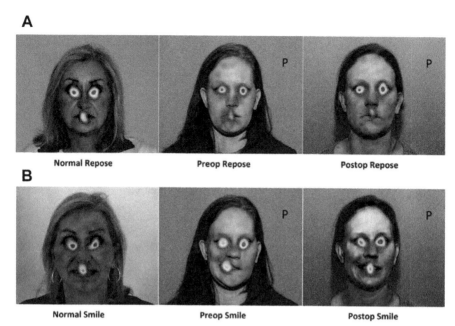

| Normal Repose | Preop Repose | Postop Repose |

B

| Normal Smile | Preop Smile | Postop Smile |

Fig. 5. Heat maps of visual fixation illustrate the distribution of attention given to a normal face and a paralyzed face (P) before and after reanimation surgery. The faces are presented in repose (*A*) and smiling (*B*). Heat maps plot the average gaze data from all observers who looked at each image, with the areas of greatest attention colored red, followed by orange, yellow, green, and blue for areas that received less attention. For normal faces, the mouth and nose have similar amounts of visual fixation. However, in the heat maps, the nose is not as bright because fixation is more evenly distributed on the nose as opposed to the mouth, where attention is centrally focused. Postop, postoperative; Preop, preoperative. (*From* Dey JK, Ishii LE, Byrne PJ, et al. Seeing is believing: objectively evaluating the impact of facial re-animation surgery on social perception. Laryngoscope 2014;124(11):2491; with permission.)

expressions could serve as a proxy for layperson assessment, forming a standard against which smile reanimation outcomes should be compared. Furthermore, such tools solve the practical and privacy concerns of undertaking layperson assessments.

Automated machine learning analysis (2018)

Recent advances in machine learning technology have enabled automated assessment of emotion expression in faces of normal individuals. Our center used commercially available software (Affdex, Affectiva, Boston, MA) to analyze voluntary smile efforts of all smile reanimation patients, before and after surgery, along with ten normal subjects. Preoperatively, positive emotion expression was significantly reduced when smiling, and negative emotion expression was significantly increased. Following smile reanimation, these findings were reversed, showing 160% improvement. Although the results were dramatic in patients with flaccid facial palsy, synkinetic patients showed near-normal levels of positive emotion expression preoperatively. However, smile reanimation was still effective, showing a significant reduction in negative emotion expression postoperatively[7].

SPONTANEOUS SMILE ASSESSMENT

Although voluntary smiles are fairly easy to simulate and measure, involuntary smiles can be more difficult. Also known as a true, emotional, or spontaneous smile, an involuntary smile is usually considered the most desirable outcome of smile reanimation surgery by both surgeons and patients.

Clinician Reported

Numerous studies have been conducted to define a spontaneous smile,[77] to determine its central neural origin,[78] and to determine its ideal peripheral neural source.[79–81] However, no standardized assessment of spontaneous smile has been developed because it is difficult both to elicit and to measure. Clinicians' personal preferences for eliciting a spontaneous smile are usually based on their ability to make a patient laugh. Chuang and colleagues[82] from Taiwan have recommended the so-called tickle test. Although there may be some consistent techniques for eliciting a spontaneous smile, there is no objective method for its measurement. Many investigators report that they are able to determine the presence of spontaneity during patient conversation.[79,80,82,83] However, there are many confounding factors that may influence this eyeball assessment. Any preexisting facial movement, synkinesis, or jaw movement may be able to confound the assessor as to whether the surgical intervention has been effective at increasing spontaneity. More importantly, clinicians may be subject to confirmation bias.

Spontaneous Smile Assay (2015)

It has been well recognized in studies of affective psychology that watching video clips of various humorous stimuli can evoke a spontaneous smile.[84] In 2015, our center validated a 1.5-minute series of video clips that generated at least one spontaneous smile in more than 95% of normal subjects (n = 95) and patients with facial palsy (n = 25).[77] Although this set of videos is reliably able to elicit a spontaneous smile, it has not solved the quantification problem.

Emotional Expressivity of Spontaneous Smile

Time stamping and synchronicity (2017)

In 2017, our center developed a rigorous technique of manual spontaneous smile assessment.[85] Two blinded assessors analyzed videos of spontaneous smile assays taken at least four months following surgery. Initially, only the lower face of the normal side was visible, and the assessor was instructed to time-stamp the video at each point when a normal side commissure movement was elicited. The blackout was then reversed so that only the lower face of the affected side was visible and oral commissure movements were time-stamped for a second time. These outputs were correlated to give an overall measure of synchronicity.

Automated machine learning analysis (2018)

It is clear that manual time stamping of videos is laborious and impractical in routine clinical practice. The authors have developed an automated technique of measuring spontaneous smile. Using two machine learning models, Emotrics, and a freely available software, Affdex (Affectiva, Boston, MA), the spontaneous smile assay of each patient was automatically analyzed to determine time-points of normal commissure movement and correlate these with affected side movement to give a synchronicity measurement. Frames where synchronous movements were detected were automatically analyzed to determine whether there was a concurrent significant increase in positive emotion expression. This tool has been used to quantify levels of spontaneous emotion expression when smiling in gracilis free functional muscle transfers using either the cross-face nerve graft, nerve to masseter, or dual innervated techniques (unpublished results).

SUMMARY

What is needed in facial palsy is a universal panel of tools that can assess severity, guide management, and ultimately measure outcomes. PROMs will remain a feature of this multimodal outcome panel in facial palsy to aid understanding of the patient-reported experience of disease and the effects of any treatment. As machine learning techniques improve, clinicians may be able to move away from clinician-graded assessments of severity, toward an automated and objective assessment system.

Rapid advances in information technology have given many insights into the negative facial perception afforded to patients with facial palsy by laypersons. For instance, laypersons have rated patients with facial palsy significantly lower in attractiveness scores and with an overall negative facial perception, whereas smile reanimation surgery had a positive effect on attractiveness and reducing negative facial perception.[73] Recent machine learning advances have allowed clinicians to scale up layperson assessment of facial expression into a robust, objective, and sensitive model of emotion expression yielding markedly similar results.[7] It has also been possible for this tool to objectively quantify spontaneous smiling.

In summary, the ultimate outcome measure panel in facial palsy should include:

1. PROMs
2. Automated and clinician-graded facial palsy grading systems
3. Layperson assessment equivalent
4. Spontaneous smile analysis

REFERENCES

1. Fattah AY, Gurusinghe ADR, Gavilan J, et al. Facial nerve grading instruments: systematic review of the literature and suggestion for uniformity. Plast Reconstr Surg 2015;135(2):569–79.
2. Guarin D, Dusseldorp JR, Hadlock TA, et al. Automated facial measurements in facial palsy: a machine learning approach. JAMA Facial Plast Surg 2018;20(4): 335–7.
3. Ishii L, Dey J, Boahene KDO, et al. The social distraction of facial paralysis: objective measurement of social attention using eye-tracking. Laryngoscope 2016;126(2):334–9.
4. Dey JK, Ishii LE, Byrne PJ, et al. Seeing is believing: objectively evaluating the impact of facial reanimation surgery on social perception. Laryngoscope 2014; 124(11):2489–97.
5. Ishii L, Godoy A, Encarnacion CO, et al. Not just another face in the crowd: society's perceptions of facial paralysis. Laryngoscope 2012;122(3):533–8.
6. Lyford-Pike S, Helwig NE, et al. Predicting perceived disfigurement from facial function in patients with unilateral paralysis. Plast Reconstr Surg, in press.
7. Dusseldorp JR, Guarin DL, Van Veen M, et al. In the eye of the beholder: changes in perceived emotion expression after smile reanimation. Plast Reconstr Surg, in press.
8. Hadlock TA, Urban LS. Toward a universal, automated facial measurement tool in facial reanimation. Arch Facial Plast Surg 2012;14(4):277–82.

9. Coulson SE, O'Dwyer NJ, Adams RD, et al. Expression of emotion and quality of life after facial nerve paralysis. Otol Neurotol 2004;25(6):1014–9.
10. Kleiss IJ, Beurskens CHG, Stalmeier PFM, et al. Quality of life assessment in facial palsy: validation of the Dutch Facial Clinimetric Evaluation Scale. Eur Arch Otorhinolaryngol 2015;272(8):2055–61.
11. Lindsay RW, Bhama P, Hadlock TA. Quality-of-life improvement after free gracilis muscle transfer for smile restoration in patients with facial paralysis. JAMA Facial Plast Surg 2014;16(6):419.
12. Fattah AY, Gavilan J, Hadlock TA, et al. Survey of methods of facial palsy documentation in use by members of the Sir Charles Bell Society. Laryngoscope 2014; 124(10):2247–51.
13. Ho AL, Scott AM, Klassen AF, et al. Measuring quality of life and patient satisfaction in facial paralysis patients: a systematic review of patient-reported outcome measures. Plast Reconstr Surg 2012;130(1):91–9.
14. Mehta RP, WernickRobinson M, Hadlock TA. Validation of the synkinesis assessment questionnaire. Laryngoscope 2007;117(5):923–6.
15. VanSwearingen JM, Brach JS. The Facial Disability Index: reliability and validity of a disability assessment instrument for disorders of the facial neuromuscular system. Phys Ther 1996;76(12):1288–98 [discussion: 1298–300]. Available at: http://www.ncbi.nlm.nih.gov/pubmed/8959998.
16. Volk GF, Steigerwald F, Vitek P, et al. Facial Disability Index and Facial Clinimetric Evaluation Scale: validation of the German versions. Laryngorhinootologie 2015; 94(3):163–8 [in German].
17. Pavese C, Cecini M, Camerino N, et al. Functional and social limitations after facial palsy: expanded and independent validation of the Italian version of the Facial Disability Index. Phys Ther 2014;94(9):1327–36.
18. Gonzalez-Cardero E, Infante-Cossio P, Cayuela A, et al. Facial Disability Index (FDI): adaptation to Spanish, reliability and validity. Med Oral Patol Oral Cir Bucal 2012;17(6):1006–12.
19. Marsk E, Hammarstedt-Nordenvall L, Engström M, et al. Validation of a Swedish version of the Facial Disability Index (FDI) and the Facial Clinimetric Evaluation (FaCE) scale. Acta Otolaryngol 2013;133(6):662–9.
20. Kahn JB, Gliklich RE, Boyev KP, et al. Validation of a patient-graded instrument for facial nerve paralysis: the FaCE scale. Laryngoscope 2001;111(3):387–98.
21. Luijmes RE, Pouwels S, Beurskens CHG, et al. Quality of life before and after different treatment modalities in peripheral facial palsy: a systematic review. Laryngoscope 2017;127(5):1044–51.
22. Li YY. Quality of life survey on patients with peripheral facial paralysis by using Chinese version of the FaCE scale. Zhonghua Er Bi Yan Hou Tou Jing Wai Ke Za Zhi 2013;48(1):11–6 [in Chinese].
23. Linstrom CJ, Silverman CA, Colson D. Facial motion analysis with a video and computer system after treatment of acoustic neuroma. Otol Neurotol 2002; 23(4):572–9.
24. Yanagihara N. Grading of facial nerve palsy. In: Fisch U, editor. Facial nerve surgery, proceedings: third international symposium on facial nerve surgery. Birmingham (AL): Aesculapius Publishing; 1977. p. 533–5.
25. Hato N, Fujiwara T, Gyo K, et al. Yanagihara facial nerve grading system as a prognostic tool in Bell's palsy. Otol Neurotol 2014;35(9):1669–72.
26. Hato N, Matsumoto S, Kisaki H, et al. Efficacy of early treatment of Bell's palsy with oral acyclovir and prednisolone. Otol Neurotol 2003;24(6):948–51.

27. Ikeda M, Nakazato H, Hiroshige K, et al. To what extent do evaluations of facial paralysis by physicians coincide with self-evaluations by patients: comparison of the Yanagihara method, the House-Brackmann method, and self-evaluation by patients. Otol Neurotol 2003;24(2):334–8.
28. Berg T, Jonsson L, Engström M. Agreement between the Sunnybrook, House-Brackmann, and Yanagihara facial nerve grading systems in Bell's palsy. Otol Neurotol 2004;25(6):1020–6.
29. House JW, Brackmann DE. Facial nerve grading system. Otolaryngol Head Neck Surg 1985;93(2):146–7.
30. Burres S, Fisch U. The comparison of facial grading systems. Arch Otolaryngol Head Neck Surg 1986;112(7):755–8.
31. Lewis BI, Adour KK. An analysis of the Adour-Swanson and House-Brackmann grading systems for facial nerve recovery. Eur Arch Otorhinolaryngol 1995; 252(5):265–9.
32. Saito H. A simple objective evaluation and grading for facial paralysis outcomes. Acta Otolaryngol 2012;132(1):101–5.
33. House JW. Facial nerve grading systems. Laryngoscope 1983;93(8):1056–69.
34. Coulson SE, Croxson GR, Adams RD, et al. Reliability of the "Sydney," "Sunnybrook," and "House Brackmann" facial grading systems to assess voluntary movement and synkinesis after facial nerve paralysis. Otolaryngol Head Neck Surg 2005;132(4):543–9.
35. Reitzen SD, Babb JS, Lalwani AK. Significance and reliability of the House-Brackmann grading system for regional facial nerve function. Otolaryngol Head Neck Surg 2009;140(2):154–8.
36. Lee HY, Moon SP, Byun JY, et al. Agreement between the facial nerve grading system 2.0 and the House-Brackmann grading system in patients with Bell palsy. Clin Exp Otorhinolaryngol 2013;6(3):135–9.
37. Smith IM, Murray JAM, Cull RE, et al. A comparison of facial grading systems. Clin Otolaryngol Allied Sci 1992;17(4):303–7.
38. Lazarini P, Mitre E, Takatu E, et al. Graphic-visual adaptation of House-Brackmann facial nerve grading for peripheral facial palsy. Clin Otolaryngol 2006;31(3):192–7.
39. Kanerva M, Poussa T, Pitkäranta A. Sunnybrook and House-Brackmann facial grading systems: intrarater repeatability and interrater agreement. Otolaryngol Head Neck Surg 2006;135(6):865–71.
40. Croxson G, May M, Mester SJ. Grading facial nerve function: House-Brackmann versus Burres-Fisch methods. Am J Otol 1990;11(4):240–6.
41. Ross BG, Fradet G, Nedzelski JM. Development of a sensitive clinical facial grading system. Otolaryngol Head Neck Surg 1996;114(3):380–6.
42. Henstrom DK, Skilbeck CJ, Weinberg J, et al. Good correlation between original and modified House Brackmann facial grading systems. Laryngoscope 2011; 121(1):47–50.
43. Kanerva M, Jonsson L, Berg T, et al. Sunnybrook and House-Brackmann systems in 5397 facial gradings. Otolaryngol Head Neck Surg 2011;144(4):570–4.
44. Ahrens A, Skarada D, Wallace M, et al. Rapid simultaneous comparison system for subjective grading scales grading scales for facial paralysis. Am J Otol 1999; 20(5):667–71.
45. Kayhan FT, Zurakowski D, Rauch SD. Toronto facial grading system: interobserver reliability. Otolaryngol Head Neck Surg 2000;122(2):212–5.
46. Hu WL, Ross B, Nedzelski J. Reliability of the Sunnybrook facial grading system by novice users. J Otolaryngol 2001;30(4):208–11.

47. Neely JG, Cherian NG, Dickerson CB, et al. Sunnybrook facial grading system: reliability and criteria for grading. Laryngoscope 2010;120(5):1038–45.
48. Terzis JK, Noah ME. Analysis of 100 cases of free-muscle transplantation for facial paralysis. Plast Reconstr Surg 1997;99(7):1905–21.
49. Biglioli F, Frigerio A, Rabbiosi D, et al. Single-stage facial reanimation in the surgical treatment of unilateral established facial paralysis. Plast Reconstr Surg 2009;124(1):124–33.
50. Brichacek M, Sultan B, Boahene KD, et al. Objective outcomes of minimally invasive temporalis tendon transfer for prolonged complete facial paralysis. Plast Surg (Oakv) 2017;25(3):200–10.
51. Balaji S. Temporalis pull-through vs fascia lata augmentation in facial reanimation for facial paralysis. Ann Maxillofac Surg 2016;6(2):267.
52. Allevi F, Motta G, Colombo V, et al. Double-bellied latissimus dorsi free flap to correct full dental smile palsy. BMJ Case Rep 2015;2015 [pii:bcr2015210436].
53. Ahuja R, Chatterjee P, Gupta R, et al. A new paradigm in facial reanimation for long-standing palsies? Indian J Plast Surg 2015;48(1):30.
54. Gordin E, Lee TS, Ducic Y, et al. Facial nerve trauma: evaluation and considerations in management. Craniomaxillofac Trauma Reconstr 2015;8(1):1–13.
55. Leckenby J, Grobbelaar A. Smile restoration for permanent facial paralysis. Arch Plast Surg 2013;40(5):633–8.
56. Labbè D, Bussu F, Iodice A. A comprehensive approach to long-standing facial paralysis based on lengthening temporalis myoplasty. Acta Otorhinolaryngol Ital 2012;32(3):145–53.
57. Vrabec JT, Backous DD, Djalilian HR, et al. Facial nerve grading system 2.0. Otolaryngol Head Neck Surg 2009;140(4):445–50.
58. Lee LN, Susarla SM, Hohman MH, et al. A comparison of facial nerve grading systems. Ann Plast Surg 2013;70(3):313–6.
59. Banks CA, Bhama PK, Park J, et al. Clinician-graded electronic facial paralysis assessment. Plast Reconstr Surg 2015;136(2):223e–30e.
60. Banks CA, Jowett N, Hadlock TA. Test-retest reliability and agreement between in-person and video assessment of facial mimetic function using the eFACE facial grading system. JAMA Facial Plast Surg 2017;19(3):206–11.
61. Banks CA, Jowett N, Hadlock CR, et al. Weighting of facial grading variables to disfigurement in facial palsy. JAMA Facial Plast Surg 2016;18(4):292–8.
62. Banks CA, Jowett N, Azizzadeh B, et al. Worldwide testing of the eFACE facial nerve clinician-graded scale. Plast Reconstr Surg 2017;139(2):491e–8e.
63. Kleiss IJ, Eviston TJ, Hadlock TA. Quantitative assessment of facial function in patients with peripheral facial palsy: a systematic review. In: Assessment of facial function in peripheral facial palsy. Nijmegen (Netherlands): Radboud University Nijmegen; 2015. p. 97–122.
64. Frey M, Jenny a, Giovanoli P, et al. Development of a new documentation system for facial movements as a basis for the international registry for neuromuscular reconstruction in the face. Plast Reconstr Surg 1994;93(7):1334–49.
65. Frey M, Giovanoli P, Gerber H, et al. Three-dimensional video analysis of facial movements: a new method to assess the quantity and quality of the smile. Plast Reconstr Surg 1999;104(7):2032–9.
66. Hontanilla B, Aubá C. Automatic three-dimensional quantitative analysis for evaluation of facial movement. J Plast Reconstr Aesthet Surg 2008;61(1):18–30.
67. Sforza C, Galante D, Shirai YF, et al. A three-dimensional study of facial mimicry in healthy young adults. J Craniomaxillofac Surg 2010;38(6):409–15.

68. Sforza C, Guzzo M, Mapelli A, et al. Facial mimicry after conservative parotidectomy: a three-dimensional optoelectronic study. Int J Oral Maxillofac Surg 2012; 41(8):986–93.

69. Verhoeven T, Xi T, Schreurs R, et al. Quantification of facial asymmetry: a comparative study of landmark-based and surface-based registrations. J Craniomaxillofac Surg 2016;44(9):1131–6.

70. Codari M, Pucciarelli V, Stangoni F, et al. Facial thirds–based evaluation of facial asymmetry using stereophotogrammetric devices: application to facial palsy subjects. J Craniomaxillofac Surg 2017;45(1):76–81.

71. McDuff D, El Kaliouby R, Senechal T, et al. Affectiva-MIT facial expression dataset (AM-FED): naturalistic and spontaneous facial expressions collected "in-the-wild." IEEE Computer Society Conference on Computer Vision and Pattern Recognition Workshops. Portland (OR), 23-28 June 2013. p. 881–8. https://doi.org/10.1109/CVPRW.2013.130.

72. Helwig NE, Sohre NE, Ruprecht MR, et al. Dynamic properties of successful smiles. PLoS One 2017;12(6):1–17.

73. Dey JK, Ishii M, Boahene KDO, et al. Changing perception: facial reanimation surgery improves attractiveness and decreases negative facial perception. Laryngoscope 2014;124(1):84–90.

74. Hadlock T. Standard outcome measures in facial paralysis getting on the same page. JAMA Facial Plast Surg 2016;18(2):85–6.

75. Surakka V, Hietanen JK. Facial and emotional reactions to Duchenne and non-Duchenne smiles. Int J Psychophysiol 1998;29(1):23–33.

76. Hall JA, Carter JD, Horgan TG. Gender differences in nonverbal communication of emotion. In: Fischer A, editor. Gender and emotion: social psychological perspectives. New York: Cambridge University Press; 2000. p. 97–117. https://doi.org/10.1017/CBO9780511628191.006.

77. Iacolucci CM, Banks C, Jowett N, et al. Development and validation of a spontaneous smile assay. JAMA Facial Plast Surg 2015;17(3):191–6.

78. Buendia J, Loayza FR, Luis EO, et al. Functional and anatomical basis for brain plasticity in facial palsy rehabilitation using the masseteric nerve. J Plast Reconstr Aesthet Surg 2016;69(3):417–26.

79. Biglioli F, Bayoudh W, Colombo V, et al. Double innervation (facial/masseter) on the gracilis flap, in the middle face reanimation in the management of facial paralysis: a new concept. Ann Chir Plast Esthet 2013;58(2):89–95 [in French].

80. Cardenas-Mejia A, Covarrubias-Ramirez JV, Bello-Margolis A, et al. Double innervated free functional muscle transfer for facial reanimation. J Plast Surg Hand Surg 2015;49(3):183–8.

81. Watanabe Y, Akizuki T, Ozawa T, et al. Dual innervation method using one-stage reconstruction with free latissimus dorsi muscle transfer for re-animation of established facial paralysis: simultaneous reinnervation of the ipsilateral masseter motor nerve and the contralateral facial nerve to improve the quality of smile and emotional facial expressions. J Plast Reconstr Aesthet Surg 2009;62(12): 1589–97.

82. Chuang DCC, Lu JCY, Anesti K. One-stage procedure using spinal accessory nerve (XI)-innervated free muscle for facial paralysis reconstruction. Plast Reconstr Surg 2013;132(1):117e–29e.

83. Sforza C, Frigerio A, Mapelli A, et al. Double-powered free gracilis muscle transfer for smile reanimation: a longitudinal optoelectronic study. J Plast Reconstr Aesthet Surg 2015;68(7):930–9.

84. Ekman P, Friesen WV, Hager JC. Facial action coding system. A technique for the measurement of facial action. Palo Alto (CA): Consulting Psychologists Press; 1978.

85. Dusseldorp JR, Van Veen M, Quatela O, et al. Dually innervated gracilis in smile reanimation. Presented at the International Facial Nerve Symposium. Los Angeles, August 3-6, 2017.

Medical Management of Acute Facial Paralysis

Teresa M. O, MD, MArch

KEYWORDS

- Acute facial paralysis • Bell palsy • Facial paresis • Medical therapy
- Corticosteroids • Antiviral therapy • Physical therapy

KEY POINTS

- Acute facial paralysis occurs within hours to days, and the most common cause is viral-associated Bell palsy, which is a diagnosis of exclusion.
- A complete history and physical examination are essential to making a diagnosis.
- Therapy is multimodal and multidisciplinary; medical therapy, meticulous eye care, and physical therapy are important. Depending on the etiology, surgery also plays a role.
- High-dose corticosteroids are the cornerstone of medical therapy.
- Absence of recovery after 4 months should prompt further diagnostic workup.

Acute facial paralysis (FP) describes acute onset of partial or complete weakness of the facial muscles innervated by the facial nerve. Acute FP occurs within a few hours to days. Bilateral acute FP is possible, but rare. The differential diagnosis (**Table 1**) of acute FP is broad; however, the most common cause is viral-associated Bell palsy (BP).[1] A comprehensive history (age, time course, associated symptoms, and medical history) and physical examination are essential in arriving at a diagnosis.

HISTORY

The importance of a thorough history cannot be overstated. Acute FP is a devastating event that causes aesthetic, functional, and psychological issues. Patients are very precise in the time/date or date range during which paralysis occurred. They will also be able to relay any events leading up to or after the paralysis.

Viral-associated acute FP (BP) is the most common cause and may be associated with a prodrome and fully evolve over 1 to 3 days. Any history of recent travel, infection, or tick exposures may suggest other infectious causes. Recent head trauma and

Disclosure Statement: The author has nothing to disclose.
Facial Nerve Center, Vascular Birthmark Institute of New York, Department of Otolaryngology-Head and Neck Surgery, Manhattan Eye, Ear, and Throat Hospital, Lenox Hill Hospital, 210 East 64th Street, 7th Floor, New York, New York, 10065, USA
E-mail address: to@vbiny.org

Otolaryngol Clin N Am 51 (2018) 1051–1075
https://doi.org/10.1016/j.otc.2018.07.004
0030-6665/18/© 2018 Elsevier Inc. All rights reserved.

Table 1
Differential diagnosis of acute facial paralysis

Diagnosis Category	Diagnosis	Clinical Signs/Symptoms	Etiology	Diagnostics	Acute Management
Infectious	Bell palsy	Fully progresses to flaccid facial paralysis (FFP) within 72 hours Viral prodrome	Herpes simplex virus (HSV) reactivation	No serology Consider ENoG and EMG	Eye care: lubricants, shield Physical therapy: eyelid stretch Medications: High-dose steroids: Prednisone 60 mg × 5 days, followed by a 5-d taper Antiviral: Valacyclovir 1 g BID × 7d
	Ramsay Hunt syndrome	Otalgia, vestibulocochlear symptoms Vesicles	Varicella zoster virus (VZV)	Audiogram	Per BP
	Lyme disease	Headache, fatigue, fever, arthritis "Erythema migrans" (bull's eye) rash, outdoors activity	Bacterium: *Borrelia burgdorferi* via tick bite	Serum and cerebrospinal fluid antibodies	Eye care: lubricants, shield PT: eyelid stretch Doxycycline 100 mg PO BID 10–21 d or Cefuroxime 500 mg PO BID, 14–21 d or Amoxicillin 500 mg PO BID, 14–21 d Per recent CDC guidelines ± steroids
	HIV	Viral symptoms, early (seroconversion) or late stages	Human immunodeficiency virus	Serology	*Antiviral, steroids Highly active antiretroviral therapy (HAART)

Congenital				
Birth trauma	Known history	Blunt trauma, forceps	None	Eye care
Geniculate ganglion vascular malformation	Recurrent FP, vestibulocochlear symptoms if impinging on other CN	Venous malformation	Magnetic Resonance Imaging (MRI), Computed Tomography (CT) Temporal bones	Neurotology evaluation
Pontine vascular malformation	Headache, seizure, and/or focal neuro deficit	Arteriovenous or venous malformation	MRI/MRA, angiogram	Surgery, embolization, or sclerotherapy or combined (sclerotherapy + surgery)
Pontine developmental venous anomaly (DVA)	FP, CVA symptoms, (typically asymptomatic)	Hemorrhage of DVA	MRI, angiogram	Embolization
Otologic				
Infectious				
Acute otitis media	Otalgia, hearing loss, ± otorrhea	Bacteria, virus	MRI with gadolinium CT temporal bones audiogram, culture	*Directed IV antibiotic therapy high-dose steroids Myringotomy ± mastoidectomy ± facial nerve decompression
Malignant otitis externa	Otalgia, otorrhea, +/- hearing loss (HL)	*Pseudomonas*, Methicillin-resistant Staphylococcus Aureus	MRI with gadolinium CT temporal bones audiogram, culture	Rule out osteomyelitis and carcinoma, consider biopsy Treatment similar to OM Screen for diabetes
Cholesteatoma	History of OM	Nonneoplastic keratinizing squamous epithelium	MRI/CT, audiogram	Transmastoid surgery

(continued on next page)

Table 1
(continued)

Diagnosis Category	Diagnosis	Clinical Signs/Symptoms	Etiology	Diagnostics	Acute Management
Intracranial tumor	Vestibular Schwannoma	Vestibulocochlear symptoms, FP	Schwann cell tumor of CNVIII	MRI with gadolinium	Neurology evaluation
	Facial nerve Schwannoma	FP common, other vestibulocochlear symptoms	Schwann cell tumor of CNVII	CT temporal bones vestibulocochlear tests	Neurology evaluation XRT or surgery
	Leptomeningeal carcinomatosis	Pain, seizure, headache	Metastatic carcinoma to meninges cerebral, cranial nerve, spinal root	MRI with gadolinium, cerebrospinal fluid cytology	Chemo/radiotherapy, supportive
Trauma	Temporal bone fracture	Known history of blunt head trauma	Fracture transverse or parallel to facial nerve	CT temporal bones ENoG, EMG audiologic testing	*High-dose steroids possible decompression within 3–14 d
	Penetrating trauma	Known history	Foreign body or knife		Explore, *
	Birth trauma	Known history	Blunt trauma, forceps	None	Eye care
Iatrogenic	Parotid or soft tissue surgery or orthognathic surgery	Immediate FP after surgery	Direct transection or neuropraxia of FN.		Exploration Primary coaptation Interposition graft *
	Otologic surgery	Known history Delayed reactivation	Reactivation of virus (BP)		Same as BP
Malignant tumors	Parotid CA	Acute or slowly progressive FP	Tumor infiltration or compression	MRI + contrast	Eye care High dose steroids Antiviral
	Head & neck CA				Surgical excision + FN reconstruction +/- adjuvant therapy

Systemic autoimmune	Sarcoidosis	Any organ system - fatigue, weight loss, lung symptoms	Systemic granulomatous disease	Diagnosis of exclusion: Angiotensin converting enzyme (ACE), Chest Xray	Steroids, anti-metabolites, immune suppressants
	Melkersson-Rosenthal syndrome	Recurrent FP, orofacial edema, fissured tongue (usually asynchronous)	Neuromucocutaneous granulomatous disease, fibrosis with nonnecrotizing perivascular granulomatous infiltrate	CSF (elevated protein) CT/MRI face, r/o other	*High-dose steroids
	Guillain-Barre	Ascending muscle weakness, viral prodrome	Demyelinating disease	IgG antibody	IVIG, plasmapharesis*
	Multiple sclerosis	Fatigue, diplopia, paresthesias, weakness	Demyelinating disease	Blood test, MRI, Lumbar puncture, Imaging	Corticosteroids, plasmapharesis, immunomodulators
	Amyloidosis	Nonspecific, fatigue, raccoon eyes, all organs	Amyloid proteins	Biopsy, Congo red stain	Corticosteroids, immunomodulators, stem cell
	Wegener granulomatosis	Usually lung and kidney symptoms	Necrotizing vasculitis	MPO, PR3	High-dose steroids ± Rituxan *
	Sjögren syndrome	Sicca syndrome-dry eyes, mouth, arthralgia	Lymphocytic infiltrate	Salivary gland biopsy Anti-SSA, RF	BP treatment Immunomodulators
	Systemic lupus erythematosus (SLE)	Fever, rash, joint pain	Vasculitis, autoantibodies	ANA, depends on organ	BP treatment Immunomodulators
	Behçet disease	Oral, genital ulcers, arthritis	Vasculitis	Clinical diagnosis ANCA, PR3	High-dose pulsed steroids Immunomodulators
Metabolic	Hypothyroidism			Thyroid Function Tests (TFTs)	Synthroid, endocrine consult, *BP treatment • Discuss risks/benefits
	Pregnancy		Bell's Palsy		

(continued on next page)

Table 1
(continued)

Diagnosis Category	Diagnosis	Clinical Signs/Symptoms	Etiology	Diagnostics	Acute Management
Vascular	Brainstem cerebrovascular accident (CVA)	FP, vertigo, hearing loss	Occlusion of vessel, ischemia to tissues or hemorrhage	MRI/CT/angio MRI diffusion	Neurology consult Interventional radiology (IR) Consider thrombolytics or thrombectomy Supportive medical management
	Central CVA	Unilateral weakness, multiple cranial nerves	Hemispheric stroke	MRI/CT/angio	Neurology consult Interventional radiology (IR) Consider thrombolytics or thrombectomy Supportive medical management
Other risk factors for acute FP	Diabetes mellitus		Glucose metabolism small vessel vasculitis	Glucose, HgA1c	Treat hyperglycemia lifestyle - diet, exercise
	Hypertension		Small vessel vasculitis or thrombosis	Physical examination, vitals	Treat hypertension high-dose steroids (may exacerbate hypertension)
					*NB: In all acute FP, consider meticulous eye care and Bell Palsy medical management.

Abbreviations: * Bell Palsy medical therapy; ANA, antinuclear antibody; ANCA, antineutrophil cytoplasmic antibodies; BID, twice a day; BP, Bell palsy; CDC, Centers for Disease Control and Prevention; CN, cranial nerve; CSF, cerebrospinal fluid; CT, computed tomography; CVA, cerebrovascular accident; EMG, electromyography; ENoG, electroneurography; FFP, flaccid FP; FP, facial paralysis; HIV, human immunodeficiency virus; Ig, immunoglobulin; IV, intravenous; IVIG, intravenous immunoglobulin; MPO, myeloperoxidase; MRA, magnetic resonance angiography; MRSA, methicillin-resistant *Staphylococcus aureus*; OM, otitis media; PO, per os; PR3, proteinase 3; PT, physical therapy; SSA, Sjögren's-syndrome-related antigen A.

hearing loss may indicate temporal bone trauma. A past medical history of immune disorders or other systemic disorders may be important, especially if associated with a bilateral or recurrent paralysis.

The patient's age at presentation is important. Traumatic congenital FP presents at birth and is noticed with the first cry or grimace. The time course of FP is also important (**Fig. 1**) and may point to a diagnosis. BP classically evolves over the first 72 hours

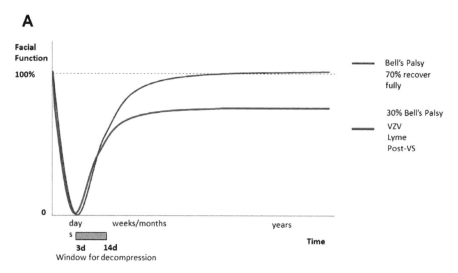

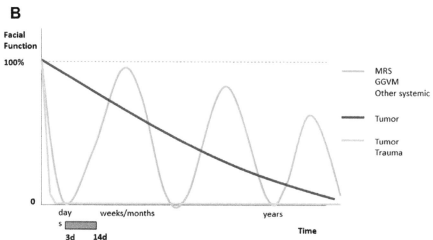

Fig. 1. Natural history of various etiologies of acute FP. (*A*) Graph shows BP with earliest recovery and return to baseline facial function. Red line depicts a minority of BP, VZV, or Lyme, or post-vestibular schwannoma resection. Note incomplete recovery. Shaded bar shows window of possible surgical decompression between 3 and 14 days. (*B*) Green line shows waxing and waning pattern evident in Melkersson-Rosenthal Syndrome (MRS), geniculate ganglion vascular malformation (GGVM), or other systemic causes. Note progressive loss of facial function over time. Red line shows tumor-related FP with slowly progressive FP. Yellow line shows tumor-related FP with sudden FP and no recovery. (*Courtesy of* Tessa A. Hadlock, MD, Boston, MA; *Modified by* Teresa MO, MD, New York, NY.)

with varying degrees of hemifacial paresis. Recovery of facial tone and movement occurs within 4 months; severe cases may see ongoing changes in facial function for a period of 12 to 18 months following onset. Approximately 70% of patients will fully recover, whereas the remainder will demonstrate varying degrees of aberrant regeneration with facial synkinesis. Zoster-associated FP is more prevalent in the older age group and may take longer to recover with a higher percentage of postrecovery residual weakness and synkinesis.

PHYSICAL EXAMINATION

The physician should note the patient's age, ethnicity, and geographic location. A complete head and neck examination should be performed, including a complete cranial nerve examination. The facial nerve function on the paralyzed side should be compared with that of the nonparalyzed side of the face. An ear examination together with tuning fork evaluation can rule out otologic causes. Palpation of the parotid area and skin will rule out parotid masses. A fissured tongue may suggest a diagnosis of Melkersson-Rosenthal syndrome (recurrent facial palsy, fissured tongue, recurrent orofacial edema, typically asynchronous). The skin examination may show a rash, nodules (systemic, autoimmune, Lyme, skin cancer) or vesicles (zoster). A directed cranial nerve examination also gives information about any other related nerve deficit and other systemic, infectious, or neoplastic causes.

The face is evaluated in horizontal thirds and compared with the nonparalytic side (**Fig. 2**). In the upper third, one notes the presence or absence of forehead wrinkles and the position of the eyebrow. Symmetry of the upper third may indicate a central cause of FP and the need for further imaging to rule out a central cause.

Care must be taken to evaluate the eye and periocular complex. One evaluates eye closure and corneal reflex, as well as the presence of a Bell phenomenon (protective superior rotation of the globe). Schirmer tear test evaluates the viability of the tear film and its ability to keep the eye moist. The vertical height of the medial palpebral fissure will be increased in flaccid paralysis. The position of the lower eyelid relative to the iris

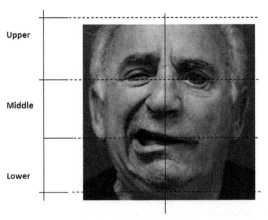

Fig. 2. Physical evaluation of patient with acute FP. Horizontal zonal approach to the paralyzed face. Note the horizontal thirds and comparison of left and right face. In upper zone, note left ptotic eyebrow, retracted upper eyelid, and lower lid ectropion. In the midface, the nasolabial fold is effaced with ptosis of the malar fat pad and inferomedial alar rotation, ptosis of the oral commissure. Lower face shows lack of lower lip depressor and platysma function.

and a snap test of the lower eyelid skin will evaluate the elasticity of the lower eyelid skin, which is an indication of the tone of the orbicularis oculi muscle. Advancing age will diminish lower eyelid skin tone and so, comparison with the nonparalyzed side is essential.

In the presence of paralysis, the middle third of the face will show flaccid ptosis of the mid cheek and fat pad. The nasal ala may also be displaced inferomedially and the philtrum pulled to the contralateral side. External nasal valve obstruction of the para-lyzed side is often present. The nasolabial fold on the affected side will be effaced. In the lower third, the oral commissure may be inferiorly displaced and there may be weakening of the lower lip with oral incompetence.

One should take note of the type of paralysis: completely flaccid, partially flaccid, or a combination of flaccidity and synkinesis. This will be helpful in determining the cause as well as a possible treatment.

DOCUMENTATION

Documentation with photography and videography is performed at the first and rele-vant follow-up visits. Still photographs of prescribed facial expressions are taken to show the range of facial movement. A short video clip of the same expressions is also performed. This allows for ongoing evaluation as the patient recovers or as inter-ventions are performed.

OUTCOME MEASURES

Patient-reported and physician-reported outcome measures are also completed. Patient-reported questionnaires include the FaCE instrument (Facial Clinimetric Eval-uation Scale), FDI (Facial Disability Index), and NOSE instrument (Nasal Obstruction and Septoplasty Effectiveness Scale). Physician-reported scales include the Sunny-brook Facial Grading Scale and the eFACE assessment (electronic clinician-graded facial function scale). These measures are useful in assessing the patients temporally as well as providing a comparison after future interventions.

ETIOLOGY OF ACUTE FACIAL PARALYSIS

The most common cause of acute FP is BP.[1–4] However, this is always a diagnosis of exclusion and should be given only after all other diagnoses have been entertained (see **Table 1**).

BP is named after Sir Charles Bell, who described idiopathic FP.[5] Although Frie-drich[6] first described the disorder 23 years prior, Bell's name is ascribed to the phe-nomenon.[1,2] BP is by far the most common cause of acute FP and accounts for up to 70% of cases. Depending on the population studied, the second most common etiol-ogy is congenital FP followed by Ramsay Hunt syndrome (RHS).[1] Clinically, patients will experience a viral prodrome with post/auricular pain, ipsilateral tongue numbness, or loss of taste. The FP will progress over 3 days.

The incidence of BP has been variously reported to be between 18 and 40 cases per 100,000 persons annually.[1,7] The largest studies with 1000 to 2000 patients show an average incidence of 29 per 100,000.[1,3,8,9] The wide variability is attributed to the various heterogeneous populations and ethnicities studied. Patients 30 to 45 years old are most commonly affected.[8] There is a slight increase in the winter months,[10] but no gender predilection.

The etiology of BP is thought to be viral reactivation of latent herpes simplex virus (HSV)[10–15] or varicella zoster virus (VZV) or human herpes virus 6.[16] After primary infection via saliva, the virus becomes latent in the sensory ganglia. Viral insult causes inflammation of the facial nerve, thought to result in ischemia centered at the labyrinthine segment of the facial nerve within the temporal bone.[17,18] VZV is more virulent and associated with delayed recovery compared with HSV-associated FP. Gadolinium-enhanced MRI shows unilateral enhancement of the facial nerve at the meatal region,[18,19] a physiologic bottleneck where inflammation compresses and causes ischemia to the nerve.

Seventy-one percent of patients with BP recover completely without treatment.[1] An improved prognosis is seen in cases of incomplete paralysis, age younger than 14 years, intact taste, intact stapedius reflex, intact tearing, absence of postauricular pain, and signs of recovery within 3 weeks. Poor prognostic indicators include diabetes, pregnancy, advanced age (>60), hypertension, and complete facial flaccidity at onset.

OTHER ACQUIRED CAUSES OF ACUTE FACIAL PARALYSIS

BP is the most common cause of acute FP. After this designation, the literature varies on the next common causes depending on the center and their referral patterns.[1,2] The following is a general sampling of other causes of FP.

Other Infectious Causes

Varicella zoster virus

VZV–associated FP represents one form of viral FP.[1] Herpes zoster oticus or RHS has a poor prognosis with delayed recovery compared with BP. RHS is characterized by unilateral FP, pain, cochleovestibular symptoms (sensorineural hearing loss), and vesicles in a segmental pattern (**Fig. 3**). Patients older than 45 years are more commonly affected and will have a more complete facial palsy. Vesicles are typically located in the concha or external ear canal; however, any distribution including cranial nerves 5, 9, and 10 and cervical nerves are possible. The vesicles may not appear simultaneously with the palsy. Zoster sine herpete occurs with an absence of vesicles and may make the diagnosis more difficult. Treatment includes high-dose corticosteroid and antiviral medication. Without treatment, only 21% will fully recover.[1]

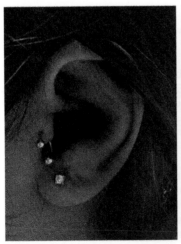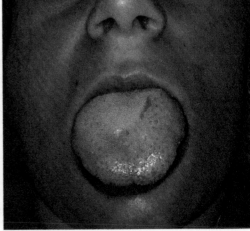

Fig. 3. RHS with left ear conchal vesicles, erythema, and edema and left tongue edema in patient with herpes zoster infection and left acute FP. She also has ipsilateral acute sensorineural hearing loss.

Lyme disease is another infectious cause. It is caused by the spirochete *Borrelia burgdorferi*, which is transmitted to humans by ticks. Although named after a town in the northeast, it is present across the entire United States. The diagnosis requires a high level of suspicion, as patients often do not recall a tick bite or rash, and serology can demonstrate false negatives early in the course of disease. Bilateral FP may occur. Patients may also report fatigue and severe headache. The differentiation from BP or other viral-associated FP is important because steroids may be associated with worse prognosis and postparalytic synkinesis.[20] Diagnostic testing includes serum and cerebrospinal fluid testing for *Borrelia* antibodies. Corticosteroid monotherapy is thought to increase the spirochete load in neural tissues. Medical treatment follows current Centers for Disease Control and Prevention (CDC) guidelines (https://www.cdc.gov/lyme/). Antibiotics, such as doxycycline, cefuroxime, or amoxicillin, are prescribed for a 10-day to 21-day course. An antiviral (valacyclovir) may also be added because facial nerve inflammation may theoretically lead to viral reactivation. Adjuvant corticosteroid therapy has not demonstrated benefit in Lyme disease–associated facial palsy and their role remains unclear.[20]

Human immunodeficiency virus

Human immunodeficiency virus (HIV)-related acute FP occurs during early or late-phase HIV infection. Patients may present with unilateral or bilateral FP.[21] In the early phase of the disease, the etiology of FP is similar to the general population and most likely related to BP. However, in the later stages, lymphoma and other secondary causes are more common.[22] Diagnostic testing includes HIV antigen and antibody tests. During seroconversion (early stages), treatment is similar to BP and corticosteroid and antiviral therapy with/without antiretroviral therapy is used. Treatment for HIV follows current CDC guidelines (www.cdc.gov/hiv/).

Nonmalignant Otologic Disease

Acute otitis media (AOM) and rarely cholesteatoma may result in acute FP.[23] In AOM, patients may present with otalgia, otorrhea, hearing loss, fever, and abnormal otoscopy findings. Broad-spectrum parenteral antibiotics and steroids should be given. Depending on the case, myringotomy with or without mastoidectomy may be indicated. Initially broad-spectrum antibiotics are used and then refined based on the bacterial culture.

Chronic otitis media causing FP is most likely due to cholesteatoma in 60% to 80% of cases.[24,25] Cholesteatoma is a nonneoplastic, keratinizing squamous lesion composed of a proliferation of epithelium and may be congenital or acquired.[26,27] In acquired cholesteatoma, one theory suggests that negative middle ear pressure causes a retraction pocket and trapped epithelial components. Secondary infection leads to accumulation of debris, immunogenic cells, and lytic enzymes. The enzymes contribute to osteolysis. Although pathologically nonmalignant, the lesion may be locally destructive. Patients commonly present with otalgia, otorrhea, and hearing loss. Three percent of patients with cholesteatoma may present with sudden or gradual FP. In this subset, most patients had acute FP, labyrinthitis, hearing loss, and bony destruction of the cranial fossa. The treatment of cholesteatoma is primarily surgical with adjuvant medical therapy (antibiotics and steroids). Surgical findings may include bony defects in the fallopian canal, bony labyrinth with exposure of the semicircular canals and vestibule, and cranial base.[24]

MALIGNANT OTITIS EXTERNA

Malignant otitis externa usually begins as an otitis externa of the external auditory canal. The infection progresses to an osteomyelitis of the temporal bone and the skull base with risk to adjacent neural and cranial structures. The facial nerve is the cranial nerve most commonly involved. Patients usually present with auricular pain, otorrhea, and hearing loss. Risk factors include diabetes mellitus, previous radiation therapy, advanced age, and an immunocompromised state. The white cell count may be normal or raised but the ESR (erythrocyte sedimentation rate) is always raised. Ear culture is positive for *Pseudomonas aeruginosa* in most cases. If squamous carcinoma of the temporal bone is suspected, a biopsy should be done. Imaging should include a computed tomography (CT) scan of the temporal bones and an MRI. If results are equivocal, technetium or gallium scans may also aid diagnosis. Treatment includes control of the diabetes, antibiotic ear drops, long-term intravenous antibiotics, and debridement. Progress may be followed clinically, as well as with serial ESR.

PREGNANCY-ASSOCIATED BELL PALSY

It is not clear whether pregnancy increases the risk of FP over the general population; however, it occurs more frequently during the third trimester in pregnant patients. The etiology is likely the same as in typical BP with viral reactivation.[28] Most cases are unilateral FP; however, bilateral may also be possible. BP during the third trimester carries a worse prognosis compared with a cohort of nonpregnant women of the same age.[29] Medical treatment is the same as for BP. Steroids and antivirals are recommended. The risk-to-benefit ratio in conjunction with the age of the fetus should be weighed and discussed with the patient. It is believed that steroids have higher risk for the fetus in the first trimester, including adrenal suppression, low birth weight, and developmental defects.[28] However, a recent literature review showed that these risks were taken from long-term administration of the drug in cases such as rheumatoid arthritis, whereas the dosing for acute FP is short.[30] The conclusion is that steroids for acute FP are safe in pregnancy, especially in the third trimester.[30] Antiviral medications are low risk to the mother and fetus and are used during late pregnancy.

TUMORS
Benign

Vestibular schwannomas are the most common benign intracranial tumors. FP is typically caused by treatment of these lesions; resection or radiation, both of which can result in facial nerve injury. A very large vestibular schwannoma can also cause FP, although less likely acute FP. Facial nerve schwannomas may also cause FP, as they slowly grow and expand, and may rarely present with acute FP (see Drs Alicia M. Quesnel and Felipe Santos' article, "Evaluation and Management of Facial Nerve Schwannoma," and Drs Vivian Kaul and Maura K. Cosetti's article, "Management of Vestibular Schwannoma (including NF2) - Facial Nerve Considerations," in this issue, for further details.)

Malignant

Head and neck tumors, such as parotid malignancies, can present with acute or slowly progressive FP. MRI with contrast will delineate the tumor and any facial nerve involvement. Treatment of the tumor will depend on the clinical and pathologic stage. Acute management focuses on eye care and antibiotic and steroid medical therapy. Planned surgical extirpation with facial nerve (FN) reconstruction will depend on the extent of the tumor as well as patient factors.

TRAUMA

Blunt or penetrating trauma to the head may result in acute FP secondary to intratemporal or extratemporal bone injury. In blunt force trauma, the area of injury may be investigated with imaging. A fine-cut, noncontrast temporal bone CT may demonstrate a fracture oriented transverse or longitudinal to the petrous segment. Transverse fractures are less common but have a higher risk of FN injury.[31] Displaced fractures may result in bony impingement of the nerve, whereas nondisplaced fractures may result in perineural inflammation and subsequent neural ischemia. These patients are typically treated with parenteral steroids and antiviral agents. The mode of FN injury and timing of paralysis, as well as the imaging and electrophysiological testing results will determine whether or not the patient will benefit from FN decompression[32,33] (see Dr. Daniel Q. Sun and colleagues' article, "Surgical Management of Acute Facial Palsy," in this issue, for further details.)

In cases of penetrating trauma to the soft tissues of the head and neck with acute FP, immediate surgical exploration and debridement are warranted. Depending on the FN deficit, a partial or full FN exploration is performed. Early exploration is important because within 1 to 3 days after the event, the distal nerve branches are still able to be stimulated with a nerve stimulator. The nerve continuity is checked and any transected segment is repaired. Ideally, a primary coaptation is performed. If necessary, an interposition graft is placed.

Birth trauma (ie, forceps delivery) can affect 1 or more branches of the facial nerve and is evident with the first cry. The mastoid bone is not fully developed until 2 years of age, thus exposing the FN. Risks of birth trauma include forceps delivery, birthweight more than 3.5 kg, and primiparity.[34] Fortunately, most infants recover fully without intervention.

IATROGENIC CAUSES

Soft tissue or mandibular surgery distal to the stylomastoid foramen can cause facial nerve injury. This includes surgery of the temporomandibular joint or other orthognathic procedures, and parotid, masseter, or other soft tissue excision. Certain otologic procedures also carry a risk of facial nerve injury. FP noticed immediately after surgical intervention should be explored.

Autoimmune or systemic causes

In patients with recurrent FP or bilateral involvement, the likely cause is autoimmune. A medical and family history of autoimmune disease or other symptomatology, such as an unexplained rash or facial swelling should be investigated.

Guillain-Barre (GBS)[35,36] is an uncommon cause of FP. GBS is a postinfectious inflammatory demyelinating polyradiculoneuropathy of motor and sensory nerves. Approximately a third of patients with GBS will present with FP. Typically, patients have a history of a viral prodrome.[37] Therapy includes plasmapheresis and intravenous immunoglobulin therapy.

Multiple sclerosis is a chronic inflammatory demyelinating disease of the central nervous system and may present with unilateral or recurrent FP.[38] Diagnosis may involve blood tests, lumbar puncture and imaging (MRI).

Amyloid disease is associated with the deposition of amyloid proteins that can directly infiltrate the facial nerve.[39,40] An autosomal dominant Finnish type of amyloidosis is also associated with progressive bilateral FP (BFP).[41] Congo red staining and a polarizing microscopic examination of tissue biopsies is diagnostic for amyloidosis.

Granulomatosis with polyangiitis (GPA), Wegener granulomatosis[42] is a multisystem inflammatory disease, characterized by necrotizing vasculitis of vessels (small and medium size) with multinucleated giant cells and microabscess formation. It most commonly affects the lungs and kidneys. FP is thought to be secondary to vasculitis of the vasa nervosum or a temporal bone abscess adjacent to the facial nerve. Antimyeloperoxidase (MPO) and proteinase 3 antineutrophil cytoplasmic antibodies (PR3 ANCA) testing aids the diagnosis. Treatment includes high-dose steroids and/or Rituxan.

Melkersson-Rosenthal syndrome (MRS) is a rare neuromucocutaneous granulomatous disorder characterized by the triad of orofacial edema (most common), facial palsy, and lingua plicata (fissured tongue).[43–45] Typically, the symptoms present at different times making the diagnosis more difficult. The etiology is unknown. Cerebrospinal fluid (CSF) examination may show elevated protein levels.[45] A biopsy of involved tissue may reveal fibrosis with nonnecrotizing perivascular and perilymphatic granulomatous infiltrates with intralymphatic involvement. Steroids are a mainstay of medical therapy. Also, prophylactic FN decompression for patients with appropriate electrophysiological changes may be considered to prevent recurrence.

Systemic Lupus Erythematosus

Systemic lupus erythematosus (SLE) is a chronic autoimmune disorder that can affect any organ system. A classic presentation includes fever, malar rash, and joint pain in a young woman. Although rare, SLE and FP has been described in the literature.[46] Theories regarding the pathophysiology of FP include immune dysregulation with activation of latent virus, presence of autoimmune antibodies to nerve antigen, or thrombotic vasculopathy.[47] The diagnosis is based on clinical and laboratory studies, such as antinuclear antibodies (ANA). Medical therapy includes nonsteroidal anti-inflammatory drugs and immune suppressants, such as corticosteroids, azathioprine, cyclophosphamide, and cyclosporine. Given the unknown etiology of FP, antivirals are also given.

Behçet Disease

Behçet disease is a relapsing autoimmune vasculitis of unknown etiology and involves any organ system: ocular inflammation, oral ulceration, genital ulceration, arthropathy, cutaneous lesions, vasculitis, and also neural tissues.[48] Although rare, patients may also present with acute or recurrent FP.[49] The diagnosis is clinical; however, diagnostic testing may include ESR, leukocyte count, and immunoglobulin evaluation. Laboratory tests for vasculitis include ANCA and PR3 to predict relapse. Imaging may be determined by the clinical picture. Treatment involves high-dose steroids and other immunosuppressant medications.

Sjögren Disease

Sjögren syndrome is an autoimmune disease characterized by dry eyes, dry mouth, fatigue, and arthropathy.[50] It can be associated with unilateral or bilateral FP and also affect any organ system.[51,52] The diagnosis is based on abnormal immunologic laboratory tests, such as serum anti-SSA antibodies (anti-Sjögren's-syndrome-related antigen A) or the presence of lymphocytic sialadenitis on biopsy of labial salivary glands. Rheumatoid factor may also be positive.[50] Treatment for FP includes typical BP management as well as immunomodulators per rheumatology recommendations.

METABOLIC

Diabetes mellitus, a metabolic disorder with dysregulation of glucose metabolism may result in vasculopathy and peripheral neuropathy. Diabetes is a risk factor for worse outcomes following BP. In these patients, FP may be unilateral or bilateral.[53] Treatment involves glucose regulation with lifestyle changes and medication. Steroid and antiviral medications are indicated in the acute setting. Care should be taken to not exacerbate hyperglycemia.

VASCULAR

Hypertension increases the risk of FP.[53] The pathogenesis is not completely clear and may be related to vasculitis or thrombus formation of the vasa nervosum leading to ischemia of the nerve.

Cerebrovascular Accidents/Infarcts/Stroke-Central

Hemispheric strokes can cause multiple cranial nerve deficits as well as unilateral body weakness. Immediate neurologic evaluation with imaging is indicated. Treatment depends on the mechanism of the stroke as well as other comorbidities. Medical treatment to prevent a repeat ischemic event should be initiated. If an embolic or ischemic stroke occurs within a window of 4 to 6 hours in a larger vessel, thrombectomy or medical thrombolytics may be used.

Cerebrovascular Accidents/Infarcts/Stroke-Brainstem

Although very rare, infarcts of the dorsal pons can lead to isolated FN palsy.[54–56] Risk factors for these isolated dorsal pons infarcts include diabetes and hypertension.[56] Other cranial nerves in the local vicinity also may be involved. The intrapontine segment of the seventh cranial nerve is primarily supplied by branches of the long penetrating basilar artery. There is also collateral circulation from the circumflex pontine arteries and the anterior inferior cerebellar artery. A thrombotic or embolic event of the basilar artery may solely affect the seventh nerve because other areas may be perfused by collateral circulation.[56] Diffusion MRI will help locate small vessel occlusion. Treatment is similar to central strokes and includes medical as well as endovascular intervention.

CONGENITAL (VASCULAR)

Although congenital etiologies are typically not considered in a discussion of the causes of acute FP, there are several congenital vascular malformations that are present at birth but manifest acutely later in life. The natural history of these lesions is to expand and grow throughout a patient's lifetime. Their growth may be influenced by intrinsic factors such as trauma or hormonal surges (www.ISSVA.org/classification).[57]

Geniculate ganglion venous malformations (previously known as geniculate ganglion "hemangiomas")

Congenital intraosseous venous malformations of the temporal bone adjacent to the geniculate ganglion or the intraosseous facial nerve characteristically enlarge throughout the patient's life and can exert direct pressure on the nerve. Imaging reveals expanded bone with bony spicules adjacent to the nerve. These patients may present with acute or recurrent FP.[58] Because the natural history of all vascular malformations is to expand over time, surgical exploration is warranted in the presence of FP. Excision with facial nerve continuity may often be achieved.[59] If this is not possible, a cable graft or combined nerve substitution procedure is indicated.

Pontine Vascular Malformations

Vascular malformations, including arteriovenous malformations (AVMs) or venous malformations (VMs) may be located in the brainstem. These lesions expand over a patient's lifetime and may cause compression or hemorrhage with resultant neurologic deficit or mortality (headache, seizure, focal deficit). Brainstem AVMs are high-flow lesions that may remain asymptomatic until an acute hemorrhagic event. In patients with syndromes associated with AVMs, such as hereditary hemorrhagic telangiectasia, capillary malformation–AVM, or a PTEN mutation, MRI screening may lead to an earlier diagnosis. VMs, on the other hand, are low-flow vascular malformations. Expansion, especially in the cerebellopontine angle, can cause FP.

Treatment for AVMs will depend on the size and extent of the lesion and includes observation, surgery, embolization, or a combined embolization and surgery, or radiation.[60,61] In general, the brainstem is very sensitive to radiation effects and therefore this is not a favored option. Treatment for VMs also includes observation, surgery, sclerotherapy, or a combined approach.

FAMILIAL

There is an association with paralysis of multiple facial nerve branches and specific alleles 3q21 to 22 with autosomal dominant transmission. However, no gene has yet been identified.[62] There are also known families with an history of BP and no identified gene defect. This may be related to a structural narrowing of the intraosseous facial nerve canal that predisposes these individuals to BP.

PEDIATRIC CONSIDERATIONS

The most common cause of pediatric acute FP is also BP[63] followed by other infectious causes (zoster, otitis media), and trauma. In a study of 975 patients at a large Korean medical center, the most common causes in pediatric and adult cases were the same. However, children had a better prognosis than adults.

BILATERAL FACIAL PARALYSIS

BFP represents 0.2% to 3% of all cases of FP.[21,64] The paralysis may occur simultaneously or in succession. The most common cause of BFP is BP followed by Lyme disease. Regarding timing of paralysis, the most common cause of simultaneous BFP is Lyme disease, followed by posterior fossa tumors, trauma, immune-mediated GBs, central nervous system lymphoma, and HIV infection. In asynchronous cases, BP was the most common, followed by NF-2–associated vestibular schwannoma and MRS.[64–66]

ACUTE RECURRENT FACIAL PARALYSIS

Recurrent FP warrants investigation into other diagnoses apart from BP. An MRI should be considered to rule out tumor as well as diagnostic laboratory studies for endocrine, metabolic, autoimmune, or other systemic causes.

DIAGNOSTIC TESTING
Laboratory Testing

Laboratory testing should be tailored to the individual history and physical examination. Patients with a history and physical consistent with BP do not require diagnostic testing, except for those in Lyme-endemic areas where serology should always be sent. In cases of bilateral FP, or if there is suspicion for other autoimmune or infectious causes, targeted laboratory testing (eg, HIV, ANA, ESR), or CSF testing should be done.

Imaging

Acute FP with a history and physical consistent with BP does not require imaging. If the paralysis does not resolve or improve within 4 months, CT or MRI with contrast should be ordered to rule out a facial nerve tumor.

Electrodiagnostic Testing

Electrodiagnostic testing may be considered in patients with acute and complete flaccid FP secondary to BP or nondisplaced temporal bone fractures. Testing consists of electroneuronography (ENoG) and electromyography (EMG). Acute surgical decompression is indicated for patients with ENoG showing more than 90% decrease in the maximum amplitude of a suprathreshold evoked compound muscle action potential in comparison with the healthy side and absent voluntary motor unit action potentials on EMG within 4 to 14 days of FP onset (see Dr. Daniel Q. Sun and colleagues' article, "Surgical Management of Acute Facial Palsy," in this issue, for further details.)

MEDICAL THERAPY FOR BELL PALSY

The medical treatment plan for patients with acute FP should be multimodal and multidisciplinary (**Fig. 4, Table 2**).

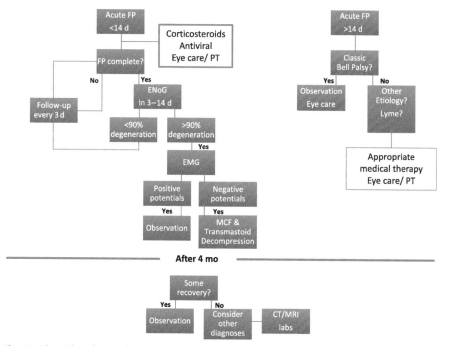

Fig. 4. Algorithm for evaluation of patient with acute FP. CT, computed tomography; FP, facial paralysis; f/u, follow-up; MCF, middle cranial fossa; MRI, magnetic resonance imaging; PT, physical therapy; Q, every.

Table 2
Summary of medical treatment of acute facial paralysis (Bell palsy)

Strong Evidence	Moderate Evidence	Low Evidence
• Corticosteroids	• Antiviral	• Acupuncture • Electrical stimulation (possibly harmful) • Physical therapy (higher for chronic facial paralysis)

Corticosteroids

Given the scientific evidence in support of neural inflammation and secondary ischemia resulting in neural blockade of the facial nerve that leads to FP, corticosteroids are a mainstay in acute therapy. A recent Cochrane review[67] compared steroids with a placebo and showed high-quality evidence from randomized controlled trials in support of a beneficial effect of the use of corticosteroids. Moderate-quality evidence revealed less motor synkinesis and crocodile tears at 6-month follow-up versus the placebo group. Lower-quality evidence suggested that there was no difference in disabling persistent sequelae. No serious adverse effects were noted. One study by Sullivan and colleagues,[68] with 496 patients, was a randomized double-blind, placebo-controlled trial that included patients within 72 hours of their paralysis. A total of 496 patients were included in 4 treatment arms. At follow-up at 3, 6, and 9-months, patients receiving prednisolone showed statistically significant improvement versus those receiving placebo (3 months: 83% vs 63.6%, 9 months: 94.4% vs 81.6%, $P<.001$) or antiviral (acyclovir) medication alone (antiviral vs placebo, 3 months: 71.2% vs 75.7%, 9 months: 85.4% vs 90.8%). Combined therapy showed improvement of 79.7% and 92.7% (3 and 9 months, $P<.001$). Another large randomized placebo-controlled study by Engstrom and colleagues[69] compared prednisone and valacyclovir: 829 patients were placed into 4 treatment arms. Time to recovery was significantly shorter in those receiving steroid therapy ($P<.001$).

The typical prednisolone dosing in most studies was 60 mg per day for 5 days followed by a 5-day taper.[69,70] In children, weight-based dosing, such as prednisone 1 to 2 mg/kg per day for 10 days with a 3-day to 5-day taper is used[71] or prednisolone 0.5 to 1.0 mg/kg per day.[72] Although intravenous delivery is an option, this is not common.[73] Recent American Academy of Otolaryngology–Head and Neck Surgery (AAO-HNS) clinical practice guidelines for BP recommend a 10-day course of oral corticosteroids with at least 5 days at a high dose (prednisolone 50 mg for 10 days or prednisone 60 mg for 5 days with a 5-day taper). Steroids should be started within 72 hours of the onset of symptoms. Although there are no high-quality data in support of steroid use in children, given that the disease process is similar and the low risk/benefit ratio of the drug, oral steroids should be considered for children.[74]

Although steroids are associated with a range of possible side effects, this short-term dosing (10 days) is typically well tolerated.[67] During steroid therapy, patients should receive H_2 receptor blockade to prevent dyspepsia and gastric ulceration. Steroids should be prescribed with caution in patients with a medical history of diabetes mellitus, gastric or duodenal ulcer, poorly controlled hypertension, renal or hepatic disease, glaucoma, pregnancy, recent head trauma, or psychiatric disease. A rare but devastating side effect of steroids is avascular necrosis of the femoral head.

Antiviral Medication

There is evidence to show that viral reactivation causes facial nerve inflammation and secondary ischemia. There are reports of reactivation after local dental, orofaciomaxillary,[75,76] and facial resurfacing[77] procedures or trauma.

Antiviral drugs have thus been used as adjuvant treatment of acute BP. Valacyclovir, the L-valine ester prodrug of acyclovir undergoes rapid and extensive first-pass metabolism to acyclovir after oral administration. Oral bioavailability of valacyclovir is threefold to fivefold higher than oral acyclovir.[78] Acyclovir is the active antiviral component.[79,80] Contraindications to antiviral therapy include liver or kidney dysfunction, pregnancy, or an immunocompromised state.

There is no role for antiviral monotherapy. In studies in which steroids were compared with antiviral agents, there was a clear benefit to steroids. Furthermore, according to a recent Cochrane review,[81] there was a benefit in combining antivirals with steroids when compared with steroids alone for patients with varying degrees of paralytic severity. This study included 10 randomized controlled trials (RCTs) with 293 participants. There was a decrease in incomplete recovery rates (low-quality evidence due to heterogeneity), as well as long-term sequelae, such as motor synkinesis and crocodile tears (moderate quality evidence).[69,82] There was also no significant difference in adverse events.[68,69,78]

Although there is a benefit to antiviral therapy, there has not been a study evaluating the ideal dosage. The studies included in the Cochrane review include acyclovir, valacyclovir, or famciclovir. The dosages also range from 1.6 to 3.0 g acyclovir per day for 5 to 7 days, or 1.0 to 3.2 g valacyclovir per day for 5 to 7 days. We recommend valacyclovir 1 g orally, twice a day for 7 days or famciclovir 1 g orally daily for 5 days.

Side effects are gastrointestinal related and include nausea, vomiting, and diarrhea. More severe but rare side effects include allergic reactions, bronchospasm, angioedema, and organ failure.[83] Antivirals have also not been widely studied in the pediatric population.

Eye Care

Patient education regarding meticulous eye care cannot be overstated. Lagophthalmos or the inability to close the upper eyelid as well as lower eyelid ectropion leads to an inability to protect the cornea. Paralysis of the orbicularis oculi muscle leads to unopposed retraction of the levator palpebrae superioris (LPS), which is innervated by the oculomotor nerve. For these reasons, the eye does not close fully. Ocular complications, such as corneal abrasion, exposure keratitis, or ulceration, may result. Typically, patients complain of a dry or watery eye and the inability to blink. The lacrimal system may also be inhibited. Prophylactic eye care consists of protective glasses, frequent administration of natural tears (preservative-free artificial tears) during the day, as well as a thicker ointment during sleep. Extra protection is afforded by a moisture chamber or a plastic eye shield. Eye patching or taping may be used, with care taken that the cornea does not become exposed under the tape.

Eyelid stretching exercises also aid in full closure of the eye. The upper eyelashes are grasped and pulled inferiorly over the lower eyelid. Countertension is placed superiorly at the midbrow to passively stretch the LPS muscle. This mechanically disrupts the myosin chain cross-linking of the LPS from the opposite orbicularis oculi muscle. The stretch is held for 30 seconds and repeated every 8 hours.[84]

Poor prognostic factors for eye injury include lack of Bell phenomenon, advanced age, an only seeing eye, no resolution after 3 months, scleral irritation, a decreased corneal reflex, or pain and vision changes. These patients will benefit from further eye evaluation and earlier surgical intervention. Temporary tarsorrhaphy, punctal plugs, or early consideration for a reversible lid loading procedure may be considered.

Adjuvant Therapy

Physical therapy for Bell palsy

Various physical therapy interventions have been proposed for acute FP, including thermal treatment, electrotherapy, acupuncture, massage, transcutaneous electrical nerve stimulation, electrical neural muscular stimulation, facial exercises, and biofeedback.[85] Physical therapy is integral to the rehabilitation of the patient with FP in both acute and chronic patients. Initial education of the normal facial musculature and its associated movement helps the patient have mental awareness of the flaccid hemiface as well as the overt contralateral pull of the other side.

Exercises

In the acute setting, soft tissue mobilization and massage are thought to increase blood flow and oxygenation to tissues. It is especially useful in the contralateral face where excess tightness and pain results from unopposed pulling. Also, active hand-assistive exercises help contraction of target muscles until voluntary movement returns.[86] Again, eye protection is crucial and gentle eyelid stretch exercises can help to facilitate eye closure.

Facial neuromuscular retraining is the most common physical therapy technique used when movement begins.[87] Mime therapy combines many of the previously described techniques with a mirror-stimulation of facial expression, functional movements, relaxation techniques, and breathing control.[88] The goal is to promote facial symmetry during movement and repose. A Cochrane review (2012) found that there was no therapy that significantly affected the outcome in cases of acute FP.[85,89] There was no statistically significant difference in synkinesis or recovery. However, the studies did suggest that early tailored facial exercises could help improve function in cases of moderate paralysis or chronic cases by decreasing recovery time and residual long-term paralysis. Overall, the studies lacked methodological consistency, appropriate duration of treatment (up to 6 months), and risk profile (see Mara Wernick Robinson and Jennifer Baiungo's article, "Facial Rehabilitation: Evaluation and Treatment Strategies for the Patient with Facial Palsy," in this issue, for further details).

Acupuncture

Acupuncture is widely practiced in China and is a part of Traditional Chinese medicine. The technique uses fine needles inserted into the skin to stimulate specific "pressure points" that are thought to regulate bodily processes or networks. Theories include the ability to promote nerve regeneration, nerve excitability, increasing muscle contraction, or blood circulation. It is known to be relatively safe; however, side effects have not routinely been reported in the Chinese literature.[90] Currently, there are no well-designed clinical trials to advocate for the use of acupuncture. A Cochrane review by Chen and colleagues[91] evaluated 6 RCTs with a total of 537 patients. Although the studies suggested a beneficial effect from acupuncture, the overall quality of the evidence was poor. The studies were limited by a lack of consistency with research methodology, heterogeneous interventions, outcomes analysis, and short study duration. Further meta-analyses echoed these findings.[92,93] The AAO-HNS also makes no recommendation for acupuncture based on poor-quality trials and an indeterminate risk/benefit ratio.[74]

Electrical stimulation

FP deprives the facial muscles of neural input. External electrical stimulation (E-stim) uses electrical impulses to promote muscle tone and to inhibit atrophy. Animal studies show that after crush injury, stimulation of a motor nerve proximal to the injury improves recovery.[94] At this time, there is no evidence to suggest that E-stim is beneficial in acute FP.[87] Some studies show a decreased time to recovery with no difference after 6 months. Overall, there was a trend toward more motor synkinesis (not statistically significant)[85] and thus E-stim is not currently recommended.

Psychological counseling

Many patients with FP suffer some element of distress and depression.[95] Our faces and facial expressions are intimately tied to how we perceive ourselves and how others perceive us. Alongside the functional and aesthetic changes, there is also uncertainty and grief in the acute setting. Patients may benefit from individual counseling or a FP support group.

REFERENCES

1. Peitersen E. Bell's palsy: the spontaneous course of 2,500 peripheral facial nerve palsies of different etiologies. Acta Otolaryngol Suppl 2002;(549):4–30.
2. Hohman MH, Hadlock TA. Etiology, diagnosis, and management of facial palsy: 2000 patients at a facial nerve center. Laryngoscope 2014;124(7):E283–93.
3. Adour KK, Byl FM, Hilsinger RL Jr, et al. The true nature of Bell's palsy: analysis of 1,000 consecutive patients. Laryngoscope 1978;88(5):787–801.
4. Devriese PP, Schumacher T, Scheide A, et al. Incidence, prognosis and recovery of Bell's palsy. A survey of about 1000 patients (1974-1983). Clin Otolaryngol Allied Sci 1990;15(1):15–27.
5. Bell C. On the nerves; giving an account of some experiments on their structure and functions, which lead to a new arrangement of the system. Philos Trans R Soc Lond 1821;111:398–424.
6. Bird TD, Nicolaus A. Friedreich's description of peripheral facial nerve paralysis in 1798. J Neurol Neurosurg Psychiatry 1979;42(1):56–8.
7. Vrabec JT. The facial nerve. In: Slattery WH, Azizzadeh B, editors. Medical treatment of bell palsy. New York: Thieme; 2014.
8. De Diego JI, Prim MP, Madero R, et al. Seasonal patterns of idiopathic facial paralysis: a 16-year study. Otolaryngol Head Neck Surg 1999;120(2):269–71.
9. Yanagihara N. Incidence of Bell's palsy. Ann Otol Rhinol Laryngol Suppl 1988; 137:3–4.
10. Campbell KE, Brundage JF. Effects of climate, latitude, and season on the incidence of Bell's palsy in the US Armed Forces, October 1997 to September 1999. Am J Epidemiol 2002;156(1):32–9.
11. Adour KK, Bell DN, Hilsinger RL Jr. Herpes simplex virus in idiopathic facial paralysis (Bell palsy). JAMA 1975;233(6):527–30.
12. Murakami S, Hato N, Mizobuchi M, et al. Role of herpes simplex virus infection in the pathogenesis of facial paralysis in mice. Ann Otol Rhinol Laryngol 1996; 105(1):49–53.
13. Murakami S, Mizobuchi M, Nakashiro Y, et al. Bell palsy and herpes simplex virus: identification of viral DNA in endoneurial fluid and muscle. Ann Intern Med 1996; 124(1 Pt 1):27–30.
14. Furuta Y, Fukuda S, Suzuki S, et al. Detection of varicella-zoster virus DNA in patients with acute peripheral facial palsy by the polymerase chain reaction, and its use for early diagnosis of zoster sine herpete. J Med Virol 1997;52(3):316–9.
15. McCormick DP. Herpes-simplex virus as a cause of Bell's palsy. Lancet 1972; 1(7757):937–9.

16. Murakami S. Bell palsy and Ramsay Hunt syndrome. In: Slattery WH, Azizzadeh B, editors. The facial nerve. New York: Thieme Medical Publishers, Inc.; 2014. p. 70–80.

17. Schwaber MK, Larson TC 3rd, Zealear DL, et al. Gadolinium-enhanced magnetic resonance imaging in Bell's palsy. Laryngoscope 1990;100(12):1264–9.

18. Engstrom M, Thuomas KA, Naeser P, et al. Facial nerve enhancement in Bell's palsy demonstrated by different gadolinium-enhanced magnetic resonance imaging techniques. Arch Otolaryngol Head Neck Surg 1993;119(2):221–5.

19. Fisch U, Esslen E. Total intratemporal exposure of the facial nerve. Pathologic findings in Bell's palsy. Arch Otolaryngol 1972;95(4):335–41.

20. Jowett N, Gaudin RA, Banks CA, et al. Steroid use in Lyme disease-associated facial palsy is associated with worse long-term outcomes. Laryngoscope 2017; 127(6):1451–8.

21. Sathirapanya P. Isolated and bilateral simultaneous facial palsy disclosing early human immunodeficiency virus infection. Singapore Med J 2015;56(6):e105–6.

22. Komolafe MA, Fatusi OA, Alatise OI, et al. The role of human immunodeficiency virus infection in infranuclear facial paralysis. J Natl Med Assoc 2009;101(4): 361–6.

23. Popovtzer A, Raveh E, Bahar G, et al. Facial palsy associated with acute otitis media. Otolaryngol Head Neck Surg 2005;132(2):327–9.

24. Ikeda M, Nakazato H, Onoda K, et al. Facial nerve paralysis caused by middle ear cholesteatoma and effects of surgical intervention. Acta Otolaryngol 2006; 126(1):95–100.

25. Savic DL, Djeric DR. Facial paralysis in chronic suppurative otitis media. Clin Otolaryngol Allied Sci 1989;14(6):515–7.

26. Maniu A, Harabagiu O, Perde Schrepler M, et al. Molecular biology of cholesteatoma. Rom J Morphol Embryol 2014;55(1):7–13.

27. Kuo CL. Etiopathogenesis of acquired cholesteatoma: prominent theories and recent advances in biomolecular research. Laryngoscope 2015;125(1):234–40.

28. Vrabec JT, Isaacson B, Van Hook JW. Bell's palsy and pregnancy. Otolaryngol Head Neck Surg 2007;137(6):858–61.

29. Phillips KM, Heiser A, Gaudin R, et al. Onset of Bell's palsy in late pregnancy and early puerperium is associated with worse long-term outcomes. Laryngoscope 2017;127(12):2854–9.

30. Hussain A, Nduka C, Moth P, et al. Bell's facial nerve palsy in pregnancy: a clinical review. J Obstet Gynaecol 2017;37(4):409–15.

31. Patel A, Groppo E. Management of temporal bone trauma. Craniomaxillofac Trauma Reconstr 2010;3(2):105–13.

32. Gordin E, Lee TS, Ducic Y, et al. Facial nerve trauma: evaluation and considerations in management. Craniomaxillofac Trauma Reconstr 2015;8(1):1–13.

33. Chang CY, Cass SP. Management of facial nerve injury due to temporal bone trauma. Am J Otol 1999;20(1):96–114.

34. Falco NA, Eriksson E. Facial nerve palsy in the newborn: incidence and outcome. Plast Reconstr Surg 1990;85(1):1–4.

35. Wakerley BR, Yuki N. Isolated facial diplegia in Guillain-Barre syndrome: bifacial weakness with paresthesias. Muscle Nerve 2015;52(6):927–32.

36. Jasem J, Marof K, Nawar A, et al. Guillain-Barré syndrome as a cause of acute flaccid paralysis in Iraqi children: a result of 15 years of nation-wide study. BMC Neurol 2013;13:195.

37. Ansar V, Valadi N. Guillain-Barre syndrome. Prim Care 2015;42(2):189–93.

38. Critchley EP. Multiple sclerosis initially presenting as facial palsy. Aviat Space En-viron Med 2004;75(11):1001–4.
39. Hornigold R, Patel AV, Ward VM, et al. Familial systemic amyloidosis associated with bilateral sensorineural hearing loss and bilateral facial palsies. J Laryngol Otol 2006;120(9):778–80.
40. Braganza RA, Tien R, Hoffman HT, et al. Amyloid of the facial nerve. Laryngo-scope 1992;102(12 Pt 1):1372–6.
41. de Souza PVS, Bortholin T, Naylor FGM, et al. Familial progressive bilateral facial paralysis in Finnish type hereditary amyloidosis. Pract Neurol 2017;17(5):408–9.
42. Gomez-Torres A, Tirado Zamora I, Abrante Jimenez A, et al. Wegener's granulo-matosis causing bilateral facial paralysis and deafness. Acta Otorrinolaringol Esp 2013;64(2):154–6.
43. Rivera-Serrano CM, Man LX, Klein S, et al. Melkersson-Rosenthal syndrome: a facial nerve center perspective. J Plast Reconstr Aesthet Surg 2014;67(8):1050–4.
44. Lin TY, Chiang CH, Cheng PS. Melkersson-Rosenthal syndrome. J Formos Med Assoc 2016;115(7):583–4.
45. Liu R, Yu S. Melkersson-Rosenthal syndrome: a review of seven patients. J Clin Neurosci 2013;20(7):993–5.
46. Gupta DK, Atam V, Chaudhary SC. Recurrent lower motor neuron type facial palsy: an unusual manifestation of SLE. BMJ Case Rep 2011;2011 [pii: bcr1220103564].
47. Kazzaz NM, El-Rifai R. Unusual aetiology of isolated lower motor neuron facial palsy: systemic lupus erythematosus presenting with cranial nerve palsy and nephritis. BMJ Case Rep 2013;2013:200378.
48. O'Duffy JD, Carney JA, Deodhar S. Behcet's disease. Report of 10 cases, 3 with new manifestations. Ann Intern Med 1971;75(4):561–70.
49. Tsirogianni ES, Hatzitolios AI, Savopoulos CG, et al. Neuro-Behcet's syndrome may present with peripheral paresis of the facial nerve. J Peripher Nerv Syst 2004;9(2):59–61.
50. Mariette X, Criswell LA. Primary Sjogren's syndrome. N Engl J Med 2018;378(10):931–9.
51. Uchihara T, Yoshida S, Tsukagoshi H. Bilateral facial paresis with Sjogren's syn-drome. J Neurol 1989;236(3):186.
52. Rousso E, Noel E, Brogard JM, et al. Recurrent facial palsy, primary Gougerot-Sjogren's syndrome and vitamin B12 deficiency. Presse Med 2005;34(2 Pt 1):107–8 [in French].
53. Yanagihara N, Hyodo M. Association of diabetes mellitus and hypertension with Bell's palsy and Ramsay Hunt syndrome. Ann Otol Rhinol Laryngol Suppl 1988;137:5–7.
54. Oh SI, Kim EG, Jeong HW, et al. Teaching neuroimages: isolated peripheral facial palsy due to ipsilateral pontine infarction. Neurology 2015;85(1):e1–2.
55. Ahn SK, Hur DG, Jeon SY, et al. A rare case of pontomedullary infarction present-ing with peripheral-type facial palsy. Auris Nasus Larynx 2010;37(6):747–9.
56. Thomke F, Urban PP, Marx JJ, et al. Seventh nerve palsies may be the only clinical sign of small pontine infarctions in diabetic and hypertensive patients. J Neurol 2002;249(11):1556–62.
57. O TM, Waner M, Fay A. Hemangiomas and vascular malformations of the head and neck. Sataloff's comprehensive textbook of Otolaryngology: head and neck surgery, vol. VI. Philadelphia: Jaypee Brothers,Medical Publishers Pvt. Limited; 2015. p. 2015.

58. Benoit MM, North PE, McKenna MJ, et al. Facial nerve hemangiomas: vascular tumors or malformations? Otolaryngol Head Neck Surg 2010;142(1):108–14.

59. Oldenburg MS, Carlson ML, Van Abel KM, et al. Management of geniculate ganglion hemangiomas: case series and systematic review of the literature. Otol Neurotol 2015;36(10):1735–40.

60. Han SJ, Englot DJ, Kim H, et al. Brainstem arteriovenous malformations: anatomical subtypes, assessment of "occlusion in situ" technique, and microsurgical results. J Neurosurg 2015;122(1):107–17.

61. Stein KP, Wanke I, Schlamann M, et al. Posterior fossa arterio-venous malformations: current multimodal treatment strategies and results. Neurosurg Rev 2014; 37(4):619–28.

62. Alrashdi IS, Rich P, Patton MA. A family with hereditary congenital facial paresis and a brief review of the literature. Clin Dysmorphol 2010;19(4):198–201.

63. Cha CI, Hong CK, Park MS, et al. Comparison of facial nerve paralysis in adults and children. Yonsei Med J 2008;49(5):725–34.

64. Gaudin RA, Jowett N, Banks CA, et al. Bilateral facial paralysis: a 13-year experience. Plast Reconstr Surg 2016;138(4):879–87.

65. Sherwen PJ, Thong NC. Bilateral facial nerve palsy: a case study and literature review. J Otolaryngol 1987;16(1):28–33.

66. Oosterveer DM, Benit CP, de Schryver EL. Differential diagnosis of recurrent or bilateral peripheral facial palsy. J Laryngol Otol 2012;126(8):833–6.

67. Madhok VB, Gagyor I, Daly F, et al. Corticosteroids for Bell's palsy (idiopathic facial paralysis). Cochrane Database Syst Rev 2016;(7):CD001942.

68. Sullivan FM, Swan IR, Donnan PT, et al. Early treatment with prednisolone or acyclovir in Bell's palsy. N Engl J Med 2007;357(16):1598–607.

69. Engstrom M, Berg T, Stjernquist-Desatnik A, et al. Prednisolone and valaciclovir in Bell's palsy: a randomised, double-blind, placebo-controlled, multicentre trial. Lancet Neurol 2008;7(11):993–1000.

70. Austin JR, Peskind SP, Austin SG, et al. Idiopathic facial nerve paralysis: a randomized double blind controlled study of placebo versus prednisone. Laryngoscope 1993;103(12):1326–33.

71. Unuvar E, Oguz F, Sidal M, et al. Corticosteroid treatment of childhood Bell's palsy. Pediatr Neurol 1999;21(5):814–6.

72. Pitaro J, Waissbluth S, Daniel SJ. Do children with Bell's palsy benefit from steroid treatment? A systematic review. Int J Pediatr Otorhinolaryngol 2012;76(7):921–6.

73. Lagalla G, Logullo F, Di Bella P, et al. Influence of early high-dose steroid treatment on Bell's palsy evolution. Neurol Sci 2002;23(3):107–12.

74. Baugh RF, Basura GJ, Ishii LE, et al. Clinical practice guideline: Bell's palsy. Otolaryngol Head Neck Surg 2013;149(3 Suppl):S1–27.

75. Miller CS, Cunningham LL, Lindroth JE, et al. The efficacy of valacyclovir in preventing recurrent herpes simplex virus infections associated with dental procedures. J Am Dent Assoc 2004;135(9):1311–8.

76. Miller CS, Avdiushko SA, Kryscio RJ, et al. Effect of prophylactic valacyclovir on the presence of human herpesvirus DNA in saliva of healthy individuals after dental treatment. J Clin Microbiol 2005;43(5):2173–80.

77. Gilbert S, McBurney E. Use of valacyclovir for herpes simplex virus-1 (HSV-1) prophylaxis after facial resurfacing: a randomized clinical trial of dosing regimens. Dermatol Surg 2000;26(1):50–4.

78. Hato N, Yamada H, Kohno H, et al. Valacyclovir and prednisolone treatment for Bell's palsy: a multicenter, randomized, placebo-controlled study. Otol Neurotol 2007;28(3):408–13.

79. Wagstaff AJ, Faulds D, Goa KL. Aciclovir. A reappraisal of its antiviral activity, pharmacokinetic properties and therapeutic efficacy. Drugs 1994;47(1):153–205.
80. Perry CM, Faulds D. Valaciclovir. A review of its antiviral activity, pharmacokinetic properties and therapeutic efficacy in herpesvirus infections. Drugs 1996;52(5): 754–72.
81. Gagyor I, Madhok VB, Daly F, et al. Antiviral treatment for Bell's palsy (idiopathic facial paralysis). Cochrane Database Syst Rev 2015;(11):CD001869.
82. Adour KK, Ruboyianes JM, Von Doersten PG, et al. Bell's palsy treatment with acyclovir and prednisone compared with prednisone alone: a double-blind, randomized, controlled trial. Ann Otol Rhinol Laryngol 1996;105(5):371–8.
83. Baugh RF, Basura GJ, Ishii LE, et al. Clinical practice guideline: Bell's palsy executive summary. Otolaryngol Head Neck Surg 2013;149(5):656–63.
84. Lindsay RW, Robinson M, Hadlock TA. Comprehensive facial rehabilitation improves function in people with facial paralysis: a 5-year experience at the Massachusetts Eye and Ear Infirmary. Phys Ther 2010;90(3):391–7.
85. Teixeira LJ, Valbuza JS, Prado GF. Physical therapy for Bell's palsy (idiopathic facial paralysis). Cochrane Database Syst Rev 2011;(12):CD006283.
86. Skouras E, Merkel D, Grosheva M, et al. Manual stimulation, but not acute electrical stimulation prior to reconstructive surgery, improves functional recovery after facial nerve injury in rats. Restor Neurol Neurosci 2009;27(3):237–51.
87. Manikandan N. Effect of facial neuromuscular re-education on facial symmetry in patients with Bell's palsy: a randomized controlled trial. Clin Rehabil 2007;21(4): 338–43.
88. Devriese P, Bronk J. Non-surgical rehabilitation of facial expression. Facial nerve surgery. Amstelveen (The Netherlands): Kugler Medical Publ; 1977. p. 290–4.
89. Pereira LM, Obara K, Dias JM, et al. Facial exercise therapy for facial palsy: systematic review and meta-analysis. Clin Rehabil 2011;25(7):649–58.
90. He W, Zhao X, Li Y, et al. Adverse events following acupuncture: a systematic review of the Chinese literature for the years 1956-2010. J Altern Complement Med 2012;18(10):892–901.
91. Chen N, Zhou M, He L, et al. Acupuncture for Bell's palsy. Cochrane Database Syst Rev 2010;(8):CD002914.
92. Kim JI, Lee MS, Choi TY, et al. Acupuncture for Bell's palsy: a systematic review and meta-analysis. Chin J Integr Med 2012;18(1):48–55.
93. Li P, Qiu T, Qin C. Efficacy of acupuncture for Bell's palsy: a systematic review and meta-analysis of randomized controlled trials. PLoS One 2015;10(5): e0121880.
94. Foecking EM, Fargo KN, Coughlin LM, et al. Single session of brief electrical stimulation immediately following crush injury enhances functional recovery of rat facial nerve. J Rehabil Res Dev 2012;49(3):451–8.
95. Nellis JC, Ishii M, Byrne PJ, et al. Association among facial paralysis, depression, and quality of life in facial plastic surgery patients. JAMA Facial Plast Surg 2017; 19(3):190–6.

Surgical Management of Acute Facial Palsy

Daniel Q. Sun, MD[a],*, Nicholas S. Andresen, MD[a], Bruce J. Gantz, MD[b]

KEYWORDS

- Bell palsy • Temporal bone fracture • Facial nerve • Facial nerve paralysis
- Facial nerve decompression • Neurotology

KEY POINTS

- Bell palsy and traumatic temporal bone fracture are common causes of acute facial palsy.
- Patients with complete facial paralysis (House-Brackmann 6/6) should undergo electro-physiologic testing (electroneurography [ENoG], electromyography [EMG]).
- Patients with complete paralysis (House-Brackmann 6/6) within 14 days of symptom onset, greater than 90% degeneration on ENoG testing, and absent EMG activity may benefit from surgical decompression.
- The return of facial nerve should not be expected for weeks to months following decompression surgery, and may be delayed up to 12 months.

INTRODUCTION

Common causes of acute facial palsy include Bell palsy and traumatic facial nerve injury secondary to temporal bone fracture. Bell palsy accounts for 75% of acute facial palsy cases.[1] Most patients with Bell palsy regain facial nerve function with conservative treatment. However, a select group of patients has a worse prognosis and may benefit from surgical decompression of the facial nerve.[2] The evidence for the use of steroids and, in some cases, antivirals for Bell palsy has been reviewed elsewhere and is beyond the scope of this article[3–6] (see Dr Teresa M. O's article, "Medical Management of Acute Facial Paralysis," in this issue). Acute facial palsy secondary to traumatic nerve injury may also require surgical decompression and possibly nerve repair or grafting depending on the nature and extent of nerve trauma. This article uses Bell palsy as a framework to consider the work-up, indications, and techniques for the surgical management of acute facial palsy.

Disclosure: The authors have no conflicts of interest to disclose.
[a] Department of Otolaryngology–Head and Neck Surgery, Johns Hopkins University School of Medicine, 601 N. Caroline St 6th Floor, Baltimore MD, 21287, USA; [b] University of Iowa Hospitals and Clinics, 375 Newton Road, Iowa City, IA 52242, USA
* Corresponding author.
E-mail address: daniel-sun@uiowa.edu

Otolaryngol Clin N Am 51 (2018) 1077–1092
https://doi.org/10.1016/j.otc.2018.07.005
0030-6665/18/© 2018 Elsevier Inc. All rights reserved.

Other causes of acute facial palsy for which the efficacy of surgical decompression has not been shown, such as Ramsay-Hunt syndrome, are beyond the scope of this article. Ramsay-Hunt syndrome is differentiated from Bell palsy by the presence of otalgia, periauricular vesicles, hearing loss, or vestibular symptoms. Causes of subacute or recurrent facial palsy, including facial nerve neuromas and facial nerve vascular malformations, are also beyond the scope of this article.

SURGICAL APPROACH
Rationale for Middle Cranial Fossa Approach for Bell Palsy

The surgical approach for Bell palsy has evolved as the understanding of its pathophysiology has changed. Historically, the stylomastoid foramen and chorda-facial junction have both been proposed as the sites of disorder in Bell palsy.[7-10] Consequently, transmastoid decompression was initially advocated, but later found to be ineffective when performed alone.[11,12]

Increased knowledge regarding the site of nerve compression and conduction blockade in Bell palsy became available following the description of the middle cranial fossa (MCF) approach by William House in 1961.[13] The MCF approach provides access to the facial nerve from the cisternal to the proximal tympanic segments, while allowing for preservation of auditory and vestibular function. Using the MCF approach, Fisch and Esslen[14] performed facial nerve decompression on a series of patients with Bell palsy and found pronounced edema and vascular injection of nerve proximal to the geniculate ganglion in 11 out of 12 patients. In a separate part of this study, 3 patients were treated with total intratemporal exposure of the facial nerve via a combined MCF and transmastoid approach, and intraoperative evoked electromyography (EEMG) of the facial nerve from the stylomastoid foramen to the internal auditory canal (IAC) was performed. The conduction abnormality was located within the IAC, proximal to the geniculate ganglion (GG) in all 3 patients. Subsequently, this finding was corroborated in a larger series of patients.[15,16] Eighteen patients with 90% to 98% degeneration on electroneurography (ENoG) underwent decompression. Intraoperative EEMG was attempted for all patients and successfully performed for 16 patients. Of these 16 patients, 15 (94%) had a conduction block proximal to the GG and 1 had a conduction block at the origin of the chorda tympani. These data suggest that, for almost all patients with Bell palsy, the conduction block occurs proximal to the GG and decompression should therefore include the fallopian canal proximal to the GG.

Anatomic studies corroborate these intraoperative conduction findings. The labyrinthine segment of the fallopian canal is the narrowest segment along the entire course of the facial nerve, measuring 0.69 mm in diameter on average.[17] In addition, a tight arachnoid band is present at the proximal extent of the labyrinthine segment of the fallopian canal and acts as a chokepoint of constriction in the setting of edema.[17,18] Several studies have shown herpes simplex virus-1[19-22] or varicella zoster virus–associated inflammatory infiltration[23] in clinically diagnosed Bell palsy. Thus, the current understanding of the pathophysiology of Bell palsy is that viral reactivation in the GG leads to lymphocytic infiltration and perineural edema that spreads along the course of the facial nerve.[24,25] Edema in the labyrinthine segment may lead to cessation of axoplasmic flow caused by compressive pressure in the fallopian canal. Further neural edema may cause cessation of vascular flow and the onset of ischemia, and wallerian degeneration distal to the point of constriction. Surgical decompression via an MCF approach therefore offers an opportunity to restore blood flow across the point of constriction by decompression of bone and lysis of the arachnoid band while preserving inner ear function.

INDICATIONS FOR SURGICAL INTERVENTION
Principles of Electrophysiologic Testing

Electrophysiologic testing provides an objective means of assessing nerve function and is indicated for patients with complete paralysis. Those with incomplete paralysis carry a favorable prognosis and electrophysiologic testing is not indicated. Electrophysiologic testing offers prognostic value for the likelihood of poor recovery (House-Brackmann [HB] grade 3 or higher) in patients with complete paralysis, thereby identifying those who may be candidates for surgical decompression. ENoG and electromyography (EMG) are the two most accurate and reliable electrophysiologic tests currently in use.

ENoG estimates the relative proportion of nerve fibers that have undergone wallerian degeneration and is most useful 4 to 14 days after the onset of complete paralysis.[26,27] ENoG testing is not performed before the fourth day of paralysis because it takes approximately 3 days for wallerian degeneration to occur. Testing is not performed after 2 weeks of paralysis because patients who have not reached the critical degeneration threshold by that time have a high likelihood of good recovery (HB 1 or 2) and are not candidates for surgical decompression.[18]

ENoG uses an evoked, supramaximal electrical stimulus to activate the facial nerve as it exits the skull at the stylomastoid foramen (**Fig. 1**A). The technique of performing ENoG must be standardized in order to provide reliable data regarding the prognosis of facial nerve function and recovery.[26,28,29] Surface electrodes are used to record the evoked biphasic compound muscle action potential (CMAP) (**Fig. 1**B), which depends on the synchronous discharge of multiple viable nerve fibers. The maximum amplitude of the CMAP correlates with the number of remaining nerve fibers that are responsive to stimulation.[30] The CMAP from the affected side is then compared with the CMAP of the normal side, which serves as a control, and a percentage of degenerated nerve fibers is calculated.[29]

Voluntary EMG measures motor activity with needle electrodes placed in the orbicularis oris and orbicularis oculi muscle while the patient is asked to make forceful facial contractions (**Fig. 1**C). In the acute phase of paralysis, EMG is used when ENoG shows 90% or greater neural degeneration,[31] to confirm absence of muscle function. Presence of active motor units on EMG in the setting of severe degeneration on ENoG indicates a phenomenon termed deblocking, which is the asynchronous discharge of regenerating nerve fibers that fail to produce a measurable CMAP on ENoG.[31] Deblocking is a sign of nerve regeneration and portends a favorable prognosis. Therefore, patients with deblocking should not proceed to surgical decompression despite severe degeneration on ENoG.

Bell Palsy: Prognosis and Assessment of Surgical Candidacy

In the setting of acute facial nerve paralysis, the utility of surgery depends on the severity of paralysis. Approximately 90% of patients with incomplete facial nerve paralysis (HB 5 or less) show complete resolution of their symptoms with steroid therapy alone.[1,32,33] However, only ~60% of patients with complete paralysis (HB 6) recover to HB 1 or 2 without surgical intervention. Electrophysiologic testing is therefore used in this group of patients to identify those at high risk for poor recovery, who may be candidates for surgical intervention. Neural degeneration of greater than 90% on ENoG testing has been associated with increased likelihood of poor outcome.[2,18] ENoG testing is performed serially between days 4 and 14 to assess both the extent and rate of degeneration. Rapid progression to the 90% level indicates more severe neural injury (eg, neurotmesis) and less likelihood of return to normal facial function.[34]

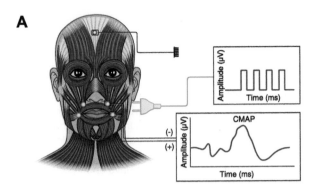

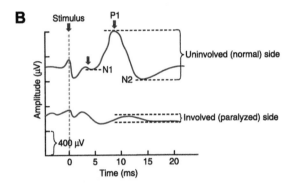

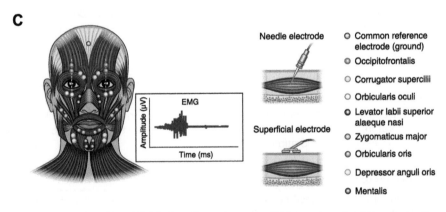

Fig. 1. ENoG/EMG testing. (*A*) ENoG testing using an evoked, supramaximal impulse to stimulate the facial nerve as it exits the stylomastoid foramen and surface electrodes placed over the orbicularis oris to measure the compound muscle action potential (CMAP). (*B*) Sample CMAPs generated during ENoG testing for facial palsy. (*C*) EMG testing with needle electrodes placed in the facial muscles.

If 90% degeneration is reached within 14 days of onset of paralysis, EMG is performed to rule out deblocking. If EMG also shows the absence of motor action potentials, the patient is a candidate for surgical decompression. If 90% degeneration is not reached by 14 days, testing is stopped because the patient is likely to have a good recovery without surgical intervention. This management algorithm is shown in **Fig. 2**.

Candidates for surgical decompression are counseled in detail on the risks and benefits of the procedure. Iatrogenic facial nerve injury, hearing loss, and/or vestibular dysfunction are rare in experienced hands. Other risks associated with MCF surgery, including cerebrospinal fluid (CSF) leak, meningitis, and complications associated with temporal lobe retraction (eg, aphasia, seizure) are also extremely rare. It is important for patients to understand that surgical decompression does not guarantee but increases the likelihood for good recovery, and that recovery is likely not to occur until several weeks to months following surgery.

Evidence supporting these surgical criteria comes from a prospective, multi-institutional, case-control study of 30 patients treated for Bell palsy during a 15-year period.[2] Criteria for inclusion were presentation within 14 days of symptom onset, complete paralysis (HB 6), greater than 90% degeneration on ENoG, and absent voluntary EMG activity. Patients meeting inclusion criteria were allowed to choose between surgery (n = 19) and oral steroid treatment (n = 11). Patients electing for steroid treatment only were considered nonsurgical controls. A second group of patients (n = 7) underwent surgical intervention 14 to 28 days after the onset of paralysis. Surgical intervention was facial nerve decompression through an MCF approach that included decompression of the distal IAC, meatal foramen, labyrinthine segment,

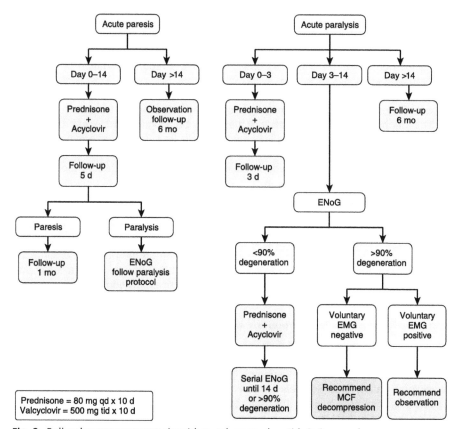

Fig. 2. Bell palsy management algorithm. qd, every day; tid, 3 times a day.

GG, and tympanic segment. For all treatment groups, a good outcome was defined as recovery to HB 1 or 2, and a poor outcome was HB 3 or worse. In the nonsurgical control group (steroids only) at 7 months' follow-up, no patients had recovered to HB 1, 4 of 11 (36%) recovered to HB 2, and 7 of 11 (64%) had only recovered to HB 3. In the cohort that underwent decompression after 14 days, 2 patients had a good outcome and 5 had a poor outcome. Of patients who underwent decompression within 14 days, 18 of 19 (94%) had a good outcome and 1 had a poor (HB 3) outcome. The benefit of surgical decompression was statistically significant (P = .0001). These findings have also been corroborated in several other studies[18,35,36] and validate the following criteria for facial nerve decompression that are currently used at our institution:

- Complete facial paralysis (HB 6)
- Presentation within 14 days of onset of paralysis
- Greater than 90% denervation on ENoG
- No voluntary EMG activity

Several previous studies have relied solely on ENoG testing to assess for surgical candidacy, choosing to forego voluntary EMG testing.[11,12,37] In these studies, no difference was observed in recovery of function for patients with greater than 90% degeneration treated with either surgery or steroids alone. It is likely that some patients treated with steroids alone may have had early deblocking of the nerve and would have shown positive voluntary EMG if tested. These patients should have been excluded from consideration for surgical decompression.

A Cochrane Review was recently performed that found insufficient evidence to recommend surgical intervention for Bell palsy, citing the lack of a randomized controlled trial.[38] An Academy of Otolaryngology– Head and Neck Surgery clinical guidelines committee on Bell palsy could not make a recommendation on whether decompression of the facial nerve was of value in Bell palsy. This decision was made on the availability of only nonrandomized clinical trials and the equilibrium of the benefit and the harm. The committee also stated that although the data supporting surgical decompression are not strong, there may be a significant benefit for a small subset of patients who meet eligibility criteria and desire surgical management. There were major differences of opinion on the committee with regard to surgical decompression. This difference of opinion is based on controversy regarding the strength of evidence (C vs D level evidence).[39,40] The estimated number of patients needed to adequately power a randomized trial for surgical intervention is 716, assuming a type I error of 0.05.[12] Given this large number of required patients, the rarity of surgical candidacy, and the ethical dilemma surrounding randomization in a surgical study, it is unlikely that a randomized trial will ever occur. Middle fossa surgery is technically demanding and requires both expertise and experience on the part of the surgeon. Therefore, the decision to proceed with surgery ought to be customized to each patient and surgeon, because the risk-benefit ratio is individualized to each surgeon's training and experience.

Traumatic Facial Nerve Palsy: Prognosis and Assessment of Surgical Candidacy

The management of acute facial paralysis secondary to traumatic temporal bone fracture carries both important similarities and differences to that of Bell palsy. Traumatic facial nerve injury may likewise cause perineural edema that leads to a similar pathophysiologic cascade as Bell palsy, resulting in nerve degeneration. Surgical decompression is directed toward the site of neural trauma based on radiographic imaging. In longitudinal fractures, the site of disruption is frequently in the perigeniculate region, similar to Bell.[41] However, unlike Bell palsy, trauma may also produce crush or penetrating injury to the nerve caused by displaced bone fragments, and sometimes even transection of the nerve. Radiologic studies (temporal bone computed tomography [CT] scans: fine-cut, axial, and coronal planes; bone window) therefore become important in assessing the likely sites of facial nerve injury (**Figs. 3–5**). Facial paresis or paralysis can present either acutely after injury or in a delayed fashion. For patients with complete facial paralysis and radiographic evidence of fracture extending to the perigeniculate region, the electrophysiologic testing algorithm is commenced much like in Bell palsy. Electrophysiologic testing may be abbreviated if imaging reveals obvious nerve displacement and transection, which represents a clear indication for surgical exploration and repair. For patients without obvious nerve transection or impingement, our institution uses the same criteria for surgical intervention as in Bell palsy. However, it should be noted that these criteria have not been studied in a specific cohort of patients who lack evidence of nerve transection or impingement on imaging.

DESCRIPTION OF SURGERY FOR ACUTE FACIAL PARALYSIS
Facial Nerve Decompression via Middle Cranial Fossa Approach

All patients undergo bone and air conduction audiometry as well as electrophysiologic testing before surgical intervention. MRI or temporal bone CT imaging may be obtained but is not necessary. A preoperative Stenver view plain radiograph may aid in determining the depth of the semicircular canal from the MCF floor.[42] The anesthesia team should be informed that long-acting paralytic agents may not be used. Endotracheal intubation is performed and the bed is rotated 180°. An arterial line, temperature probe, and urinary catheter are placed. Intraoperative hearing monitoring using auditory brainstem response is an option but is not routinely used at our institution for this procedure. Facial nerve monitoring leads are applied. Prophylactic antibiotics, corticosteroids, and mannitol (0.5 g/kg ideal weight) are given. The end-tidal carbon dioxide level is decreased to less than 30 mm Hg by hyperventilation. The head may be positioned via pinning, a horseshoe, or a circular gel headrest. At our institution, the head is rested on a circular gel headrest with the ear of the affected side facing the ceiling. If necessary, the incision site is shaved. The planned incision site is injected with local anesthetic and epinephrine. The operative site is prepared and draped.

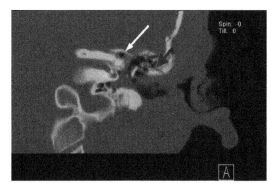

Fig. 3. Coronal-section temporal bone CT scan showing comminuted fracture (*red arrow*) of the middle fossa floor causing crush injury to the perigeniculate section (*white arrow*) of the facial nerve. This patient developed delayed facial paralysis. MCF approach was used for facial nerve decompression.

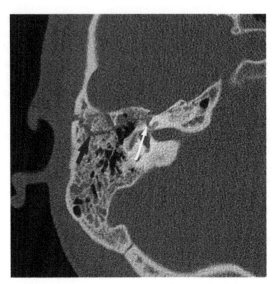

Fig. 4. Axial-section temporal bone CT scan showing longitudinal fracture (*red arrow*) of the temporal bone involving the geniculate ganglion (*white arrow*). MCF approach was used for facial nerve decompression, which was found to be anatomically intact. Facial nerve function returned to HB 1 by 6 months postoperatively.

A posteriorly based skin flap approximately 6 × 8 cm is created within the hairline above the ear. The incision is carried down to the level of the temporalis fascia and should remain posterior to the temporal hairline to avoid injury to the temporal branch of the facial nerve. The temporoparietal fascia is left attached to the skin flap. A large

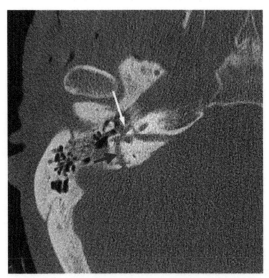

Fig. 5. Axial-section temporal bone CT scan showing transverse fracture (*red arrow*) of the temporal bone through the otic capsule resulting in injury to the perigeniculate section (*white arrow*) of the facial nerve, which was decompressed via a translabyrinthine approach.

piece of temporoparietal fascia is harvested for later use before retracting the temporalis muscle anteriorly. An anteriorly based temporalis muscle flap is elevated from the outer cortex of the skull. A 4 × 4 cm craniotomy centered over the zygomatic root is then performed with cutting and diamond burrs. The bone flap is dissected from the temporal lobe dura with attention paid to the middle meningeal artery, which may be encased within the bone.

Under magnification, the dura is elevated from the MCF floor in a posterolateral to anteromedial direction. The limits of exposure are the petrous ridge posteromedially and the foramen spinosum anteriorly; the middle meningeal artery may be sacrificed if necessary for adequate exposure or temporal lobe retraction. The arcuate eminence and greater superficial petrosal nerve (GSPN) are identified. The GG is dehiscent 5% to 15% of the time.[43–46] As elevation proceeds anteromedially along the petrous ridge, a lip of bone is usually encountered that denotes the approximate location of the porus acosticus.

A House-Urban retractor is placed to retract the temporal lobe with the retractor blade tip carefully placed at the medial margin of the petrous ridge. The superior semicircular canal (SSCC), which is always perpendicular to the petrous ridge, is identified by blue lining, taking note of the transition from the membranous bone of the mastoid to the yellow-white, dense bone of the otic capsule. Identification of the SSCC allows localization of the IAC, cochlea, GG, and tympanic cavity.

The meatal plane is then drilled to identify the IAC, which is skeletonized from medial to lateral. A rim of bone at the porus acosticus may be kept intact to prevent slippage of the retractor blade. As the dissection advances laterally, the IAC courses lateral and cephalad. Using the blue-lined SSCC as a guide, the labyrinthine segment is approached, taking care to avoid the SSCC ampulla and vestibule posteriorly and the cochlea anteriorly. Once the meatus of the labyrinthine segment has been identified at the Bill's bar, the bony canal is removed from the meatal foramen to the GG, which is triangulated by the courses of labyrinthine segment, GSPN, and tympanic segment. The tympanic segment may be visualized by opening the epitympanum with the drill, taking care to avoid injury to the head of the malleus. Bone removal over the labyrinthine segment is approximately 90° of the canal. This limited exposure provides decompression while reducing the risk of inadvertent injury to the basal turn of the cochlea, which is less than 1 mm anterior and inferior to the labyrinthine segment of the nerve, and the SSCC ampulla posteriorly. The bone over the GG is then removed (**Fig. 6**). The fallopian canal should be opened to the cochleariform process (**Fig. 7**). A very thin layer of bone should be left over the course of the nerve until the entire nerve is exposed. This entire bony layer is then removed with a small right-angled hook or Fisch nerve dissector. Following removal of bone from the nerve, a microscalpel (Beaver no. 59-10) is used to open the dura of the IAC from proximal to distal. The tight arachnoid band at the meatal foramen is then incised (**Fig. 8**).

Following nerve decompression, intraoperative EEMG is performed. A facial nerve stimulator, such as a Prass probe or Parsons-McCabe facial stimulator, is used to locate the exact site of conduction block. The scrub nurse should visualize the forehead, eye, mouth, and chin to serve as a backup to intraoperative EMG. The tympanic segment is stimulated first to ensure that a signal can be obtained distally. If so, the intracanalicular, labyrinthine, and geniculate segments are then stimulated to locate the conduction block. Although rare, stimulation failure of the proximal tympanic segment indicates a conduction block more distally. The postauricular limb of the skin incision may then be extended inferiorly and a concurrent transmastoid approach may be undertaken for decompression of the distal tympanic and descending segments.

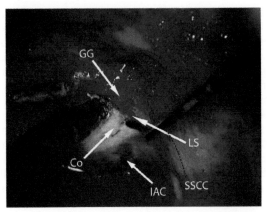

Fig. 6. Intraoperative image of decompression of the geniculate ganglion in a patient with Bell palsy. Co, cochlea; LS, labyrinthine segment of facial nerve; SSCC, superior semicircular canal (*dotted line*).

Attention is then turned to reconstruction. A free muscle graft is harvested from the undersurface of the temporalis muscle. This muscle is used to plug the dural defect in the IAC. Previously harvested temporalis fascia graft is then placed to resurface the entire middle fossa floor. A split-thickness calvarial graft is then harvested from the bone flap and placed over the epitympanum. The House-Urban retractor is removed and hemostasis confirmed around the area of the middle meningeal artery. Two dural elevation sutures are placed inferiorly in the craniotomy window and tacked to the temporalis muscle to close the space between the dura and bone flap. The temporalis muscle is then closed in a watertight fashion with interrupted absorbable suture. The subdermal layer is closed with galea/temporoparietal fascia in an interrupted fashion. The skin is closed with interrupted nylon sutures. A pressure dressing should be applied to the wound.

Surgical Approach for Traumatic Facial Nerve Injury

Surgical decompression secondary to traumatic temporal bone fracture is similar to that of Bell palsy. The segments targeted for decompression are determined by the

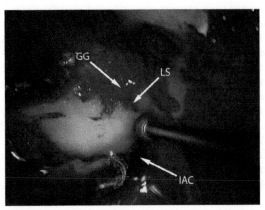

Fig. 7. Intraoperative image of decompression of the labyrinthine segment, connecting the IAC to the GG, in a patient with Bell palsy.

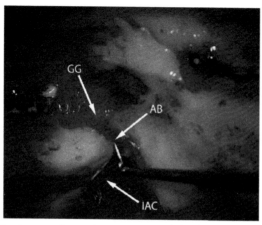

Fig. 8. Intraoperative image of complete exposure of the facial nerve with the arachnoid (dural) band being lysed, in a patient with Bell palsy. AB, arachnoid band.

most likely location of facial nerve injury based on imaging data. The perigeniculate region is the most commonly injured and surgical decompression proceeds similarly to that in Bell palsy.

Preoperative hearing assessment is crucial because, in contrast with Bell palsy, otic capsule–involving temporal bone fractures may result in profound sensorineural hearing loss, in which case a translabyrinthine approach may be undertaken. In addition, surgeons should be prepared for neurorrhaphy or interposition grafting based on intraoperative assessment of the traumatic nerve injury.

Translabyrinthine Approach

The translabyrinthine approach should only be used in patients who are confirmed to have complete hearing loss in the ipsilateral ear. Using the translabyrinthine approach to access cerebellopontine angle lesions has been described in detail elsewhere,[41] and a similar technique is used for facial nerve decompression. A complete mastoidectomy is done with identification of the middle and posterior fossa dural plates, sinodural angle, sigmoid sinus, digastric ridge, incus, and lateral semicircular canal. The vertical segment of the facial nerve can be localized using the horizontal semicircular canal, chorda tympani, and the digastric ridge. The facial recess is then opened, providing access to the tympanic segment of the nerve. The incus and head of the malleus are removed.

Labyrinthectomy is performed by removing the entire bony labyrinth; the SSCC ampulla is removed last and used as a landmark to locate the labyrinthine segment of the facial nerve. The posterior fossa is decompressed and the IAC is skeletonized. The superior trough is developed from medial to lateral and the labyrinthine segment, Bill bar, and superior vestibular nerves are identified. The labyrinthine segment is then followed to the GG.

Targeted electrical stimulation is then performed to localize the site of the conduction block. The entire intratemporal course of the nerve is inspected for traumatic injury. Focal endoneural herniation may be relieved by carefully incising the surrounding epineurium with a 59-10 blade. Frank transection requires repair via primary neurorrhaphy if a tension-free anastomosis can be achieved, or an interposition graft. Either the great auricular or sural nerve may be used for grafting. Neural coaptation is performed under the operating microscope with atraumatic technique. The ends of the nerve or graft should be freshened sharply using microscissors. Nerve ends are joined using 8-0 to 10-0 monofilament (eg, nylon or polypropylene) sutures in the epineurium at 6 and 12 o'clock positions.[26] If grafting of an intracranial portion of nerve is required, only 1 or 2 sutures are placed. Following suture approximation, a fibrin sealant may be applied.

POSTOPERATIVE CARE AND POTENTIAL COMPLICATIONS
Postoperative Care

Postoperatively, patients should be cared for in the intensive care unit overnight with frequent neurologic examinations. The pressure dressing should be changed every day to assess the skin and check for hematoma or CSF effusion. Oral narcotics usually provide adequate pain control, but intravenous narcotics may be used judiciously for breakthrough pain. Patients are kept nil per os until postoperative day 1. Eye care should be continued through the postoperative period (discussed later). Steroids (hydrocortisone or dexamethasone) are continued for 48 hours.

Eye Care

Ocular complications are the greatest source of morbidity in facial nerve palsy. Facial nerve palsy results in decreased lacrimation, upper eyelid retraction, lower eyelid paralytic ectropion, and lagophthalmos. Together these deficits result in decreased tear film and an inability to close the eye, leading to corneal exposure keratopathy that may lead to corneal ulceration and ultimately loss of vision in the affected eye. Ophthalmologic consultation is recommended if ocular symptoms are present, there is concern for decreased corneal sensation, or prolonged facial nerve paralysis is expected.

Conservative management may be divided into 5 categories: lubrication, retaining moisture, obstruction of tear outflow, improvement of tear quality, and bandage or scleral contact lenses.[47] Aggressive lubrication should be performed using artificial tears for mild cases and thicker lubricating ointments for more severe cases. The retention of moisture is aided by air humidifiers, removing fans from the environment, wearing humidification goggles, moisture release eye flow, or taping the affected eye shut. Obstruction of tear outflow is accomplished by placement of silicone punctal plugs or permanent thermal cautery in the punctum. Tear quality can be improved by increasing the lipid component of tears with warm compresses, lipid-enhanced artificial tears, oral omega-3 fatty acids, or doxycycline.[48] Bandage soft contact lenses can be placed to protect the corneal surface from exposure, but they require antibiotic prophylaxis and close follow-up to prevent infectious complications. Scleral hard lenses may also be used if a long-term solution is desired.

Temporary interventions focus on mechanically lowering the upper eyelid or temporarily sealing the eye shut. The upper eyelid may be lowered with adhesive stick-on weights, protective ptosis with botulinum toxin injection to the levator muscle, or hyaluronic acid gel injection into the upper eyelid. The eyelids may be temporarily closed using suture tarsorrhaphy. Permanent intervention most commonly includes lateral tarsorrhaphy but may also include medial or pillar tarsorrhaphy. Further surgical rehabilitation may include lifting the brow and static or dynamic interventions to rehabilitate the upper eyelid. Static interventions include the placement of a gold or platinum upper eyelid weight. Dynamic eyelid closure may be attained with a palpebral spring that attaches between the lateral orbital rim and the tarsus and forces the eyelid closed during levator inaction.

Return of Facial Nerve Function and Follow-up

For both Bell palsy and temporal bone fracture, patients should be counseled that any recovery of facial nerve function will be delayed, despite exceptional reports of immediate improvement in facial nerve function following decompression.[49–51] In most cases, there are signs of recovery 3 to 6 months postoperatively; however, synkinesis can develop up to 12 months following injury. A large number of patients with Bell palsy treated with decompression eventually experience good recovery (HB 1 or 2) of facial nerve function.[2] In cases of traumatic injury requiring primary neurorrhaphy or grafting, the restoration of facial tone and voluntary movement can be expected, albeit with synkinesis.

As facial nerve function recovers, aberrant innervation of the facial nerve may affect the ocular system in 3 ways.[47] Gustatory lacrimation, or crocodile tears, can occur as fibers to the submandibular and sublingual glands aberrantly innervate the lacrimal gland, causing tearing during chewing. Synkinesis may result from axons reinnervating different muscles than those originally served, resulting in aberrant twitching or movement of the eyelid with lower face movement, and vice versa. Hypertonicity may result in the affected side contracting at rest despite decreased dynamic function.

Complications of Facial Nerve Surgery

The potential complications of facial nerve surgery depend on the approach used. Hearing preservation via an MCF approach requires detailed knowledge of the unforgiving middle fossa anatomy. In our experience, intraoperative image guidance offers limited value because the margin of error in the navigation system is frequently larger than the margin of error afforded by the anatomy, especially in the lateral IAC. The rate of CSF leak following acoustic neuroma excision via an MCF approach is 2% to 6%[52] but is lower in cases of facial nerve decompression because the cerebellopontine angle is not widely opened. Seizure, stroke, hematoma (epidural/subarachnoid/parenchymal), and meningitis are also potential risks, albeit extremely rare. Transient aphasia has been observed only rarely over 30 years of experience at our institution, presumably from retraction on the dominant temporal lobe; full recovery occurred in each case.

SUMMARY

Bell palsy or traumatic facial nerve injury are two common causes of acute facial palsy. Bell palsy accounts for most acute facial palsy cases, and most patients with Bell palsy completely recover with medical therapy alone. However, patients with complete paralysis who meet electrophysiologic criteria have a poor prognosis with medical therapy alone and may benefit from facial nerve decompression via an MCF approach. Patients with acute facial palsy from traumatic injury may be candidates for decompression via an MCF or translabyrinthine approach based on hearing status. Available evidence suggests that, for those meeting criteria, surgical decompression improves that chance of recovery. However, detailed counseling is required for an intervention plan customized to each patient.

REFERENCES

1. Peitersen E. Bell's palsy: the spontaneous course of 2,500 peripheral facial nerve palsies of different etiologies. Acta Otolaryngol Suppl 2002;(549):4–30.
2. Gantz BJ, Rubinstein JT, Gidley P, et al. Surgical management of Bell's palsy. Laryngoscope 1999;109(8):1177–88. Available at: https://www.ncbi.nlm.nih.gov/pubmed/10443817.

3. Sullivan FM, Swan IR, Donnan PT, et al. Early treatment with prednisolone or acyclovir in Bell's palsy. N Engl J Med 2007;357:1598–607.

4. Engstrom M, Berg T, Stjernquist-Desatnik A, et al. Prednisolone and valaciclovir in Bell's palsy: a randomised, double-blind, placebo-controlled, multicentre trial. Lancet Neurol 2008;7:993–1000.

5. Hato N, Yamada H, Kohno H, et al. Valacyclovir and prednisolone treatment for Bell's palsy: a multicenter, randomized, placebo-controlled study. Otol Neurotol 2007;28:408–13.

6. Gagyor I, Madhok VB, Daly F, et al. Antiviral treatment for Bell's palsy (idiopathic facial paralysis). Cochrane Database Syst Rev 2015;(4):CD001869.

7. Balance C, Duel AB. The operative treatment of facial palsy: by the introduction of nerve grafts into the fallopian canal and by other intratemporal methods. Arch Otolaryngol 1932;15:1–70.

8. May M, Schlaepfer WM. Bell's palsy and the chorda tympani nerve: a clinical and electron microscopic study. Laryngoscope 1975;85(12):1957–75.

9. Gussen R. Pathogenesis of Bell's Palsy. Retrograde epineural edema and postedematous fibrous compression neuropathy of the facial nerve. Ann Otol Rhinol Laryngol 1977;86(4):549–58.

10. May M. Total facial nerve exploration: transmastoid, extralabyrinthine and subtemporal indications and results. Laryngoscope 1979;89(6):906–17.

11. May M, Klein SR, Taylor FH. Indications for surgery for Bell's palsy. Am J Otol 1984;5(6):503–12.

12. May M, Klein SR, Taylor FH. Idiopathic (Bell's) facial palsy: natural history defies steroid or surgical treatment. Laryngoscope 1985;95(4):406–10.

13. House WF. Surgical exposure of the internal auditory canal and its contents through the middle, cranial fossa. Laryngoscope 1961;71:1363–85.

14. Fisch U, Esslen E. Total intratemporal exposure of the facial nerve. Arch Otolaryngol 1972;95:335–41.

15. Gantz BJ, Gmür A, Fisch U. Intraoperative evoked electromyography in Bell's palsy. Am J Otolaryngol 1982;3(4):273–8.

16. Andresen NS, Clark TJE, Sun DQ, et al. Bell's palsy treated with facial nerve decompression, EyeRounds.org. 2018. Available at: http://EyeRounds.org/cases/256-Bells-Palsy.htm. Accessed May 1, 2018.

17. Ge XX, Spector GJ. Labyrinthine segment and geniculate ganglion of facial nerve in fetal and adult human temporal bones. Ann Otol Rhinol Laryngol 1981;90(suppl 85):1–12.

18. Fisch U. Surgery for Bell's palsy. Arch Otolaryngol 1981;107(1):1–11.

19. Burgess RC, Michaels L, Bale JF Jr, et al. Polymerase chain reaction amplification of herpes simplex viral DNA from the geniculate ganglion of a patient with Bell's palsy. Ann Otol Rhinol Laryngol 1994;103(10):775–9.

20. Murakami S, Mizobuchi M, Nakashiro Y, et al. Bell palsy and herpes simplex virus: identification of viral DNA in endoneurial fluid and muscle. Ann Intern Med 1996;124(1 Pt 1):27–30.

21. Furuta Y, Fukuda S, Chida E, et al. Reactivation of herpes simplex virus type 1 in patients with Bell's palsy. J Med Virol 1998;54(3):162–6.

22. Lazarini PR, Vianna MF, Alcantara MP, et al. Herpes simplex virus in the saliva of peripheral Bell's palsy patients. Braz J Otorhinolaryngol 2006;72(1):7–11.

23. Furuta Y, Ohtani F, Kawabata H, et al. High prevalence of varicella-zoster virus reactivation in herpes simplex virus-seronegative patients with acute peripheral facial palsy. Clin Infect Dis 2000;30(3):529–33.

24. Liston SL, Kleid MS. Histopathology of Bell's palsy. Laryngoscope 1989;99(1): 23–6.

25. Sugita T, Murakami S, Yanagihara N, et al. Facial nerve paralysis induced by herpes simplex virus in mice: an animal model of acute and transient facial paralysis. Ann Otol Rhinol Laryngol 1995;104(7):574–81.

26. Gantz BJ. Traumatic facial paralysis, in current therapy in otolaryngology head and neck surgery. Hamilton (ON): BC Decker; 1987. p. 112–5.

27. Fisch U. Facial nerve grafting. Otolaryngol Clin North Am 1974;7(2):517–29.

28. Sittel C, Guntinas-Lichius O, Streppel M, et al. Variability of repeated facial nerve electroneurography in healthy subjects. Laryngoscope 1998;108(8 Pt 1): 1177–80.

29. Gantz BJ, Gmuer AA, Holliday M, et al. Electroneurographic evaluation of the facial nerve. Method and technical problems. Ann Otol Rhinol Laryngol 1984; 93(4 Pt 1):394–8.

30. Krarup C. Compound sensory action potential in normal and pathological human nerves. Muscle Nerve 2004;29(4):465–83.

31. Fisch U. Maximal nerve excitability testing vs electroneuronography. Arch Otolaryngol 1980;106(6):352–7.

32. Takemoto N, Horii A, Sakata Y, et al. Prognostic factors of peripheral facial palsy: multivariate analysis followed by receiver operating characteristic and Kaplan-Meier analyses. Otol Neurotol 2011;32(6):1031–6. Available at: https://www. ncbi.nlm.nih.gov/pubmed/21725266.

33. Byun H, Cho YS, Jang JY, et al. Value of electroneurography as a prognostic indicator for recovery in acute severe inflammatory facial paralysis: a prospective study of Bell's palsy and Ramsay Hunt syndrome. Laryngoscope 2013;123(10): 2526–32. Available at: https://www.ncbi.nlm.nih.gov/pubmed/23918352.

34. Fisch U. Prognostic value of electrical tests in acute facial paralysis. Am J Otol 1984;5(6):494–8.

35. Yanagihara N, Hato N, Murakami S, et al. Transmastoid decompression as a treatment of Bell palsy. Otolaryngol Head Neck Surg 2001;124(3):282–6.

36. Cannon RB, Gurgel RK, Warren FM, et al. Facial nerve outcomes after middle fossa decompression for Bell's palsy. Otol Neurotol 2015;36(3):513–8.

37. Adour KK. Decompression for Bell's palsy: why I don't do it. Eur Arch Otorhinolaryngol 2002;259(1):40–7.

38. McAllister K, Walker D, Donnan PT, et al. Surgical interventions for the early management of Bell's palsy. Cochrane Database Syst Rev 2013;(10). CD007468. Available at: https://www.ncbi.nlm.nih.gov/pubmed/24132718.

39. Baugh RF, Basura GJ, Ishii LE, et al. Clinical practice guideline: Bell's palsy. Otolaryngol Head Neck Surg 2013;149(3 Suppl):S1–27. Available at: https://www. ncbi.nlm.nih.gov/pubmed/24189771.

40. Grogan PM, Gronseth GS. Practice parameter: steroids, acyclovir, and surgery for Bell's palsy (an evidence-based review): report of the quality standards subcommittee of the American Academy of Neurology. Neurology 2001;56(7):830–6. Available at: https://www.ncbi.nlm.nih.gov/pubmed/11294918.

41. Gantz BJ, Gubbels SP, Samy RN. Facial nerve surgery. In: Glasscock M, Shambaugh G, editors. Surgery of the ear. 6th edition. Philadelphia: WB Saunders; 2010. p. 619–42.

42. Gantz BJ, Wackym PA. Facial nerve abnormalities. In: Smith J, Bumstead R, editors. Pediatric facial plastic and reconstructive surgery. Raven Press; 1993. p. 337–47.

43. House WF, Crabtree JA. Surgical exposure of the petrous portion of the 7th nerve. Arch Otolaryngol 1965;81:506–7.

44. Rhoton AL Jr, Pulec JL, Hall GM, et al. Absence of bone over the geniculate ganglion. J Neurosurg 1968;28(1):48–53.

45. Barrs DM. Facial nerve trauma: optimal timing for repair. Laryngoscope 1991; 101(8):835–48.

46. Gidley PW, Gantz BJ, Rubinstein JT. Facial nerve grafts: from cerebellopontine angle and beyond. Am J Otol 1999;20(6):781–8.

47. Welder JD, Allen RC, Shriver EM. Facial nerve palsy: ocular complications and management. EyeRounds.org. 2015. Available at: http://www.EyeRounds.org/cases/215-facial-nerve.htm. Accessed May 1, 2018.

48. Garrigue JS, Amrane M, Faure MO, et al. Relevance of lipid-based products in the management of dry eye disease. J Ocul Pharmacol Ther 2017;33(9):647–61.

49. Yanagihara N, Gyo K, Yumoto E, et al. Transmastoid decompression of the facial nerve in Bell's palsy. Arch Otolaryngol 1979;105(9):530–4.

50. McCabe BF. Some evidence for the efficacy of decompression for Bell's Palsy: immediate motion postoperatively. Laryngoscope 1977;87(2):246–9.

51. Pulec JL. Early decompression of the facial nerve in Bell's Palsy. Ann Otol 1981; 90(6 Pt 1):570–7.

52. Weber PC, Gantz BJ. Results and complications from acoustic neuroma excision via middle cranial fossa approach. Am J Otol 1996;17(4):669–75.

Management of Flaccid Facial Paralysis of Less Than Two Years' Duration

Andrew William Joseph, MD, MPH, Jennifer C. Kim, MD*

KEYWORDS

- Facial palsy • Facial paralysis • Facial reanimation • Facial reinnervation
- Nerve grafting

KEY POINTS

- The treatment of patients with facial paralysis should involve a systematic approach.
- Treatment should be individualized based on duration of facial paralysis, accessibility and functional status of the distal and proximal facial nerve branches, as well as patient-specific factors, such as comorbidities and patient goals.
- Primary nerve repair has been shown to have the best outcome and is the preferred approach when possible.
- In cases of flaccid facial paralysis of less than 2 years' duration in which primary nerve repair is not possible, nerve substitution procedures serve as the primary modality for restoring facial tone and dynamic motion.

INTRODUCTION

The management of flaccid facial paralysis is complicated and treatment approaches are based on patient-specific and disease-specific factors. Flaccid facial paralysis can cause profound facial disfigurement and negatively affect quality of life and how strangers perceive these individuals.[1] Furthermore, patients with facial paralysis frequently have functional sequelae, with potentially catastrophic ophthalmic outcomes in patients with periocular involvement. Most patients with facial palsy screened in ophthalmology clinics demonstrate evidence of corneal abnormalities despite that few report symptoms.[2] Other functional sequelae include oral incompetence, articulation difficulty, and psychosocial isolation and distress.

Disclosure Statement: The authors have nothing to disclose.
Division of Facial Plastic and Reconstructive Surgery, Department of Otorhinolaryngology–Head and Neck Surgery, University of Michigan Medical School, Ann Arbor, MI, USA
* Corresponding author. 19900 Haggerty Road, Suite 103, Livonia, MI 48152.
E-mail address: jennkim@med.umich.edu

Otolaryngol Clin N Am 51 (2018) 1093–1105
https://doi.org/10.1016/j.otc.2018.07.006
0030-6665/18/© 2018 Elsevier Inc. All rights reserved.

Long-standing flaccid facial paralysis present for greater than 2 years will result in ultrastructural changes within the distal facial nerve branches and within the denervated facial muscles, which may preclude dynamic reinnervation of the native facial musculature. However, these structures are generally preserved in patients who present less than 1 year from the time of onset, and up to 2 years in some cases. The goal of this article is to discuss management and rehabilitation strategies for patients who present with flaccid facial paralysis of less than 2 years' duration.

EVALUATION AND INITIAL MANAGEMENT OF FACIAL PARALYSIS
Management of Acute Facial Paralysis

All practitioners who work with patients with facial paralysis should be well-versed in the workup and management of acute facial paralysis. When these patients present acutely, the cause of facial weakness is often uncertain. Some patients may be referred with the diagnosis of Bell palsy before any meaningful evaluation. Others may have undergone unnecessarily extensive and costly workups. In 2013, the American Academy of Otolaryngology–Head and Neck Surgery developed the Bell palsy clinical practice guideline, which outlines many important topics in the clinical decision-making for these patients.[3] (See Teresa M. O's article, "Medical Management of Acute Facial Paralysis," in this issue.)

Individualized Treatment Planning

The management of facial paralysis should be individualized based on several patient-specific factors that are outlined here. During initial consultation, all new patients with flaccid facial paralysis undergo a thorough history and physical. The medical history interview of the patient should focus on the onset and characteristics of the paralysis (eg, acute complete, chronic progressive), associated symptoms (eg, hearing loss, tinnitus, dysphagia, diplopia), involved facial nerve branches, and whether any perceived recovery has begun to take place. Patients should specifically be questioned about treatments that have been attempted (eg, oral steroids, electrical stimulation, surgery). Most important, patients' individual perception of their facial disability and goals of care should be solicited.

One of the most critical factors in treatment planning is determining the cause for facial paralysis. The cause can vary tremendously and includes traumatic (temporal bone fracture or traumatic transection); neoplastic (cerebellopontine angle tumor, facial nerve schwannoma, glomus tumors, salivary gland lesions); iatrogenic (inadvertent facial nerve transection or facial nerve sacrifice); and inflammatory, infectious, and congenital causes. Understanding the natural course of disease associated with the various causes will aid in determination of an optimal treatment strategy.

When planning treatments, it is extremely important to identify if other cranial nerves have been (or expected to become) affected by the disease process. Assessment of cranial nerves should be comprehensive, with a particular focus on assessment of the motor and sensory functions of the trigeminal nerve, as well as the motor functions of the contralateral (unaffected) facial nerve, glossopharyngeal nerve, spinal accessory nerve, and hypoglossal nerve. This evaluation is critical because nerve substitution procedures are among the mainstays of flaccid facial paralysis treatment when the duration of paralysis is less than 2 years.

Assessment of Affected Facial Zones

Physical examination of patients with facial paralysis should proceed in a systematic manner. The authors find it helpful to assess the affected branches of the facial nerve by considering the various facial aesthetic subunits in comparison with the contralateral (nonflaccid) hemiface. It is important to recognize that the position of structures and features of the contralateral face may also be abnormal because it is common for patients with flaccid facial paralysis to have compensatory hyperactivation within the contralateral facial musculature.

It is often advantageous to divide the face into thirds during evaluation. The upper third of the face includes the forehead and brows. The forehead, where the rhytides on the flaccid versus the nonflaccid side are evaluated, is considered first. Next, the brow positions on the flaccid versus nonflaccid side are considered. The nonflaccid brow may show elevation, which should be noted in comparison with what is commonly a depressed brow on the flaccid hemiface.

The middle third of the face is considered next. Upper eyelid position, lower eyelid position, and blink should all be assessed. During assessment, we ask patients to blink gently and then blink tightly to assess orbicularis oculi function. Patients with flaccid paralysis commonly have a less efficient blink, even if they can achieve full eye closure. Corneal sensation and Bell phenomenon are usually also assessed at this time. Finally, nasal base position is assessed and patients are questioned regarding any symptoms of nasal obstruction.

Within the lower face, nasolabial fold depth, oral commissure position at rest, and then with smile are evaluated. The contralateral lower lip depressor anguli oris and depressor labii inferioris are frequently hyperactivated, and this should be documented.

Systematic assessment of facial nerve function with standardized instruments is an indispensable part of treatment planning and outcome assessment. The eFACE instrument has been developed and validated by Banks and colleagues.[4] This instrument is easy to use and has high interrater reliability among facial nerve experts.

TREATMENT PLANNING

The goal of facial reanimation procedures is to facilitate improvement in both facial muscle tone and dynamic facial symmetry. Formerly, reanimation procedures primarily focused on restoring perioral and periocular movement; however, it has been increasingly recognized that facial muscle tone restoration is equally important and can alleviate hyperdynamic motion of the contralateral face. Most procedures developed to date have focused on restoration of midface and lower face symmetry. Most of these procedures can be grouped within 2 categories: nerve substitution procedures and muscle transfer procedures. Nerve substitution procedures involve substituting proximal motor nerve input from another cranial nerve. Conversely, muscle transfer or tendon transfer procedures use pedicled muscle flaps or free tissue transfer for reanimation of the face. When free muscle transfers are used, proximal neural input may be derived from the facial nerve (ipsilateral or contralateral) or another cranial nerve (usually masseteric and/or hypoglossal nerves).

A stepwise approach that may be used for patients with flaccid facial paralysis present for less than 2 years follows (**Fig. 1**).

Duration of Facial Paralysis

The key determinants in selecting a treatment strategy for flaccid facial paralysis are the duration and degree of facial weakness. The reason that duration of paralysis is so important is that it affects whether the end organs, namely the distal facial nerve branches and facial musculature, remain functional. Depending on the clinical scenario, patients who present less than 2 years from the onset of flaccid facial paralysis

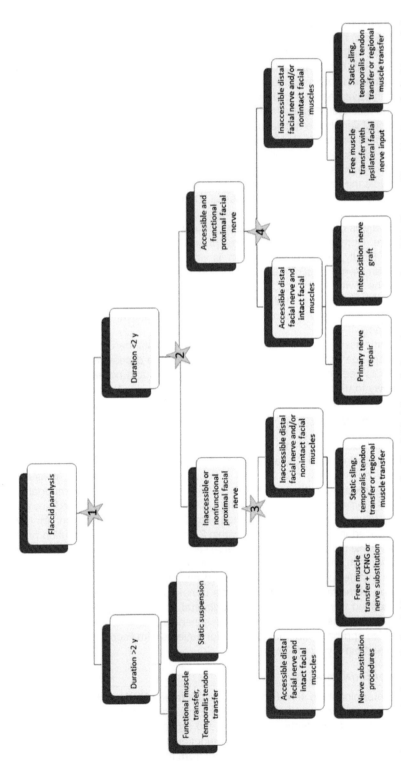

Fig. 1. Major factors in developing a management plan for flaccid facial paralysis patients presenting within 2 years. Stars denote each decision point.

may be candidates for reinnervation of the native facial musculature. Nevertheless, in the authors' experience, the best outcomes are observed when interventions take place within a year after paralysis onset. Patients who have paralysis longer than 2 years will often require functional muscle or tendon transfer to mitigate nonfunctional native facial musculature (see **Fig. 1**, decision point 1). For patients who have excessive comorbidities, or those who do not wish to undergo more invasive procedures, static facial suspension techniques may be considered.

Proximal Facial Nerve Status

The second factor used to determine the optimal treatment strategy is the functional status and accessibility of the proximal ipsilateral facial nerve (see **Fig. 1**, decision point 2). There are numerous scenarios that preclude accessibility or utilization of the proximal stump of the facial nerve, the most common of which is very proximal facial nerve sacrifice or transection at the cerebellopontine angle, making nerve grafting impossible. In other situations, the proximal facial nerve trunk is anatomically intact but presumed nonfunctional. This may occur when a patient develops dense facial paralysis following temporal bone trauma, middle cranial fossa surgery, or temporal bone surgery. Denervation may be assumed if patients have not shown any discernible functional facial nerve recovery by 12 months after the insult and electromyogram demonstrates a lack of electrophysiologic reinnervation potentials. In these cases, other cranial nerves will be required to drive motor function of the face.

Facial Musculature and Distal Facial Nerve Status

A third determinant in selecting a facial reanimation treatment strategy is the status of the distal facial nerve branches and facial musculature (see **Fig. 1**, decision points 3 and 4). It is desirable to use native facial mimetic muscles when possible because no current procedure can recreate the complex motion and vector of these muscles. Fortunately, many patients presenting with facial paralysis for less than 2 years have accessible distal facial nerve branches and facial musculature. The notable exception is in patients who have undergone radical resections of head and neck or parotid neoplasms without preservation of distal facial nerve branches. Nevertheless, it should be noted that, in the authors' experience, even in situations in which a radical parotidectomy has been performed, distal facial nerve branches are commonly still present and can be used. The more difficult scenario occurs when extirpation of head and neck neoplasms involves resection of facial mimetic muscles, which necessitates functional muscle transfer.

SURGICAL APPROACHES TO TREATMENT OF FLACCID FACIAL PARALYSIS
Dynamic Reanimation Procedures

Primary nerve repair and interposition grafting

The best dynamic outcomes (better static tone, dynamic movement, and less synkinesis) are observed when it is possible to directly repair discontinuity of the facial nerve. Nonetheless, it is very important to obtain a tension-free neurorrhaphy to ensure the best outcomes possible.[5,6] In cases in which defects are 5 to 10 mm, additional proximal facial nerve length may be obtained through mobilization within the mastoid cavity.[7,8] However, mobilization of the facial nerve may theoretically result in transient perfusion changes to the nerve, which is a risk that must be weighed in the decision-making process. In cases in which a tension-free repair cannot be accomplished but distal and proximal portions of the facial nerve are present and functional, an interposition nerve graft should be used. Common donor nerves include the sural nerve, antebrachial cutaneous nerve, and the great auricular nerve. Epineural repair is then performed in an end-to-end fashion.

Nerve substitution procedures

Most facial reanimation procedures performed for patients with flaccid facial paralysis less than 2 years in duration and without a functional (or accessible) proximal facial nerve are nerve substitution procedures. These are also known as reinnervation techniques, in which the motor input from the native facial nerve nucleus is replaced by motor nerve axons from another cranial nerve or from the contralateral functional facial nerve. The following section reviews modern nerve substitution procedures.

Hypoglossal nerve (XII–VII transfer) In many institutions, the hypoglossal nerve is the most common cranial nerve used to reinnervate the facial nerve. There are several distinct advantages in using this cranial nerve, including close proximity to the surgical site, a consistent location making surgical identification relatively uncomplicated, a robust supply of donor motor axons, and a relatively minimal donor organ deficit when using modern techniques.[9]

The hypoglossal nerve has been used as a donor nerve since the early twentieth century.[10] The original descriptions of hypoglossal to facial nerve transfers involved use of the entire hypoglossal nerve. In the classic procedure, the hypoglossal nerve was identified and then fully transected so that it could be transposed into the proximity of the distal facial nerve stump and sutured in an end-to-end fashion (crossover procedure). As might be expected, this approach results in hemilingual atrophy, resulting in dysarthria and dysphagia.[11,12]

To avoid functional deficits associated with the classic technique, several newer approaches were developed. The first was developed by May and colleagues.[12] In their technique, a perineural window was created by making an incision in the hypoglossal nerve to 50% of its diameter. Following creation of the perineural window, an interposition free nerve graft was coapted in an end-to-side fashion to the hypoglossal nerve. The distal aspect of the interposition nerve graft may then be sutured to the affected facial nerve. The use of only 50% of donor hypoglossal axons is supported by histologic studies that suggest that the hypoglossal nerve contains up to twice as many axons as the injured facial nerve.[13] Therefore, use of only half of the available hypoglossal axons is presumably appropriate. The procedure as described by May and colleagues[12] resulted in a drastically reduced risk of developing symptomatic tongue-related deficits (4%) but showed equivalent dynamic results with less synkinesis when compared with the classic technique. Some surgeons have raised the concern that the use of an interposition nerve graft may have worse outcomes due to axonal loss across 2 neurorrhaphy sites. Nonetheless, numerous reports have shown dynamic results that are equivalent to the classic end-to-end technique.[14,15]

To avoid use of an interposition nerve graft as well as to circumvent drawbacks to longitudinal nerve section, an additional technique has been described that involves rerouting of the temporal portion of the proximal facial nerve.[11,16,17] With this technique, the mastoid portion of the facial nerve distal to the second genu of the facial nerve is isolated and mobilized from the temporal bone. This technique allows enough facial nerve length to be mobilized so that a direct end-to-side neurorrhaphy between the proximal facial nerve and the hypoglossal nerve can be achieved. This technique shows efficacy similar to direct end-to-end hypoglossal to facial anastomosis but with morbidity similar to the technique by Samii and colleagues.[18] The main drawback to this technique is the requirement for mastoidectomy and facial nerve drillout.

Masseteric nerve (V–VII transfer) The motor nerve to the masseter muscle is a valuable donor nerve that has been increasingly used in facial reanimation procedures over the past 15 years. This nerve is located in close proximity to zygomatic branches of the facial nerve that controls smiling, allowing for primary neurorrhaphy for targeted bite-driven smile reanimation. Furthermore, the close proximity of this nerve and, therefore, short distance for axonal regrowth, allows for expedient clinical recovery and return of dynamic facial function, which is often as soon as 3 to 4 months following reanimation surgery. The masseteric motor nerve has been estimated to provide between 1500 and 2000 myelinated donor axons, which is a sufficient number to power the main trunk of the facial nerve or transferred free muscle tissue.[19] Another major benefit in the use of the motor nerve to masseter is that its sacrifice results in essentially no clinical deficit, which may be related to preserved innervation through undisturbed proximal masseter nerve branches, as well as compensation by other muscles of mastication.[19]

Surgical Technique

Several reports have described techniques for localizing the motor nerve to masseter.[19–21] The masseteric motor nerve crosses the caudal aspect of the zygomatic arch at an angle of approximately 50° and, after entering the masseter muscle, continues distally toward the oral commissure.[19] Dissection may be initiated approximately 3 cm anterior to the tragus and 1 cm inferior to the caudal aspect of the zygomatic arch. An alternative approach to nerve localization involves use of what has been termed the subzygomatic triangle.[20] After locating the starting point in both techniques, dissection then proceeds in a superficial to deep manner through the masseter muscle. The authors generally find it helpful to have an assistant retract muscle fibers with a Cummings or Ragnell retractor while a fine curved hemostat and bipolar cautery is used by the surgeon to carefully divide the muscle. A dominant branch of the nerve will be located 1.0 to 1.5 cm deep into the parotidomasseteric fascia.[19,20] Very often, a branch-free segment approximately 2 cm long can be located. An electrical nerve stimulator may also aid in localization of the nerve, which generally causes a strong activation of the masseter muscle. Some surgeons prefer to preserve the superomedial branch of the masseteric nerve to decrease the risk of facial hollowing associated with complete denervation. However, some evidence suggests that the first branch of the motor nerve to the masseter muscle is not visible unless the zygomatic arch is removed, suggesting that sacrifice inferior to the arch likely preserves some innervation.[19]

Contralateral facial nerve via cross-face nerve graft

The contralateral facial nerve is another important source of donor axons, which can be used in facial reanimation with a cross-face nerve graft (CFNG). The most important benefit of using the contralateral facial nerve is that spontaneous blink and emotive smile are possible. The CFNG technique relies on a contralateral (unaffected) facial nerve having significant redundancy in the distal buccal and zygomatic neural input due to significant arborization of nerve fibers among branches. Therefore, division and utilization of 1 of the distal buccal or zygomatic branches results in little or no clinical deficit.

There are, however, distinct disadvantages associated with this approach. Due to the requirement for a long interposition nerve graft, there is a significant delay of 6 to 8 months between the time a CFNG procedure is completed and the time that nerve fibers reach the distal aspect of the nerve graft and target muscle. Because many facial nerve patients present for reinnervation at 1 year or greater following the onset of paralysis, an additional period of 6 to 8 months of denervation may result in further muscle and distal nerve fibrosis, potentially limiting functional outcomes. However, in this situation, some surgeons may prefer to perform dual innervation and use a so-called babysitter nerve that may provide earlier reinnervation and thus preserve the function of native distal muscle and nerve (see later discussion of dual innervation). Additional disadvantages include the potential for weakness in the unaffected (good) facial nerve, more unpredictable results compared with other donor nerves, and fewer available donor axons compared with hypoglossal or masseteric nerves. Of note, it has been shown that an ideal donor nerve for facial reinnervation procedures should have greater than 900 axons because this results in improved functional outcomes.[22] In an elegant anatomic study, Hembd and colleagues group demonstrated that, when sampling facial nerve branches just adjacent to the anterior border of the parotid gland, there is a 90% chance of obtaining a donor buccal or zygomatic nerve branch with more than 900 axons.[23]

Surgical Technique

We begin by harvest of a sural nerve graft from the lower extremity. This procedure may be performed with or without the use of an endoscope and has been well described elsewhere.[24,25] Following harvest of the sural nerve graft, the distal end is marked with methylene blue. Next, a facelift style preauricular incision is designed on the donor side of the face and 1:100,000 epinephrine without lidocaine is injected into the proposed preauricular incision line and the subcutaneous tissue of the donor midface. A subcutaneous skin flap is raised similar to that performed with a facelift. The superficial musculoaponeurotic system (SMAS) fascia is identified and an incision is sharply made within this layer, 2 to 3 cm anterior to the tragus. Next, a sub-SMAS flap is developed and dissection proceeds in this layer anteriorly until the masseterocutaneous ligaments are identified. Just beyond these ligaments is the buccal fat pad, at which point several buccal branches of the facial nerve may be identified. The facial nerve branch to the zygomaticus major may be identified at the Zuker point, which is located halfway along a line drawn between the root of the helix and the oral commissure.[26] The branches can be followed in a retrograde fashion for a short distance to the edge of the parotid gland to obtain donor nerve segment of larger caliber and greater axonal load. We routinely use a nerve stimulator to test several candidate nerve branches. Among candidate branches that have similar caliber, we select nerve branches that have the most specificity for causing zygomaticus major activation.

After selection of a donor facial nerve branch, the sural nerve is tunneled in antidromic orientation from a stab incision in the gingivolabial sulcus to the location where the donor nerve branch was identified. Next, we use an operating microscope for neurorrhaphy, which is performed between the donor facial nerve branch and the sural nerve graft through approximation of the epineurium of the nerves with 9 to 0 nylon suture. Often, we will use a small vein graft for entubulation of the neurorrhaphy sites. Next, the neurorrhaphy is performed for the contralateral side, where a dominant facial nerve branch to the zygomaticus is usually selected. The wounds are irrigated and then closed in a routine fashion.

Dual innervation procedures

Dual innervation procedures are newer approaches to reinnervation that involve the use of donor nerve input from more than 1 cranial nerve. Each cranial nerve possesses inherent characteristics that may affect its usefulness in individual reconstructive scenarios. Characteristics that are commonly important to the facial nerve surgeon include the ability to restore resting facial tone, the capacity to produce robust dynamic motion (ie, donor nerve axonal count), the ability to achieve consistent results, ease of use, and the degree of donor site morbidity. The aim of dual innervation techniques is to use multiple donor cranial nerves with the intention of allowing the individual properties of each donor nerve to complement each other and avoid drawbacks inherent to any individual donor nerve when used on its own.

Yamamoto and colleagues[27] first reported this approach for rehabilitation of facial paralysis subject. They described the use of the hypoglossal nerve to supplement proximal facial nerve for donor nerve sources in 8 subjects with both complete and incomplete facial paralysis and salvageable facial musculature.[27] The investigators termed this approach supercharging because the donor hypoglossal nerve augmented the attenuated neural input from the damaged facial nerve. Yamamoto and colleagues[27] reported improvement from House-Brackmann grade IV–VI to grade II–III in their small case series of this technique, and did not observe any mass synkinesis associated with use of the hypoglossal donor nerve.

Use of the motor branch to the masseter muscle has gained popularity for use in facial reanimation procedures due to its ability to provide expedient regrowth of donor nerve axons and consistent dynamic motor outcomes (**Fig. 2**). However, evidence suggests that the motor nerve to masseter has limited ability to restore baseline resting tone, especially in patients with severe flaccid facial paralysis.[28] A recent report by Owusu and colleagues[29] described a series of 9 subjects who underwent immediate facial nerve repair following radical parotidectomy with concurrent cable grafting and masseteric to facial transposition. In their series, the motor branch to the masseteric nerve was coapted to a midfacial branch of the facial nerve controlling smile, whereas the cable graft was used to repair the remaining branches (**Fig. 3**A). This method of dual innervation combined the advantages of being able to restore tone to the periocular area and upper facial with the cable graft, whereas the masseteric nerve was used for restoration of dynamic motion to the oral commissure (ie, reanimate smile). All subjects were found to have return of oral commissure motion within 7 months after

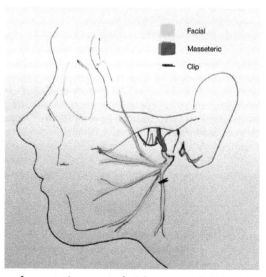

Fig. 2. Transposition of masseteric nerve to facial nerve trunk. Selective cervical branch neurectomy may be performed simultaneously to reduce synkinesis involving the platysma.

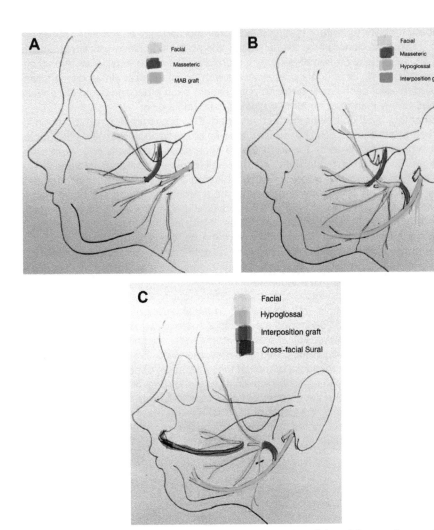

Fig. 3. Common schemes used to provide dual innervation. (*A*) Facial nerve interposition nerve graft combined with masseteric to buccal branch nerve transposition. (*B*) Partial hypoglossal to facial nerve transposition via interposition graft combined with masseteric nerve to buccal nerve branch transposition. (*C*) Partial hypoglossal to facial nerve transposition via interposition graft combined with CFNG to buccal nerve branch transposition. Cross-facial sural, cross-face sural nerve graft; Facial, facial nerve; MAB, median antebrachial cutaneous nerve; Masseteric, masseteric nerve.

surgery.[29] Furthermore, an additional benefit to the dual innervation technique was the minimal reported synkinesis, which is not often the case when cable grafts are used for multiple facial nerve branches. Similar results had been previously described by Volk and colleagues[30] with the hypoglossal nerve and a cable graft.

Dual innervation or polyinnervation procedures may be accomplished in many ways. Hypoglossal nerve transfer is well-recognized to provide good resting tone, although the smile is not as natural as with transfer of other donor cranial nerves, such as the masseteric nerve or CFNG. The hypoglossal and masseteric nerves may be used in a scenario in which the hypoglossal nerve contributes to good resting tone, whereas the masseteric nerve allows for a more natural smile with clenching, as well as reduced synkinesis (**Fig. 3**B). Finally, a partial hypoglossal nerve transfer may be used in conjunction with a CFNG coapted to a buccal nerve branch to provide a natural emotive smile, good resting tone, and reduced synkinesis (**Fig. 3**C). Beyond nerve transfer procedures, surgeons are also beginning to use dual innervation approaches with free tissue transfer, although a discussion is beyond the scope of this article.[31,32] Nonetheless, dual innervation procedures have great potential for improving facial reanimation outcomes, although more research is required to define their exact role.

Static Approaches and Adjunctive Procedures

Static procedures for facial reanimation may be used in situations in which patients are not candidates for general anesthesia due to medical comorbidities or other factors, precluding more invasive dynamic procedures. Static procedures are more commonly used in longstanding facial paralysis but may be indicated in select cases of paralysis of shorter duration to augment dynamic procedures even when partial recovery of tone and dynamic motion is expected. For example, static suspension of the oral commissure may be used to more quickly rehabilitate patients as they await recovery of facial tone. Suture techniques or suspension with fascia lata or the palmaris longus tendon are all effective and minimally invasive.

The periocular complex deserves special consideration. Patients who are expected to have expedient recovery of facial tone can often be managed with vigilant eye lubrication, moisture chamber use, and other conservative measures. In cases in which the periocular area is not expected to recover tone, eyelid loading with a platinum weight may be considered. Eyelid weights are useful when there is lagophthalmos exceeding 1 to 2 mm, poor Bell phenomenon, corneal anesthesia, or exposure keratopathy. One of the advantages of eyelid weights compared with other procedures is the reversibility and general tolerance for placing these with the patient under local anesthesia. In very severe cases, temporary lateral tarsorrhaphy may be performed. The authors prefer to defer permanent procedures until maximal recovery has been achieved, and the functional status of the periocular complex can be evaluated in that setting. Patients with lower eyelid paralytic ectropion may be candidates for canthopexy and/or the placement of a spacer graft, although this is generally deferred in patients who are expected to regain midface or periocular tone. In all cases, it is imperative to involve an ophthalmologist who can monitor corneal health throughout the recovery process.

SUMMARY

Flaccid facial paralysis is a disfiguring condition that may profoundly affect the lives of patients. For patients with paralysis of less than 2 years' duration, primary nerve repair and nerve substitution procedures serve as the primary modalities for dynamic rehabilitation. Facial nerve surgeons should seek to restore facial symmetry through restoration of not only dynamic facial motion but also resting facial tone. The authors recommend an organized approach to treatment planning based on duration and cause of paralysis, status, and accessibility of the affected facial nerve, as well as medical comorbidities and patient-specific goals.

REFERENCES

1. Goines JB, Ishii LE, Dey JK, et al. Association of facial paralysis–related disability with patient- and observer-perceived quality of life. JAMA Facial Plast Surg 2016; 18(5):363–9.

2. Joseph SS, Joseph AW, Smith JI, et al. Evaluation of patients with facial palsy and ophthalmic sequelae: a 23-year retrospective review. Ophthalmic Epidemiol 2017;24(5):341–5.

3. Baugh RF, Basura GJ, Ishii LE, et al. Clinical practice guideline: Bell's palsy. Otolaryngol Head Neck Surg 2013;149(3_suppl):S1–27.

4. Banks CA, Jowett N, Hadlock CR, et al. Weighting of facial grading variables to disfigurement in facial palsy. JAMA Facial Plast Surg 2016;18(4):292–9.

5. Spector JG. Neural repair in facial paralysis: clinical and experimental studies. Eur Arch Otorhinolaryngol 1997;254(1):S68–75.

6. Terzis JMD, Faibisoff BBA, Williams HBMD. The nerve gap: suture under tension vs. graft. Plast Reconstr Surg 1975;56(2):166–70.

7. Pillsbury HC, Price HC, Gardiner LJ. Primary tumors of the facial nerve: diagnosis and management. Laryngoscope 1983;93(8):1045–8.

8. Piza-Katzer H, Balogh B, Muzika-Herczeg E, et al. Secondary end-to-end repair of extensive facial nerve defects: surgical technique and postoperative functional results. Head Neck 2004;26(9):770–7.

9. Kunihiro T, Kanzaki J, Yoshihara S, et al. Hypoglossal-facial nerve anastomosis after acoustic neuroma resection: influence of the time of anastomosis on recovery of facial movement. ORL J Otorhinolaryngol Relat Spec 1996;58(1):32–5.

10. Stennert EI. Hypoglossal facial anastomosis: its significance for modern facial surgery. II. Combined approach in extratemporal facial nerve reconstruction. Clin Plast Surg 1979;6(3):471–86.

11. Slattery WH, Cassis AM, Wilkinson EP, et al. Side-to-end hypoglossal to facial anastomosis with transposition of the intratemporal facial nerve. Otol Neurotol 2014;35(3):509–13.

12. May M, Sobol SM, Mester SJ. Hypoglossal-facial nerve interpositional-jump graft for facial reanimation without tongue atrophy. Otolaryngol Head Neck Surg 1991; 104(6):818–25.

13. Campero A, Socolovsky M. Facial reanimation by means of the hypoglossal nerve: anatomic comparison of different techniques. Neurosurgery 2007; 61(suppl_3):41–9.

14. Guntinas-Lichius O, Streppel M, Stennert E. Postoperative functional evaluation of different reanimation techniques for facial nerve repair. Am J Surg 2006; 191(1):61–7.

15. Manni JJ, Beurskens CHG, van de Velde C, et al. Reanimation of the paralyzed face by indirect hypoglossal-facial nerve anastomosis. Am J Surg 2001;182(3): 268–73.

16. Atlas MD, Lowinger DSG. A new technique for hypoglossal-facial nerve repair. Laryngoscope 1997;107(7):984–91.

17. Martins RS, Socolovsky M, Siqueira MG, et al. Hemihypoglossal–facial neurorrhaphy after mastoid dissection of the facial nerve results in 24 patients and comparison with the classic technique. Neurosurgery 2008;63(2):310–7.

18. Samii M, Alimohamadi M, Khouzani RK, et al. Comparison of direct side-to-end and end-to-end hypoglossal-facial anastomosis for facial nerve repair. World Neurosurg 2015;84(2):368–75.

19. Borschel GH, Kawamura DH, Kasukurthi R, et al. The motor nerve to the masseter muscle: an anatomic and histomorphometric study to facilitate its use in facial reanimation. J Plast Reconstr Aesthet Surg 2012;65(3):363–6.

20. Collar RM, Byrne PJ, Boahene KDO. The subzygomatic triangle: rapid, minimally invasive identification of the masseteric nerve for facial reanimation. Plast Reconstr Surg 2013;132(1):183–8.

21. Manktelow RT, Tomat LR, Zuker RM, et al. Smile reconstruction in adults with free muscle transfer innervated by the masseter motor nerve: effectiveness and cerebral adaptation. Plast Reconstr Surg 2006;118(4):885–99.
22. Terzis JK, Wang W, Zhao Y. Effect of axonal load on the functional and aesthetic outcomes of the cross-facial nerve graft procedure for facial reanimation. Plast Reconstr Surg 2009;124(5):1499–512.
23. Hembd A, Nagarkar PA, Saba S, et al. Facial nerve axonal analysis and anatomical localization in donor nerve: optimizing axonal load for cross-facial nerve grafting in facial reanimation. Plast Reconstr Surg 2017;139(1):177–83.
24. Strauch B, Goldberg N, Herman CK. Sural nerve harvest: anatomy and technique. J Reconstr Microsurg 2005;21(02):133–6.
25. Hadlock TA, Cheney ML. Single-incision endoscopic sural nerve harvest for cross face nerve grafting. J Reconstr Microsurg 2008;24(07):519–23.
26. Dorafshar AH, Borsuk DE, Bojovic B, et al. Surface anatomy of the middle division of the facial nerve: Zuker's point. Plast Reconstr Surg 2013;131(2):253–7.
27. Yamamoto Y, Sekido M, Furukawa H, et al. Surgical rehabilitation of reversible facial palsy: facial–hypoglossal network system based on neural signal augmentation/neural supercharge concept. J Plast Reconstr Aesthet Surg 2007;60(3):223–31.
28. Chen G, Wang W, Wang W, et al. Symmetry restoration at rest after masseter-to-facial nerve transfer: is it as efficient as smile reanimation? Plast Reconstr Surg 2017;140(4):793–801.
29. Owusu JA, Truong L, Kim JC. Facial nerve reconstruction with concurrent masseteric nerve transfer and cable grafting. JAMA Facial Plast Surg 2016;18(5):335.
30. Volk GF, Pantel M, Streppel M, et al. Reconstruction of complex peripheral facial nerve defects by a combined approach using facial nerve interpositional graft and hypoglossal-facial jump nerve suture. Laryngoscope 2011;121(11):2402–5.
31. Biglioli F, Colombo V, Tarabbia F, et al. Double innervation in free-flap surgery for long-standing facial paralysis. J Plast Reconstr Aesthet Surg 2012;65(10):1343–9.
32. Watanabe Y, Akizuki T, Ozawa T, et al. Dual innervation method using one-stage reconstruction with free latissimus dorsi muscle transfer for re-animation of established facial paralysis: simultaneous reinnervation of the ipsilateral masseter motor nerve and the contralateral facial nerve to improve the quality of smile and emotional facial expressions. J Plast Reconstr Aesthet Surg 2009;62(12):1589–97.

Management of Long-Standing Flaccid Facial Palsy: Periocular Considerations

Natalie Homer, MD[a,b], Aaron Fay, MD[b,*]

KEYWORDS

- Lagophthalmos • Exposure keratopathy • Dry eye • Eyelid retraction • Ectropion
- Epiphora • Synkinesis

KEY POINTS

- Patients with facial nerve palsy require acute and chronic examination and treatment.
- Facial nerve palsy can be associated with mild, moderate, or severe ocular injury.
- Systematic examination of 4 distinct periocular regions will contribute to a logical, multi-step treatment plan.
- Corneal exposure coupled with corneal hypoesthesia is associated with an ominous prognosis and should be treated aggressively.
- Rehabilitation includes an array of interventions ranging from intermittent lubrication to major surgical reconstruction and should be staged carefully to preserve all treatment options.

INTRODUCTION

The periocular manifestations of long-standing facial nerve palsy can lead to decreased vision or even loss of the eye. Thorough evaluation of the ocular surface and ocular adnexa can help to plan the interventions necessary to prevent such damage. Just as the face is approached in a systematic manner with independent analysis of the forehead, eyes, midface, and oral region, the "eye zone" can also be considered in 4 distinct regions: eyebrow, upper eyelid, ocular surface, and lower eyelid. Proper functioning in each of these anatomic regions is needed to preserve vision. Careful attention to rehabilitate each of these synergistic structures will help to ensure protection of the eye.

Disclosure Statement: The authors have no commercial or financial disclosures.
[a] Department of Ophthalmology, Harvard Medical School, 243 Charles Street, Boston, MA 02114, USA; [b] Massachusetts Eye and Ear Infirmary, 243 Charles Street, Boston, MA 02114, USA
* Corresponding author. 5 Joseph Comee Road, Lexington, MA 02420.
E-mail address: aaronfay@gmail.com

Otolaryngol Clin N Am 51 (2018) 1107–1118
https://doi.org/10.1016/j.otc.2018.07.007
0030-6665/18/© 2018 Elsevier Inc. All rights reserved.

oto.theclinics.com

PERIORBITAL AND OCULAR SURFACE ASSESSMENT

The focused ophthalmic examination begins with assessment of facial function. Particular attention, naturally, is paid to the forehead, eyelids, ocular surface, and mid-face. The 4 distinct periorbital regions should then be independently assessed.

Eyebrow

The frontalis-orbicularis oculi antagonistic muscle complex acts as a secondary elevator of the eyelid. In contrast, the orbital portion of the orbicularis oculi along with the corrugator and procerus forms the depressors of the eyebrow. As such, this group acts to close the eyelids. All these muscles are innervated via the temporal (frontal) branch of the facial nerve. The brow normally rests at the level of the superior orbital rim in men and is arched slightly above the superior orbital rim in women. The normal eyebrow contour forms an arc laterally, with the peak at the junction at the lateral third of the brow. Dysfunction of eyebrow elevator muscles in patients with facial nerve palsy produces brow ptosis (**Fig. 1**), often more prominently laterally where the frontalis muscle is sparse and the retroorbicularis oculi fat pad is robust, with corresponding superior and temporal visual field loss (**Fig. 2**).[1] Brow descent tends to accentuate the effects of dermatochalasis, especially when tone is lost in all regions of the orbicularis oculi. The redundant skin, no longer retracted effectively by the brow, can hang over the lid margin and rub directly on the ocular surface. Over-hanging eyebrows may shed dandruff-like material into to the eye and cause consider-able irritation (**Fig. 3**).

Upper Eyelid

The upper eyelid is more dynamic than the lower eyelid and is therefore primarily responsible for protecting, lubricating, and cleaning the ocular surface. Proper posi-tion relative to the cornea optimizes visual function and ocular surface protection. When the eyelid rests too low, it protects the surface but can obscure the visual

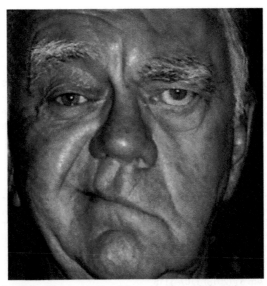

Fig. 1. Patient with left facial nerve palsy shows significant left eyebrow ptosis with attempt at biltaeral brow elevation.

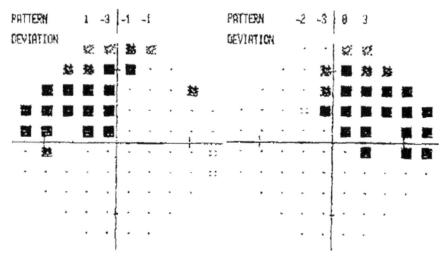

Fig. 2. Pattern deviation plot of both eyes shows bitemporal superior hemianopsia in a patient with bilateral eyebrow ptosis. (*From* Fay A, Lee LC, Pasquale LR. Dermatochalasis causing apparent bitemporal hemianopsia. Ophthalmic Plast Reconstr Surg 2003;19(2):153; with permission.)

axis; when it is too high (retracted), the visual field is expanded but the ocular surface is vulnerable. The primary retractors of the upper eyelid are the levator palpebrae superioris and Horner superior tarsal muscle. Importantly, these muscles are innervated by the oculomotor nerve and branches of the sympathetic nervous system, respectively, meaning that the eyelid retractors act unopposed in patients with facial paralysis, leaving the upper lid to rest in an abnormally elevated position. Eyelid closure, however, results from contraction of the orbicularis oculi muscle, which is directly supplied by the facial nerve. Patients with long-standing facial nerve palsy commonly have deficient eyelid closure with varying degrees of lagophthalmos, with diminished lid velocity and excursion in both reflexive blinking and voluntary eye closure (**Fig. 4**). Assessment of orbicularis strength, compared with that of the contralateral side,

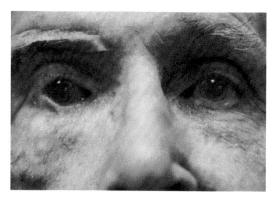

Fig. 3. Patient with right facial nerve palsy shows mild right eyebrow ptosis with overlying epidermal shedding.

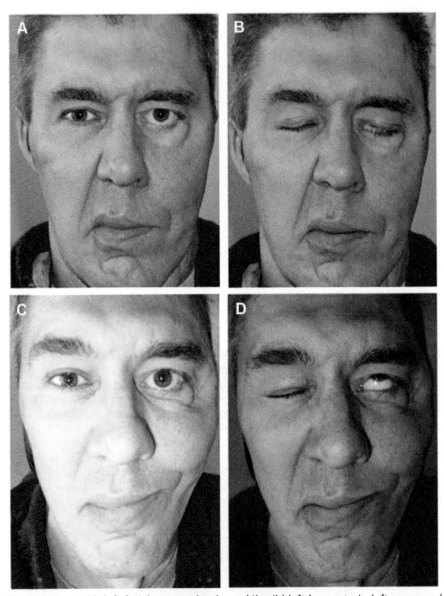

Fig. 4. Patient with left facial nerve palsy shows (*A*) mild left brow ptosis, left upper and lower eyelid retraction, and (*B*) left medial lagophthalmos with attempt at complete eyelid closure. (*C*) Patient in supine position shows exacerbation of left upper and lower eyelid retraction, and (*D*) lagophthalmos with attempts at complete eyelid closure.

should be assessed by instructing the patient to squeeze her/his eyelids closed and resist manual eyelid opening by the examiner. Unopposed retraction of the eyelid also contributes to lagophthalmos. This incomplete eyelid closure is further exacerbated when the patient is in the supine position, where the usual aid of gravity may be counterproductive (see **Fig. 4**). Thus, examiners should evaluate upper eyelid closure in both the upright and supine position in all patients with facial motor dysfunction. The degree of Bell phenomenon (reflexive upward rotation of the eyeball with eyelid closure) should also be considered.

In addition, abnormal eyelid closure impairs the lacrimal pump mechanism, driven by contraction of the sphincteric orbicularis oculi muscle. This dysfunction leads to an elevated but turbid tear lake, with poor tear distribution on the side of paralysis. The lacrimal system should be assessed by noting the tear lake height on the ocular surface, and observing for epiphora, or tear overflow, onto the cheek. Management for ocular dryness will be further discussed later within the "Ocular Surface" section of this article.

Ocular Surface

Periorbital compromise in facial nerve palsy renders the ocular surface vulnerable. Ocular surface damage may occur from upper and lower eyelid malposition, lagophthalmos, and incomplete blink reflex, with subsequent dehydration of the corneal surface. Resulting irritation of the corneal surface not only leads to blurred vision and discomfort but also increases susceptibility to corneal injury, such as abrasion, sterile or bacterial ulceration, perforation of the cornea, herniation of intraocular contents, endophthalmitis (intraocular abscess), and loss of eye. Patients with corneal hypesthesia are at particular risk of neurotrophic ulceration.

Presenting visual acuity should be documented and compared with prior measurements when possible. The ocular surface should be examined by an eye care provider and includes assessment for corneal and conjunctival dryness, aided by the use of fluorescein and lissamine green dyes. Careful assessment for signs of corneal thinning or infection should be performed.

Lower Eyelid

Although the lower lid is less mobile than the upper lid, it too helps to protect the ocular surface. The lower lid margin provides a platform against which the upper lid margin can seal during sleep and intentional closure. The lower lid retracts in downgaze to broaden the inferior visual field and rises in primary gaze to protect the inferior conjunctiva, sclera, and cornea. The lower lid margin also supports the resting tear lake and forms the inferior conjunctival fornix. Depression of the lower eyelid is controlled by the capsulopalpebral fascia and the inferior tarsus muscle, innervated by branches of the oculomotor nerve and sympathetic nerves, respectively. Superior movement of the lower eyelid to promote eyelid closure occurs from contraction of the orbicularis oculi muscle, innervated by branches of the facial nerve. In cases of facial nerve palsy, paralytic retraction from unopposed action of the lower eyelid retractors, as well as ectropion, or outward turning of the lower eyelid, may ensue (**Fig. 5**). Downward

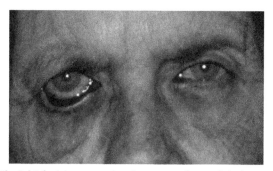

Fig. 5. Patient with right facial nerve palsy shows prominent right lower eyelid ectropion.

tension on the lower eyelid from gravitational forces on the atonic cheek also displaces the lower eyelid and causes paralytic ectropion.

Lower eyelid dysfunction causes epiphora by 2 mechanisms. Punctal ectropion, as the name implies, displaces the lower eyelid punctum from the globe surface when the eyelid margin rotates outward. The outflow tract for tears is effectively obstructed, leading to poor tear drainage and overflow onto the cheek. (This in turn can produce eczematous contraction of the skin, thereby worsening the ectropion in a positive feedback loop.) Loss of lower eyelid tone also disables the lacrimal pumping mechanism, further contributing to tear stasis and overflow.

Additional Considerations

Synkinetic eyelid movement can result from aberrant nerve regeneration in long-term facial nerve paralysis, often occurring 24 to 39 weeks after initial symptoms.[2] Abnormal eyelid movements may include the "jaw-wink" phenomenon of transient upper eyelid ptosis following oral movements. Management may be undertaken with botulinum toxin injections applied to the involved orbicularis oculi muscle.

Regenerating fibers of the chorda tympani may also aberrantly innervate the postganglionic parasympathetic secretomotor fibers of the lacrimal system, inducing the phenomenon of tearing reflexive to chewing, known as gustatory lacrimation or "crocodile tears." Management of this disorder may also be pursued with botulinum toxin injections into the palpebral lobe of the lacrimal gland.[3]

PERIORBITAL AND OCULAR SURFACE MANAGEMENT
Eyebrow

Treatment of symptomatic eyebrow ptosis involves surgical elevation of the eyebrow. A direct brow lift may be performed by removal of an ellipse of skin and muscle tissue directly superior to the brow. The brow may be surgically elevated along the entire length of the brow, or limited to the lateral half only in cases of disproportionate lateral brow ptosis. Alternatively, an internal browpexy may be performed through an upper eyelid crease incision, with securing of the subcutaneous brow tissue to the periosteum of the superior orbital rim. More extensive forehead lifts via an endoscopic, pretrichial, or coronal approach can aid in lifting the eyebrows in patients with widespread frontalis muscle weakness. Careful measures should be taken to avoid overcorrection of eyebrow ptosis, which could exacerbate upper eyelid lagophthalmos and ocular surface exposure.

Upper Eyelid

Eyelid taping
For lagophthalmos present only in the supine position, bedtime eyelid taping can be performed by manually closing the upper eyelid and placing a small piece of tape vertically across upper eyelid to maintain full eyelid closure. Careful measures to avoid inward rotation of eyelashes during taping, which could induce corneal abrasion, should be taken. This method can be limited by development of periorbital tape sensitivity, with paper tape typically best tolerated.

Botulinum toxin
In cases of mild eyelid retraction in anticipated short-term facial nerve palsy, botulinum toxin can be injected transcutaneously or subconjunctivally along the superior tarsus border to produce temporary ptosis.[2] This method may mechanically impair ocular function by limiting eyelid excursion. Repeated treatments may be required to obtain the desired amount of eyelid ptosis.

Partial tarsorrhaphy

A partial tarsorrhaphy, or surgical apposition of the upper to the lower eyelid, can be performed to shorten the vertical interpalpebral fissure height. In patients with acute facial nerve palsy with anticipated improvement, a temporary tarsorrhaphy can be performed using nonabsorbable sutures in a mattress fashion. The suture should enter partial thickness (skin and orbicularis) through the upper eyelid and exit through the eyelid margin at the gray line (distal edge of orbicularis oculi muscle), followed by a margin-to-mid lid suture pass through the lower eyelid, to appose the 2. Suture ends can be tied over bolsters made of rubber tubing or foam.

Long-standing facial nerve palsy may instead call for a permanent limited tarsorrhaphy. The tarsorrhaphy is typically performed on the lateral aspect of the eyelid, to allow for preservation of some visual function and so to not disturb the lacrimal drainage puncta in the medial eyelid. The length of tarsorrhaphy can range from the lateral one-third to one-half of the eyelid, adjusted to ensure full voluntary eyelid closure, with a 5-mm lateral tarsorrhaphy generally reducing lagophthalmos by 70% to 80%.[4] The procedure is performed under local anesthesia and requires deepithelialization of the upper and lower eyelid margins, followed by apposition of the margin edges with a mattress suture. Although designated as "permanent," delayed separation of the eyelid margins can be performed if facial function returns. Drawbacks to the tarsorrhaphy include the static nature of eyelid closure and suboptimal cosmetic result.

Upper eyelid loading

Gravity-dependent closure of the upper eyelid can be aided by upper eyelid loading with implanted weights. Historically, materials including gold, platinum, and titanium mesh have been implanted into the upper eyelid to provide this effect. Gold weights are most commonly used due to their malleable and inert qualities. Weight placement can be performed under local anesthesia and is fully reversible. The procedure is typically initiated through an external upper eyelid crease incision, and a gold implant of desired weight (typically 0.8–1.4 g) is secured over the tarsal plate of the upper eyelid (**Fig. 6**). Implants are positioned posterior to the orbicularis muscle to minimize a visible lump. Blepharoptosis of the affected eyelid is an expected outcome, with improvement of lagophthalmos. The weight is less effective in correcting

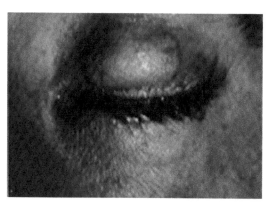

Fig. 6. Patient after surgical gold weight placement into the left upper eyelid for correction of lagophthalmos.

lagophthalmos when the patient assumes a supine position. Corneal topography studies have shown induction of refractive astigmatism in the vertical axis following weight placement, correctable with eyeglasses, and reversible following weight removal.[5] Risks of this procedure include implant extrusion and migration, suboptimal cosmetic result, and infection.

Cerclage

The eyelid cerclage procedure was first described by English and Apel[6] in 1973 for restoration of dynamic eyelid closure. This method is preferred when both the upper and lower eyelid functions are affected. This procedure is initiated through a medial canthal incision to expose the medial canthal tendon, and an additional lateral canthal incision to expose the lateral orbital rim. A small hole is drilled into the lateral orbital rim, and a silicone strap is threaded through the bony opening, across the length along the upper eyelid margin within the pretarsal plane, and anchored to the medial canthal tendon. The procedure is then repeated along the lower eyelid, thus producing a "purse-string" effect to shorten the vertical interpalpebral fissure height. Tension may be adjusted to accommodate the patient's dynamic eyelid function. Postoperative blepharoptosis with improvement of lagophthalmos is expected (**Fig. 7**). Potential complications include silicone rod extrusion, granuloma formation, infection, and lower eyelid ectropion.

Palpebral spring

Reanimation of the upper eyelid has been further optimized using the palpebral spring procedure.[4] This procedure is an excellent choice to optimize the blinking mechanism in patients unlikely to experience recovery of facial nerve. This complex procedure uses a prebent "V"-shaped orthodontic stainless-steel wire with a small apical loop, which serves as the fulcrum. The spring is surgically implanted with the superior arm fixed along the inferior concavity of the superior orbital border, and the mobile inferior arm spanning the length of the inferior eyelid margin within the tarsal plane. The apical loop fulcrum is fixated to the lateral orbital rim periosteum.[7] This procedure has been augmented back-looping of the terminal wire ends, enveloping the palpebral wire arm in Dacron mesh, and anchoring this arm to the tarsal plate to limit implant extrusion.[8,9] Nickel-based implants can be preferentially used in patients with need for MRI surveillance (eg, those with facial palsy secondary to vestibular schwannoma extirpation) to allow for this imaging modality.[9] Disadvantages of this technique include its technical complexity, difficulty in obtaining the proper spring tension, induction of blepharoptosis of the upper eyelid, and postoperative risk of extrusion and infection.

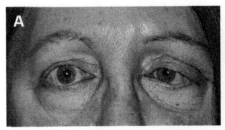 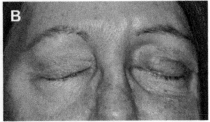

Fig. 7. Patient with left facial nerve palsy after left upper and lower eyelid cerclage procedure shows postoperative (A) improved left upper eyelid retraction with mild left upper eyelid ptosis and (B) complete resolution of left lagophthalmos.

Tendon transfer and facial reanimation

A temporalis tendon transfer or facial nerve reinnervation procedure, including facial nerve grafting or hypoglossal-facial nerve anastomosis, can improve upper eyelid closure as part of the overall restoration of hemifacial movement (**Table 1**).

Table 1 Lagophthalmos management			
	Indication	**Pros**	**Cons**
Eyelid taping	Primarily night-time lagophthalmos in facial nerve palsy expected to improve	• Noninvasive • Reversible	• Temporary • No daytime globe protection • Risk of accidental corneal injury
Botulinum toxin	Constant corneal exposure from mild eyelid retraction and lagophthalmos	• Minimally invasive • Temporary	• Induces noncosmetically pleasing ptosis • Nondynamic
Partial tarsorrhaphy	Constant lagophthalmos in facial nerve palsy	• Minimally invasive • Simple procedure • Reversible or permanent	• Suboptimal aesthetic outcome • Decreased visual field • Nondynamic
Gold weight eyelid loading	Constant lagophthalmos in long-term facial nerve palsy	• Technically simple • Able to remove if facial movement improves	• Suboptimal aesthetic outcome • Risk of infection, allergy, implant extrusion • Risk of induction of refractive astigmatism
Cerclage	Constant lagophthalmos in long-term facial nerve palsy	• Shortens interpalpebral height from upper and lower eyelid • Tailorable to specific patient needs • Adjustable	• Specialized procedure • Risk of silicone rod extrusion, granuloma formation, infection • May induce lower eyelid ectropion • Nondynamic
Palpebral spring	Constant lagophthalmos and impaired blink in long-term facial nerve palsy	• Improved lagophthalmos and dynamic blink • Tailorable to specific patient needs	• Complex procedure • Risk of spring extrusion, infection • Induction of blepharoptosis of the upper eyelid
Temporalis tendon transfer	Significant facial movement asymmetry	• Improvement of facial symmetry and function, including dynamic eyelid movement	• Invasive procedure with associated postoperative risks
Facial nerve reinnervation (facial nerve grafting or hypoglossal-facial nerve anastomosis)	Significant facial movement asymmetry	• Improvement of facial symmetry and function, including dynamic eyelid movement	• Invasive procedure with associated postoperative risks

---

Box 1
Ocular lubrication strategies

- Artificial tears (preservative-free)
- Artificial tear ointment (at bedtime)
- Nighttime eyelid taping
- Nighttime moisture chamber
- Lacrimal punctal plugs
- Lacrimal punctal cauterization
- Soft contact lens

Ocular Surface

Various strategies to lubricate and protect the ocular surface are advocated when facial nerve palsy prevents complete eyelid closure (**Box 1**). Tear substitutes without preservatives should be administered frequently to replace the compromised tear film. Petroleum-based ointments may also be used at bedtime to prevent corneal dehydration during sleep.[4] Ophthalmic ointment may additionally be used during the daytime in severe cases. Notable supine lagophthalmos may require taping eyelids at bedtime, by manually closing the eyelid and placing a small piece of tape vertically to appose the upper and lower eyelid margins. A "moisture chamber" may alternatively be used in severe lagophthalmos, in which copious ophthalmic ointment is applied to the ocular surface, and the entire periorbital area is covered in Tegaderm or alternative nonabrasive dressing. Careful measures should be taken to avoid accidental corneal injury from improper bedtime eyelid taping or covering techniques.

Silicone or collagen plugs can be inserted into the upper and lower eyelid punctas to obstruct nasolacrimal drainage and maintain an elevated tear lake over the globe surface. More definitive punctal closure can be accomplished with electrocauterization. In severely symptomatic corneal irritation not relieved by topical lubricants, a soft "bandage" contact lens can be worn on the eye under careful surveillance by an eye care provider, because risk for lens-related infection is high (see **Box 1**).

Lower Eyelid

Lower eyelid malposition and ectropion can be surgically managed with lower eyelid horizontal tightening procedures (**Table 2**). A lateral tarsal strip operation can elevate and anchor the lower eyelid into the desired position by inducing lateral lid traction. This procedure is initiated with a lateral canthotomy and lysis of the inferior lateral canthal tendon, followed by isolation, deepithelialization and truncation of the lateral

---

Table 2
Lower eyelid malposition management

Problem	Recommended Procedure
Lateral lower eyelid malposition	Lateral tarsal strip procedure
Medial lower eyelid malposition	Medial spindle procedure
Paralytic lower eyelid retraction	Anterior lamellar graft with or without midface resuspension

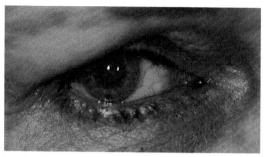

Fig. 8. Right eye after Jones tube implantation within the medial canthus for symptomatic right epiphora.

portion of the lower eyelid tarsus, and reattachment of the tarsus to the lateral orbital rim. This procedure can be further augmented by placement of a middle lamellar spacer between the lower tarsal border and the lower lid retractors using autologous cartilage or acellular porcine dermis.[10]

Medial lower lid malposition is more challenging to treat. A medial spindle procedure can be performed to promote posterior rotation of the medial eyelid by removal of a small "diamond" of conjunctiva on the internal surface of the lower eyelid, followed by suturing of the inferior tarsus to the superior lower eyelid retractors in a spiraling fashion, and externalization of the sutures to rotate the eyelid posteriorly. This inward rotation can reappose the lower lid lacrimal puncta to the ocular surface and improve tear drainage into the nasolacrimal duct.

In the case of paralytic cicatricial ectropion of the lower eyelid, lengthening of the anterior lamella (skin and orbicularis) may need to be facilitated with a full-thickness skin graft. Potential donor sites include the contralateral upper eyelid (as skin removal from the ipsilateral upper eyelid may worsen upper eyelid retraction), postauricular, supraclavicular, and inner brachial areas. The paralytic ectropion repair is initiated through a subciliary lower eyelid incision, followed by measuring of desired graft size, graft harvesting, and suturing of the graft into position. Pressure should be applied over the graft site for a minimum of 5 days following surgery.

A midface resuspension procedure to elevate the cheek can also restore lower eyelid height.

Following full correction of eyelid malposition, a small proportion of patients continues to experience symptomatic epiphora, likely due to the compromised orbicularis oculi–driven lacrimal pumping system. Tear outflow can be further facilitated in these patients by nasolacrimal bypass procedures, including dacryocystorhinostomy or a conjunctivorhinostomy with Jones tube placement (**Fig. 8**).[10,11]

SUMMARY

Significant ocular compromise can result from facial nerve paralysis. Thorough periorbital examination with rehabilitation to the 4 interrelated anatomic areas (eyebrow, upper eyelid, ocular surface, and lower eyelid) can help to ensure comprehensive ocular protection.

REFERENCES

1. Fay A, Lee LC, Pasquale LR. Dermatochalasis causing apparent bitemporal hemianopsia. Ophthalmic Plast Reconstr Surg 2003;19(2):151–3.

2. Rahman I, Sadiq SA. Ophthalmic management of facial nerve palsy: a review. Surv Ophthalmol 2007;52:121–44.

3. Alsuhaibani AH. Facial nerve palsy: providing eye comfort and cosmesis. Middle East Afr J Ophthalmol 2010;17(2):142–7.

4. Kumar K. Management of facial nerve paralysis. Kerala J Ophthalmol 2011;23(4): 332–6.

5. Mavrikakis I, Beckinsale P, Lee E, et al. Changes in corneal topography with upper eyelid gold weight implants. Ophthalmic Plast Reconstr Surg 2006;22(5): 331–4.

6. English FP, Apel JVT. Cerclage technique for dynamic eyelid closure in facial paralysis. Br J Ophthalmol 1973;57:750–2.

7. Morel-Fatio D, Lalardrie JP. Palliative surgical treatment of facial paralysis: the palpebral spring. Plast Reconstr Surg 1964;33:446–56.

8. Demerci H, Frueh BR. Palpebral spring in the management of lagophthalmos and exposure keratopathy secondary to facial nerve palsy. Ophthalmic Plast Reconstr Surg 2009;25(4):270–5.

9. Levine RE, Fay A. Re: "Palpebral spring in the management of lagophthalmos and exposure keratopathy secondary to facial nerve palsy". Ophthalmic Plast Reconstr Surg 2010;26(6):499–500.

10. Sohrab M, Abugo U, Grant M, et al. Management of the eye in facial paralysis. Facial Plast Surg 2015;31:140–4.

11. Madge SN, Malhotra R, Desousa J, et al. The lacrimal bypass tube for lacrimal pump failure attributable to facial palsy. Am J Ophthalmol 2010;149(1):155–9.

Management of Long-Standing Flaccid Facial Palsy: Midface/Smile

Locoregional Muscle Transfer

James A. Owusu, MD[a],*, Kofi Derek Boahene, MD[b]

KEYWORDS

- Masseter muscle transfer • Temporalis tendon transfer • Facial paralysis

KEY POINTS

- Locoregional muscle transfer is an effective means of improving facial symmetry and smile in flaccid paralysis.
- Muscle transfer has the advantage of being a single-stage procedure with quick recovery of function.
- The procedure should be guided by the principles and biomechanics of muscle transfer in order to optimize outcome.

INTRODUCTION

Facial expression plays a crucial role in communication and social interactions. It provides a nonverbal means of expressing emotions and reflects overall well-being. These complex facial movements are orchestrated by the facial muscles directed by the facial nucleus through a network of the facial nerve and its branches. Injury to any of these components of facial animation can result in partial or complete paralysis of the face with devastating implications. Loss of facial muscle function over time results in laxity and drooping of the affected side of the face creating a deformed appearance. In addition to physical appearance, difficulties with speech, eye closure, and eating can arise as a result of the loss of function of the eye and oral sphincters. Many patients with facial paralysis suffer psychological effects in addition to the physical and functional deficits. Impaired facial expression and facial deformity often lead to social isolation

Financial Disclosure: None.

Conflicts of Interest: None.

[a] Department of Head and Neck Surgery, Mid-Atlanatic Permanente Medical Group, 8008 Westpark Drive, McLean, VA 22102, USA; [b] Department of Otorhinolaryngology, The Johns Hopkins Hospital, 601 North Caroline Street, Baltimore, MD 48109, USA

* Corresponding author.

E-mail address: james.a.owusu@kp.org

and depression. Patients afflicted with facial paralysis are often erroneously judged by observers as unattractive or expressing negative emotions even when smiling. This psychosocial impact can result in an overall decrease in quality of life.[1]

The aim of facial paralysis rehabilitation is to restore facial symmetry at rest as well as spontaneous and coordinated function of the facial muscles. When the facial muscles are viable, the best results can be achieved using reinnervation techniques to restore facial muscle function. Reinnervation techniques include nerve repair, nerve grafting, and nerve transfer. In long-term facial paralysis, the facial muscles are irreversibly paralyzed. The prolonged period of denervation results in fibrosis and atrophy of the facial musculature and degeneration of the motor endplates, which precludes reinnervation. Restoring facial animation in long-term paralysis requires recruitment of functional muscle to replace the function of the paralyzed facial muscles. Functional muscle can be recruited through free micro-neurovascular muscle transfer (FMMT) or locoregional muscle transposition. FMMT is considered by many to be the gold standard for facial reanimation in long-term facial paralysis. However, this is typically an extensive procedure and may require multiple stages and a prolonged recovery period. Patients with long-standing facial paralysis who are not candidates for FMMT due to personal preference or comorbidities may benefit from locoregional muscle transfer for reanimation. Locoregional muscle transfer can improve facial symmetry and provide dynamic reanimation by repurposing a muscle tendon unit (MTU) to replace or augment the function of a paralyzed facial muscle. Both masseter and temporalis muscles have been described for smile reanimation in long-term facial paralysis. The temporalis is the more popular choice because it provides a better vector of excursion. The masseter muscle creates a more horizontal smile vector that is suboptimal. Compared with FMMT, MTU transfer is a less complicated procedure with faster recovery and minimal donor site morbidity making it the ideal option in select cases. Recent advances in techniques of locoregional muscle transfer are discussed in this article.

BIOMECHANICS OF MUSCLE TRANSFER

Muscle contraction is required to restore dynamic support of the paralyzed facial tissue in MTU transfer. To achieve dynamic results, the transferred MTU needs to maintain a normal and unrestricted ability to contract. Myofibrils, the contractile elements of skeletal muscles, are composed mainly of actin, myosin proteins. The interaction between actin and myosin generates the mechanical force to create muscle contraction. This highly coordinated actin-myosin interaction is impacted by the tension placed on the muscle fibers. To maintain normal contraction ability and achieve maximum excursion, the transferred MTU needs to be set close to its pretransfer resting tension. Overstretching the transferred MTU distorts actin-myosin interaction and reduces contraction force resulting in reduced excursion.[2]

PRINCIPLES OF MUSCLE TENDON UNIT TRANSFER

Many factors can affect the outcome of MTU transfer, including patient comorbidities and prior treatment. However, there are key principles to be taken into consideration when planning MTU transfer for facial paralysis rehabilitation. These principles have been discussed in detail by Boahene[3] in 2016 and are summarized in later discussion.

MUSCLE TENDON UNIT SELECTION

The selected MTU should be dispensable. Loss of function of the selected MTU should be associated with minimal donor morbidity. The temporalis and masseter muscles are the primary MTU's used in midface rehabilitation. Both of these muscles can be transposed with minimal donor site morbidity. The function of the temporalis muscle is to elevate and retrude the mandible. The masseter muscle elevates and protrudes the mandible. The pterygoid muscle duplicates the actions of these muscles, and as a result, there is minimal donor site morbidity from loss of function of either one or both temporalis and masseter muscles.

The selected muscle for MTU transfer should also be functional and have adequate contraction to achieve the desired excursion. No single muscle can substitute the function of the upper lip elevators that normally produces a multivector smile. However, the selected muscle should have enough strength to suspend and elevate the paralyzed oral commissure. It is particularly important to preoperatively test the function of the muscle in patients with prior history of trauma, prior radiation therapy, or surgical resection.

SUITABLE SOFT TISSUE BED

Normal muscles glide smoothly in a plane created by the surrounding muscle fascia, myomesium, and paratenon. It is crucial to maintain a gliding plane for the transferred muscle. The buccal fat pad can be used to decrease scarring and provide a soft tissue-gliding plane for the transferred MTU. Scarring between the transposed MTU and the surrounding tissue will reduce translation of the muscle contraction to commissure excursion.

FLEXIBILITY OF THE ORAL COMMISSURE

To achieve dynamic excursion of the oral commissure in MTU transfer, the paralyzed lip musculature and surrounding soft tissue need to be supple. MTU transfer will be less effective if the lip and surrounding soft tissue are fibrosed and stiff. In cases where the lip tissue is stiff, such as postradiation and extensive scarring, measures should be taken to improve the flexibility before the MTU transfer.

A firm fixation of the transferred MTU at the modiolus is crucial for effective oral commissure excursion. The oral musculature becomes atrophic after a period of paralysis and may not support the tension generated by the transferred resulting in the dehiscence of the transferred tendon at the insertion point. A fascia graft can be placed to strengthen the fixation point during the MTU transfer or several weeks before the procedure to create a firm and stable fixation point.

PATIENT EVALUATION

Evaluation of a patient with facial paralysis begins with a comprehensive history and physical examination to determine the cause, extent, duration, and prognosis for recovery. Reanimation options are ultimately determined by the status of the facial muscles that are the functional end organ for facial expression. The transposed muscles in MTU transposition are innervated by cranial nerves other than the facial nerve. A thorough cranial nerve examination is essential to determine the status of the muscle to be transposed. The action of the temporalis and masseter muscle can be palpated during clenching of the jaw. The type of smile should be noted during the preoperative evaluation (**Fig. 1**). The insertion point of the transferred MTU is chosen based on the type of smile to closely match the normal side.[4,5]

TEMPORALIS TENDON TRANSFER

The temporalis muscle has been used in rehabilitation of facial paralysis for almost a decade. Gillies[6] initially described use of the temporalis muscle for smile rehabilitation

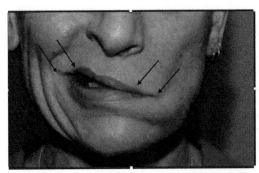

Fig. 1. Marking the site of tendon insertion along the lip margin based on the vector of the dominant smile on the function contralateral side. Arrows indicate smile vector on the normal side and the ideal vector on the paralyzed.

in 1934. In the classic description, the entire temporalis muscle belly or a portion of the muscle belly is transposed over the zygomatic arch to suspend the paralyzed lip using a fascia lata extension. This approach creates an obvious bulge over the zygomatic arch and a hollowing defect at the temple donor site. Several modifications of temporalis transfer have subsequently been described to minimize donor site morbidity and improve smile excursion. In 1949, McLaughlin[7] described the use of the temporalis muscle in an orthodromic fashion for smile rehabilitation. In McLaughlin's description, a coronoidectomy is performed to release the temporalis MTU that is transposed to support the paralyzed lip using fascia lata extension. McLaughlin's approach improves on the classic description by avoiding the temporal hallowing deformity. Labbè and colleagues[5,8] described the lengthening temporalis myoplasty that eliminates the need for a fascia graft. In lengthening myoplasty, the muscle belly is released from the temporal fossa, a coronoidectomy is performed, and the muscle tendon is released and transposed to the paralyzed lip. Technique modifications have also been described to minimize access incisions using the minimally invasive approaches to MTU transfer.[9]

ANATOMY

The temporalis is a fan-shaped muscle that originates from the temporal fossa and inserts onto the coronoid process of the mandible. The broad muscle belly fills the entire temporal fossa. The temporalis muscle elevates and retracts the mandible. The muscle is composed of 3 parts: superficial, zygomatic, and deep. The zygomatic part originates from the zygomatic arch to insert into the superficial part as it inserts onto the lateral surface of the coronoid process. The deep part contains muscle fibers that originate from the temporal fossa and inserts onto the medial aspect of the coronoid process and retromolar triangle down to the buccinators line.[10] The temporalis muscle is innervated by the deep temporal branch of the mandibular division of the trigeminal nerve. The blood supply of the temporalis muscle arises from the deep temporal branch of the internal maxillary artery.

SURGICAL TECHNIQUE

Preoperatively, the desired smile vector is determined and marked. In unilateral cases, the chosen smile vector should match that of the normal side for symmetry. The procedure is performed under general anesthesia with the patient in the supine position. Oral intubation with the tube secured to the teeth or nasotracheal intubation is used to prevent distortion of the lip and allow assessment of lip symmetry during the procedure. Long-acting neuromuscular blockade should be avoided to allow for muscle stimulation during the procedure. The entire face and temporal scalp should be included in the surgical preparation.

The coronoid process may be approached through an intraoral or external incision. In patients with deep melolabial folds, external melolabial incision may be used with the advantage of avoiding oral contamination. In younger patients and those with less defined melolabial creases, an intraoral incision placed under the lip provides wide exposure of the orbicularis muscle for tendon insertion and direct access to the buccal space and coronoid process. Intraoral incisions avoid facial scars but expose the surgical bed to oral contaminants, increasing the risk for infection. Placing a passive drain for a few days may be helpful.

Dissection through the buccal space is mostly blunt and is facilitated by the use of malleable retractors. The parotid duct should be protected. Buccal fat should be preserved as a cushion against tendon scarring. As the malleable retractors are advanced deep, the anterior edge of the mandibular ramus and the coronoid process is exposed.

To protect the temporalis tendon from shredding, subperiosteal elevation of the fascia-periosteum tendon complex is performed on the medial aspect of the coronoid beginning from the retromolar area and extending superiorly to the level of the sigmoid notch. A Kocher is then placed on the coronoid, and a right-angled hemostat is passed between the coronoid bone and the elevated tendon into the sigmoid notch. The right angle hemostat acts as a retractor and guide for coronoidectomy. It is important to keep a Kocher firmly secured on the coronoid before detaching the tendon to avoid retraction into the infratemporal fossa. A small reciprocating saw is used to osteotomize the coronoid. The tendon on the medial aspect of the coronoid is separated from any attachments to the medial pterygoid muscle and the lateral aspect from masseter muscle attachments. The tendon is then carefully freed laterally from the masseter muscle and medially from the medial pterygoid muscle. At this point, the tendon is divided as low as possible for length and transposed through the buccal space toward the modiolus. If necessary, additional mobilization for length may be achieved by freeing the attachment of the temporalis muscle from the undersurface of the zygomatic arch. This is done carefully, staying close to the undersurface of the zygomatic bone to preserve a fat layer between the arch and the muscle thereby preserving a fatty glide plane.

After transposing the temporalis tendon through the buccal space toward the modiolus, the temporalis muscle is electrically stimulated with transcutaneous or needle electrodes placed into the temporalis muscles. With traction of the Kocher, the tension on the released tendon is manually varied while electrically stimulating the muscle. At the point of maximum force contraction, a marker is placed on the Kocher clamp to represent the ideal traction tension and muscle length for maximal excursion. The marked Kocher is used to guide the degree of traction needed to ideally position the temporalis tendon for insertion. The tendon is then inserted at the determined optimal length (tension) based on the intraoperative excursion measurements.

GAINING TENDON LENGTH

Fundamental to the temporalis MTU procedure is mobilization of the temporalis tendon from the mandible for reinsertion into the orbicularis oris muscle around the oral commissure. To gain tendon reach, Labbé and Huault[8] described the temporalis tendon lengthening myoplasty procedure. In their original description, the temporalis muscle is exposed through a scalp incision and the posterior third of the muscle is released and elevated from its periosteal attachment. The zygomatic arch is osteotomized to gain access to the coronoid process for tendon release. By sliding the released muscle inferiorly, the muscle fibers are redistributed and fixated inferiorly, thereby allowing the released coronoid with the attached temporalis tendon to reach the lip. When releasing the temporalis muscle, care is taken to avoid injury to the neurovascular supply deep to the muscle. In addition, the released muscle should be refixated at the appropriate tension. Recent modifications by Labbé avoid osteotomy of the zygomatic arch and approach the coronoid through the buccal space similar to the minimally invasive temporalis tendon transfer procedure.[5,9] The extent of incisions, dissection, and temporalis MTU mobilization described in the classic lengthening procedure disrupts the multiple glide planes at the level of the muscle belly and transition under the zygomatic arch, introduces external scars, but yields 4 cm or more of tendon transposition.

Tendon length may also be gained by extension with fascia or donor tendon without mobilization of the muscle belly. Tendon extenders introduce a noncontractile element into the MTU transfer and can reduce the effectiveness of the contraction. The longer tendon extenders have a more negative impact on the effectiveness of the contraction.[11]

Given the options available to gain tendon reach, it may be confusing when to select one method over another. First, the temporalis MTU should always be inserted close to its optimal passive length at which point there is maximal contraction. For optimal contraction, overstretching should be avoided. Second, the temporalis MTU should be disturbed as little as possible to avoid scarring and disruptions of glide planes. Based on these principles, it is recommended to use intraoperative electrical stimulation and tension variation to help determine optimal length and tension at which to insert the mobilized tendon and the need for tendon lengthening. When the ideal tension is determined, if the tendon reaches the orbicularis oris muscle, it is secured without extension. If the tendon at the optimal tension is within 1 to 2 cm of the orbicularis oris muscle, it is extended with fascia. When the tendon is more than 2 cm from the orbicularis oris muscle, the entire temporalis MTU should be released and advanced under the zygomatic arch toward the lip for insertion (**Fig. 2**).

INSERTION SITE

The upper lip elevators include the zygomaticus major insert and interdigitate with fibers of the orbicularis oris around the modiolus. The transposed temporalis tendon should be inserted as close to the lip margin as possible to mimic the insertion of the zygomaticus muscles. In this position, a natural melolabial fold develops, and contraction of the temporalis muscle translates to movement of the mobile lip, dental show, and smile restoration. Insertion of the tendon in the melolabial fold results in a deep fold and muscle contractions that do not translate well into lip excursion.

MASSETER MUSCLE TRANSFER

The use of masseter muscle for smile rehabilitation was described before that of the temporalis muscle. However, the temporalis muscle is a more popular choice given its superior results. Lexer and Eden[12] described masseter muscle transfer for facial paralysis rehabilitation at the turn of the century. When transposed to the lip, the masseter muscle creates a horizontal suboptimal smile vector. As a result, it has remained second choice to the temporalis as an option for regional muscle transfer for smile rehabilitation. In the classic description, the masseter

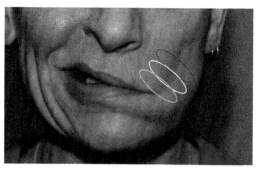

Fig. 2. Guide to the use of fascia extension versus lengthening myoplasty in temporalis MTU procedure. Tendon in the red zone requires lengthening myoplasty (>2 cm) from the target insertion point, in the yellow zone requires fascia extension, and in the green zone can be directly inserted.

muscle or a portion of it is released from its insertion at the mandibular angle and transposed to oral commissure. Compared with the temporalis muscle, the masseter muscle produces limited excursion of the commissure and also leaves a hallowing deformity over the mandible when transposed. Several modifications of masseter muscle transfer have been described to improve smile vector and donor site morbidity. Technique modifications described to improve the smile vector and reduce donor site morbidity include pedicled masseter muscle transfer (PMMT) described by Matic and Yoo.[13] In PMMT, the masseter muscle is released from its origin and insertion leaving the muscle pedicled on its neurovascular bundle. The pedicled muscle is transposed in an orientation parallel to the zygomaticus major muscle resulting in a more natural smile vector (**Fig. 3**). Shinohara and

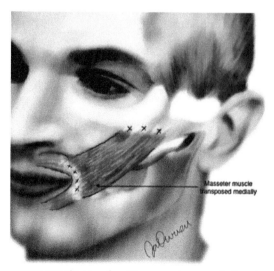

Fig. 3. Pedicled masseter muscle transfer. The masseter muscle is released from both its insertion and origin and left pedicled on its neurovascular bundle. The entire muscle is transposed medially and refixated in an orientation parallel to the zygomaticus major. (*Courtesy of* James A. Owusu, MD, McLean, VA.)

colleagues[14] described combining masseter muscle with a strip fascia lata using the zygomatic arch as a pulley to create a dynamic sling. In this technique, a segment of the masseter muscle is released from its origin at the anterior portion of the zygomatic arch. A fascia lata sling is sutured to the released tendinous insertion of the muscle. The fascia sling is passed under and over the zygomatic arch and sutured to the oral commissure to create a dynamic sling (**Fig. 4**). MTU transfer typically generates a single smile vector; combining both temporalis MTU and masseter muscle transfer provides as opportunity to create a multivector smile with locoregional flaps.

Despite recent technique refinement for masseter muscle transfer, it remains an unpopular choice for smile reanimation. Literature on the use of masseter muscle for smile reanimation is sparse with most papers reporting on a few case series. Further research is needed to fully realize the potential of the masseter muscle for smile reanimation.

ANATOMY

The masseter is a rectangular-shaped muscle that overlies the mandibular ramus and angle. Similar to the temporalis muscle, the masseter consists of 3 parts: superficial, middle, and deep. The larger superficial portion originates from the anterior-inferior aspect zygomatic arch and the zygomatic process of the maxilla. The fibers of the superficial part travel in a posterior-oblique orientation to insert into the lower aspect of the mandibular ramus and angle. The middle part originates from the deep surface of the anterior zygomatic arch and the lower border of the posterior zygomatic arch and inserts along the middle third of the ramus. The deep part of the muscle arises from the inferior aspect of the posterior third of the zygomatic arch. The fibers of the deep portion have an anterior oblique orientation and insert on the superior aspect of the ramus and the lateral surface of the coronoid process. The primary action of the masseter muscle is to elevate and protrude the mandible. The masseter muscle is innervated by the masseteric branch of

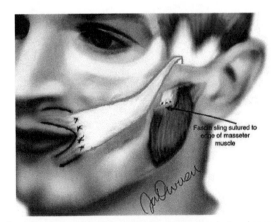

Fig. 4. Masseter dynamic sling. The anterior half of the muscle is released from its origin at the zygomatic arch. A fascia graft is sutured to the released margin of the muscle and passed around the zygomatic arch to suspend the lip. The arch acts as a pulley. (*Courtesy of* James A. Owusu, MD, McLean, VA.)

the mandibular division of the trigeminal nerve. The masseteric nerve passes through the posterior aspect of the sigmoid notch accompanied by the masseteric artery posterior to the insertion of the temporalis muscle on the coronoid process.[15] The masseteric neurovascular bundle enters the deep surface of the masseter muscle and arborizes in an anteroinferior trajectory to innervate the muscle. The location of the masseteric neurovascular bundle should be considered during dissection of the muscle to avoid injury.

SURGICAL TECHNIQUE

Masseter muscle transposition can be performed using an intraoral incision along the ascending ramus or externally using a parotidectomy type incision. The external approach is preferred due to the superior exposure it provides. Patient preparation is similar to that described for temporalis tendon transfer. If the parotid gland is in place, it will need to be mobilized to expose the masseter muscle. Once the masseter muscle is exposed, it is elevated off the mandibular ramus. Preserving a deep fascia layer provides a secure tissue for anchoring sutures. The anterior half of the muscle is released from its insertion at inferior aspect of the mandible. The posterior portion of the muscle is preserved to prevent the depression at the angle of the mandible that is typically created when the entire muscle is transposed. The released muscle segment is mobilized off the mandible with care to avoid injury to the neurovascular bundle on the deep aspect of the muscle. A glide plane tunnel is dissected through the buccal fat pad to nasolabial fold. An incision is made in the nasolabial fold to connect the glide plane tunnel. Dissection is continued medial around the commissure and the upper and lower lip margin. The mobilized muscle is tunneled through the glide plane and split into 2 slips. The muscle slips are sutured to the orbicularis incorporating the dermis around the upper and lower lip and commissure. The muscle is inserted close to its resting tension; this can be determined using electrical stimulation as discussed in the procedure for temporalis MTU transfer.

PHYSIOTHERAPY

Muscle-retraining exercises are essential in optimizing the outcome of any muscle transfer procedure. In the preoperative period, it is helpful for patients to work with a physical therapist on specific exercises to strengthen the temporalis and masseter muscles and to identify isolated jaw movements that are essential in contracting the muscles. After the first 2 postoperative weeks, active mobilization of the transposed MTU should be initiated followed by muscle-strengthening exercises. The main goal of the therapy is to systematically rehabilitate smile, speech, and articulation function by transferring labial functions to the transferred muscle.

SUMMARY

Locoregional muscle transposition provides a means for restoring facial symmetry and smile after facial paralysis. Although effective, outcomes are generally inferior to that of FMMT. Intraoperative assessment with electrical stimulation to determine the tension of the MTU is necessary to improve results. The best outcomes are achieved through proper patient selection, and observing the principles and biomechanics of muscle contraction.

REFERENCES

1. Ishii L, Godoy A, Encarnacion CO, et al. Not just another face in the crowd: society's perceptions of facial paralysis. Laryngoscope 2012;122(3):533–8.
2. Boahene KD. Principles and biomechanics of muscle tendon unit transfer: application in temporalis muscle tendon transposition for smile improvement in facial paralysis. Laryngoscope 2013;123(2):350–5.
3. Owusu Boahene KD. Temporalis muscle tendon unit transfer for smile restoration after facial paralysis. Facial Plast Surg Clin North Am 2016;24(1):37–45.
4. Rubin LR. The anatomy of a smile: its importance in the treatment of facial paralysis. Plast Reconstr Surg 1974;53(4):384–7.
5. Labbè D, Bussu F, Iodice A. A comprehensive approach to long-standing facial paralysis based on lengthening temporalis myoplasty. Acta Otorhinolaryngol Ital 2012;32(3):145–53.
6. Gillies H. Experiences with fascia lata grafts in the operative treatment of facial paralysis: (section of otology and section of laryngology). Proc R Soc Med 1934;27(10):1372–82.
7. McLaughlin CR. Surgical support in permanent facial paralysis. Plast Reconstr Surg (1946) 1953;11(4):302–14.
8. Labbé D, Huault M. Lengthening temporalis myoplasty and lip reanimation. Plast Reconstr Surg 2000;105:1289–97.
9. Boahene KD, Farrag TY, Ishii L, et al. Minimally invasive temporalis tendon transposition. Arch Facial Plast Surg 2011;13:8–13.
10. Sedlmayr JC, Kirsch CF, Wisco JJ. The human temporalis muscle: superficial, deep, and zygomatic parts comprise one structural unit. Clin Anat 2009;22: 655–64.
11. Brunner R. Changes in muscle power following tendon lengthening and tendon transfer. Orthopade 1995;24:246–51.
12. Lexer E, Eden R. Uber die chirurgische behandlung der peripheren facialisliihmung. Beitr Klin Chir 1911;73:116.
13. Matic DB, Yoo J. The pedicled masseter muscle transfer for smile reconstruction in facial paralysis: repositioning the origin and insertion. J Plast Reconstr Aesthet Surg 2012;65:1002–8.
14. Shinohara H, Matsuo K, Osada Y, et al. Facial reanimation by transposition of the masseter muscle combined with tensor fascia lata, using the zygomatic arch as a pulley. Scand J Plast Reconstr Surg Hand Surg 2008;42:17–22.
15. Hontanilla B, Qiu SS. Transposition of the hemimasseteric muscle for dynamic rehabilitation of facial paralysis. J Craniofac Surg 2012;23:203–5.

Free Gracilis Transfer and Static Facial Suspension for Midfacial Reanimation in Long-Standing Flaccid Facial Palsy

Nate Jowett, MD*, Tessa A. Hadlock, MD

KEYWORDS

- Facial palsy • Free flap • Gracilis • Facial reanimation • Facial nerve • Fascia lata
- Static suspension

KEY POINTS

- Free muscle transfer for smile reanimation is indicated in cases of long-standing flaccid facial palsy.
- Knowledge of gracilis anatomy facilitates harvest and thinning of the flap to avoid facial bulk through a small incision.
- Muscle transfer may be combined with static suspension of the midface to open the nasal airway, reestablish a nasolabial fold, and improve esthetic outcomes.

 Video content accompanies this article at https://www.oto.theclinics.com/.

INTRODUCTION

The smile is an evolutionary adaptation facilitating successful interaction in complex social groups.[1] Smiling conveys increased intelligence,[2] happiness,[3] and social status.[4] Rehabilitation of the smile is a principal focus of facial reanimation. Since first reported by Sir Harold Gillies,[5] functional muscle transfer remains a central technique for smile reanimation. Free functional muscle transfer for smile reanimation has become the favored technique for long-standing facial palsy in many institutions, since first described by Harii and colleagues[6] more than 40 years ago. Herein, the authors

Disclosure Statement: The authors have no commercial or financial conflicts to disclose.
Division of Facial Plastic and Reconstructive Surgery, Department of Otolaryngology, Massachusetts Eye and Ear Infirmary, Harvard Medical School, 243 Charles Street, Boston, MA 02114, USA
* Corresponding author.
E-mail address: nate_jowett@meei.harvard.edu

Otolaryngol Clin N Am 51 (2018) 1129–1139
https://doi.org/10.1016/j.otc.2018.07.009
0030-6665/18/© 2018 Elsevier Inc. All rights reserved.

present an approach to midfacial reanimation by functional free gracilis muscle transfer and static facial suspension.

INDICATIONS

Since the introduction of targeted transfer of the nerve-to-masseter to zygomatic branches of the facial nerve for reanimation of native smile musculature (ie, V-VII transfer),[7] indications for muscle transfer are principally limited to cases whereby native facial musculature is presumed nonreceptive to innervation. Common clinical scenarios requiring free muscle transfer include absence of native facial musculature (congenital or postablative), facial muscle myopathy, or long denervation periods. Although no definitive criteria exist, evidence from case series suggests facial musculature remains receptive to reinnervation up to 24 months following denervation in adults[8–11] and possibly longer in children. Muscle transfer should be considered in the setting of radical parotidectomy where extensive perineural infiltration of distal facial nerve branches occurs.

Contrary to regional temporalis and nerve-to-masseter transfers that provide a bite-activated volitional smile, free muscle may be innervated by contralateral facial nerve branches for reanimation of spontaneous smile in patients with hemifacial palsy. Because of the longer regeneration distances required, higher failure rates occur with cross-facial innervation techniques, especially in older patients. Although the added value of spontaneity with respect to the increased risk of failure has yet to be well characterized, cross-facial innervation (via direct hook-up to paralyzed side musculature or to free muscle) may be considered as a first-line option in children (for whom the procedure carries a good chance of success) even where V to VII transfer is thought likely to succeed. Free muscle transfer by cross-facial innervation may also be used as an adjunctive option to add spontaneity to the smile in adults who have previously undergone successful V to VII transfer. Smile reanimation outcomes may be further enhanced by midfacial static sling procedures to open the nasal airway and reestablish the resting tone of the nasolabial fold.

SURGICAL TECHNIQUES

Free muscle transfer for smile reanimation may be innervated by branches of the trigeminal nerve (nerve-to-masseter or deep temporal[6]) or in select cases by ipsilateral zygomatic branches of the facial nerve (for instance, in facial muscle myopathy) in a 1-stage procedure. Cross-facial innervation may be achieved in a single stage using the latissimus dorsi flap, as the thoracodorsal nerve is of sufficient length to cross the face.[12] The gracilis muscle remains widely used for smile reanimation; its use permits a 2-team approach that minimizes the duration of general anesthesia. When gracilis muscle transfer with cross-facial innervation is planned, a 2-stage approach is typically used with antecedent cross-face nerve grafting to minimize the ultimate time required for flap innervation.[13]

Sural Nerve Harvest and Cross-Facial Grafting

Cross-facial innervation of free muscle is an excellent choice in young patients with hemifacial palsy. Because of its low donor site morbidity and length, the sural nerve is most commonly used for cross-facial nerve grafting. The common sural nerve is identified deep to the lesser saphenous vein through a small incision posterior to the lateral malleolus. An endoscope may be used to facilitate the harvest through a single incision (Video 1).[14–16] The common sural nerve is traced proximally, and its lateral and medial components are identified. The lateral component is a branch of the peroneal nerve coursing through the subcutaneous plane, whereas the medial component branches from the tibial nerve and travels between the two heads of the gastrocnemius muscle deep to its enveloping fascia. In most cases, the medial component is of larger caliber and is preferentially harvested.[17]

Donor nerve branches controlling the smile on the healthy side of the face are accessed through an extended Blair incision. A sub–superficial musculoaponeurotic system (SMAS) flap is elevated off the parotidomasseteric fascia, and midfacial branches of the facial nerve are identified at the anterior border of the parotid through meticulous blunt dissection. A tetanic nerve stimulator is used to assess associated facial displacements; one or more branches producing an ideal smile vector with minimal blink are selected and sharply transected following confirmation of redundancy. A fascia passer is used to inlay the sural nerve graft in the deep plane of the face across the upper lip for future coaptation to the nerve-to-gracilis. Short graft lengths (ie, terminating in the upper lip on the paralyzed side) are thought to result in stronger innervation for the subsequently transferred muscle.[18]

Functional Gracilis Muscle Flap Harvest

One of several thigh adductor muscles, the gracilis is readily harvested without reported functional morbidity.[19] To minimize neural regeneration distance, the flap is harvested ipsilateral to the paretic side except where innervation is by a short cross-face nerve graft; in the latter case, use of the contralateral gracilis results in a more favorable nerve position (**Fig. 1**). Flap lengths of up to 16 cm of in situ resting tension may be readily harvested though a 7-cm incision in the medial thigh; the incision is positioned longitudinally, one or two fingerbreadths posterior to the pubic tubercle, extending from 4 cm to 11 cm below the inguinal crease. The gracilis muscle is identified following dissection through the subcutaneous tissues and fascia overlying the adductor compartment. The neurovascular pedicle is identified coursing superficial to the adductor magnus muscle, approximately 8 cm below the inguinal crease. The anterior branch of the obturator nerve (AON) courses obliquely from the obturator foramen toward the gracilis muscle. The vascular pedicle typically comprises an arterial branch of the profunda femoris with its 2 venae comitans coursing transversely inferior to the nerve. In rare cases, the dominant vascular pedicle originates more superiorly from the medial circumflex femoral vessels deep to the adductor longus or from the femoral vessels coursing superficial to the adductor longus muscle.

With the neurovascular pedicle identified, the gracilis muscle is mobilized. The fascia overlying the adductor magnus muscle superior to the AON and inferior to the

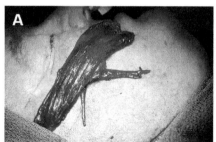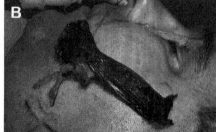

Fig. 1. Laterality of the gracilis flap. (*A*) Where the nerve-to-masseter muscle is used, harvest of the ipsilateral gracilis results in more favorable superolateral orientation of the nerve to gracilis. (*B*) Where innervation is by a short cross-face nerve graft, use of the contralateral gracilis muscle results in a more favorable inferomedial location of the nerve to gracilis.

vascular pedicle is released toward the anteromedial surface of the gracilis muscle, with care to avoid disruption of critical superior and inferior branches of the nerve (**Fig. 2**). The cutaneous branch of the obturator nerve, which courses from the deep to the superficial aspect of the adductor longus muscle often crossing superficial to the vascular pedicle, is identified and preserved. Elevation of the gracilis muscle off the medial aspect of the adductor magnus muscle is achieved using blunt finger dissection superior, inferior, and deep to the neurovascular pedicle between its tendinous origin and the desired in situ resting length (typically 12–16 cm). At its inferior extent, the muscle is divided into an anterior segment comprising the flap and a posterior segment left in situ. The anterior segment (typically 2–3 cm wide) is released transversely at the inferior aspect of the incision using bipolar scissors and bluntly dissected from the posterior segment. Continuing branches of the neurovascular pedicle to the posterior segment are identified and suture ligated. A locking 2-0 polyglactin suture is run across the cut edge of the inferior aspect of the flap, and the muscle is thinned in situ to a target weight of 15 to 20 g in adults and 10 to 15 g in children to avoid facial bulk (**Fig. 3**). The superior tendinous muscle attachment is released, and the neurovascular pedicle is meticulously dissected toward the profunda femoris vessels.

Nerve-to-Masseter Dissection

The nerve-to-masseter is commonly used to drive free muscle for smile reanimation. Blunt dissection through masseter muscle fibers is used to identify the nerve as it courses through the sigmoid notch inferior to the zygoma or alternatively more inferiorly 5 cm anterior to the auricular attachment. When accessed proximally, it is often identified deep to and between 2 large zygomatic facial nerve branches (one traveling toward the lower eyelid and the other to the zygomaticus muscle) at the level of the transverse facial vessels. The nerve is meticulously circumferentially dissected over a long length, transected, and reflected out of the dissection pocket for coaptation to the flap nerve. Medial branches of the nerve-to-masseter are preserved whenever possible to prevent denervation atrophy of the muscle and resulting loss of facial contour.

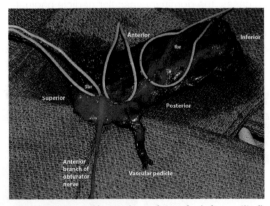

Fig. 2. Gracilis flap neural anatomy. The undersurface of a left gracilis flap is pictured, with critical superior (Sbr) and inferior (Ibr) branches labeled (*blue vessel loops* and *black arrowheads*). The inferior branch is particularly important, as it provides the bulk of the innervation to the anterior segment of the gracilis muscle (ie, the portion comprising the flap) in the authors' experience. It courses over and enters the muscle far inferior to the vascular pedicle.

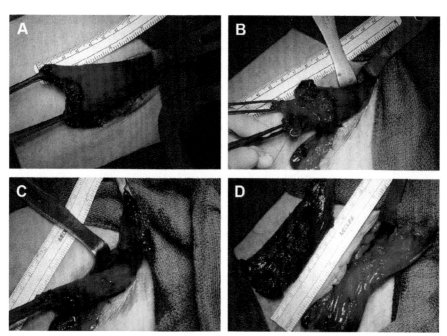

Fig. 3. Gracilis thinning in situ. (*A*) The flap may be readily harvested through a 7-cm incision. Following dissection of the anterior segment and inferior release, the muscle is brought out through the wound. (*B*) A locking 2-0 polyglactin 910 suture is run along the inferior aspect of the flap to function as a pseudotendon following partial dissection of the superficial half of the muscle off the deep aspect. (*C, D*) Blunt dissection of the superficial half thickness of the muscle is completed up to the tendinous origin. The target weight of the flap is 15 to 20 g for adults and 10 to 15 g for children.

Flap Inset

The paralyzed hemiface is opened via an extended Blair incision extending from the temporal hairline to the angle of the mandible. Superior to the zygoma, the facial flap is elevated in the subcutaneous plane superficial to the temporoparietal fascia. Below the zygoma, a thick facial flap is elevated in the sub-SMAS plane atop the parotidomasseteric fascia, extending medially to the modiolus and nasolabial fold immediately superficial to the zygomaticus major muscle (ie, the deep plane of the face[20]). The temporoparietal and innominate fasciae are sharply incised posterior to the course of the temporal branch of the facial nerve to expose the true temporalis fascia. The superficial temporal vessels are preserved. When present, the facial vessels are preferred over the superficial temporal vessels as donors for their larger caliber, favorable position, and lower propensity for spasm. Inset of the flap along the dermis of the nasolabial fold may result in a more natural looking smile but carries higher risk of dehiscence. An alternative option is inset of the flap to remnant fibers of the orbicularis oris and upper lip about the modiolus; such fibers are robust and often present even in congenital and long-standing flaccid facial palsy. Five or more heavy absorbable sutures (0 polyglactin) are parachuted into position and secured sequentially around the pseudotendon of the flap. Microvascular anastomosis is performed, and the flap is perfused. The opposite edge of the muscle is secured under neutral tension to the true temporalis fascia; overcorrection of static oral commissure position is avoided, as subsequent lateralization may result. Neural coaptation is then completed; when innervation is by a short cross-face nerve graft, the nerve is passed deep to the muscle into the upper lip through a labial mucosal incision following identification of the tip of the graft and neuroma resection. Inset of the gracilis flap to the modiolus and upper lip may be combined with static suspension of the nasolabial fold for improved esthetics (**Figs. 4** and **5**); in these cases, the gracilis flap lays deep to the fascia lata.

Static Facial Suspension and Fascia Lata Harvest

Static facial suspension may be achieved using sutures, allografts (eg, acellular dermis), or autografts (fascia lata, palmaris longus tendon). Alloplastic materials are ill advised, as they carry higher risk of infection and extrusion. Presently, the authors favor the use of fascia lata in static facial suspension for its strength, broad width, resistance to reabsorption, low rates of infection, and low donor site morbidity. In the midface, fascia lata strips may be used to correct external nasal valve collapse, reestablish the nasolabial fold, and resuspend the oral commissure to a more appropriate position. A broad graft (7 × 14 cm) may be readily harvested through two 1-in incisions in the lateral thigh (**Fig. 6**A, B). Two narrow bands are cut from the fascia (**Fig. 6**C, D). For nasal valve correction, a peri-alar incision is made and a narrow band is secured to the sesamoid cartilages (**Fig. 6**E). The other narrow band is secured to the modiolus. The nasolabial fold is marked from its origin superior to the ala at the nose-cheek junction and its terminus at the level of the oral commissure. A wide band of fascia lata may be secured to the undersurface of the nasolabial fold using double-armed straight-needle sutures tunneled in the deep dermis between adjacent stab incisions along the marked line (**Fig. 6**F–H). In older patients with low propensity for excess scarring, the nasolabial fold may be sharply incised and the fascia secured to the deep dermis under direct visualization. The lateral ends of the 3 bands are then secured to the true temporalis fascia (**Fig. 6**I); slight overcorrection is used for the nasal valve inset, whereas minimal tension is used for oral commissure correction and neutral tension for nasolabial fold suspension. When combined with free gracilis

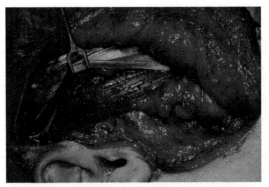

Fig. 4. Gracilis muscle inset with static facial suspension. An ipsilateral gracilis flap is inset about the modiolus medially and the true temporalis fascia above the zygoma laterally at neutral tension following microvascular anastomosis to the facial vessels. The nerve-to-gracilis was trimmed to a short length and coapted to the nerve-to-masseter. Note the thick sub-SMAS facial flap used to avoid tethering of the muscle to the facial skin. A wide band of fascia lata is secured superficial to the flap about the nasolabial fold dermis medially and the true temporalis fascia laterally. In addition to improved nasolabial fold esthetics, use of fascia lata might also optimize the gracilis gliding plane.

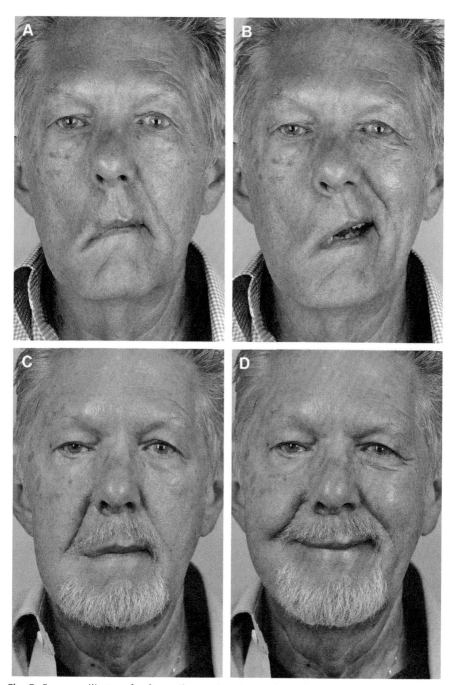

Fig. 5. Free gracilis transfer for smile reanimation with midfacial fascia lata suspension. (*A, B*) Preoperative photographs at rest and with smile effort in a patient with long-standing flaccid facial palsy. (*C, D*) Postoperative result following gracilis transfer innervated by the nerve-to-masseter, with static suspension of the external nasal valve and nasolabial fold using minimally invasive stab incisions.

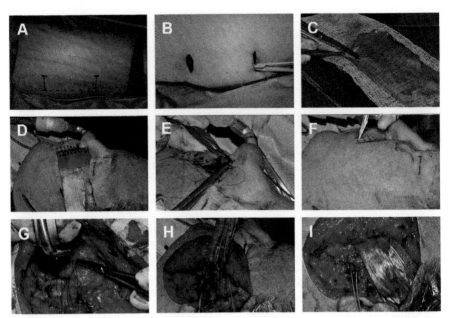

Fig. 6. Fascia lata harvest and static facial suspension. (*A, B*) Two 1-in incisions are marked on the midsection of the lateral thigh through which a large band of fascia lata (~7 × 14 cm) is bluntly dissected. (*C, D*) The fascia lata is cut into narrow and wide bands for suspension of the external nasal valve and nasolabial fold. A third narrow band may be used to suspend the oral commissure where muscle transfer for smile reanimation is not planned. (*E*) After elevation of a deep plane facelift flap, a peri-alar incision is made and a narrow band of fascia lata is secured to the sesamoid cartilages using 4-0 polypropylene sutures. (*F*) Small stab incisions are made just anterior the marked nasolabial fold, extending from the superior aspect of the alar cartilage at the nose-cheek junction to the level of the oral commissure. (*G*) Double-armed straight needles attached to 4-0 polypropylene sutures are tunneled across adjacent stab incisions in the deep dermis and sequentially passed under the facial flap and parachuted in order into the broad band of fascia lata. (*H*) The fascia lata is then passed along the parachuted sutures to the undersurface of the nasolabial fold and sutures tied on the deep surface. (*I*) The lateral aspects of the fascia lata bands are secured to the true temporalis fascia using polypropylene sutures; slight overcorrection under tension is used on the band to the external nasal valve and neutral tension is used for the wide band to the nasolabial fold. Overcorrection of the nasolabial fold is unsightly and should be avoided. When fascia lata suspension of the oral commissure is performed, neutral positioning with minimal tension is used.

transfer, static correction of the oral commissure using a narrow band of fascia lata secured to the modiolus is typically not required.

Postoperative Care and Outcomes

Patients undergoing static facial suspension alone are mobilized following surgery and discharged the following day. Patients undergoing free muscle transfer are mobilized the first postoperative day, though a 3-day hospitalization is generally required for drain management and flap perfusion monitoring by bedside Doppler ultrasound. Meaningful oral commissure excursion is achieved in approximately 90% of cases innervated by the nerve-to-masseter, with onset of movement expected within 3 to 4 months. When cross-facial innervation is used, the success rate is approximately 80%, with movement typically first noted within 6 to 9 months. Smile outcomes are optimized with facial nerve physical therapy. Weakening of the healthy-side depressor labii inferioris muscle may be used to improve smile esthetics in many patients.[21,22]

TECHNICAL AND CLINICAL PEARLS

- Donor nerve caliber and the associated facial displacement vector are critical factors in cross-facial nerve grafting. Selection of too small of a donor nerve caliber risks too few axons and ultimate underpowering of the free muscle, whereas too large a caliber risks weakening the healthy-side smile. Furthermore, selection of a donor nerve with too strong of oculi activation may ultimately yield a blink-driven cross face smile (instead of the desired spontaneous, joy-driven smile). After confirmation of redundancy, a large-caliber zygomatic nerve branch (or 2 smaller branches) at the level of the anterior border of the parotid gland that provides ideal smile vector with minimal oculi activation should be selected.
- Although some movement is expected within 6 to 12 months, smile excursion in cross-face–driven free muscle may continue to strengthen over a period of up to 2 to 4 years.
- Long cotton-tip applicators are ideal for circumferential blunt dissection of the nerve-to-masseter muscle following its identification in the sigmoid notch; veins coursing with the nerve are readily separated without injury using this technique. Time invested in obtaining a long donor nerve length is recuperated at the time of neural coaptation, when the nerve-to-masseter may be completely reflected out of the dissection pocket to facilitate microsurgery geometry
- Thinning of the gracilis muscle flap may be achieved without subsequent disruption of gliding planes and tethering of the muscle to the overlying skin if a thick facial flap (ie, sub-SMAS/deep plane) is elevated; elevation of a thin facial flap is to be avoided
- Flap thinning is optimally performed in situ while the muscle is still perfusing. Not only is the ischemia time decreased but the hematoma risk also decreases as myocutaneous perforators are readily identified and controlled.
- Overcorrection of the gracilis muscle at the inset should be avoided; subsequent lateralization of the oral commissure may result whose correction is fraught with risk. The authors typically inset the gracilis muscle under neutral tension, such that its inset length is equal to its resting length following harvest (not its resting length in situ).
- Overcorrection of the nasolabial fold with static facial suspension should be avoided. Static suspension of the nasolabial fold is intended to support the midface when patients are upright; nasolabial folds are blunted in most adults when supine; thus, one aims for subtle correction on the table using neutral tension when insetting the fascia lata to the temporalis fascia.
- In the authors' experience, postoperative hematomas are often the result of inadvertent injury to the facial or angular artery or branches thereof during the time of medial muscle inset or fascia lata inset to the nasolabial fold. Hematomas can be largely avoided by systematic examination of the distal facial/angular artery deep to the gracilis flap before closure.

SUPPLEMENTARY DATA

Supplementary data related to this article can be found online at https://doi.org/10.1016/j.otc.2018.07.009.

REFERENCES

1. Schmidt KL, Cohn JF. Human facial expressions as adaptations: evolutionary questions in facial expression research. Am J Phys Anthropol 2001;(Suppl 33): 3–24.
2. Otta E, Lira BB, Delevati NM, et al. The effect of smiling and of head tilting on person perception. J Psychol 1994;128(3):323–31.
3. Otta E, Folladore Abrosio F, Hoshino RL. Reading a smiling face: messages conveyed by various forms of smiling. Percept Mot Skills 1996;82(3 Pt 2): 1111–21.
4. LaFrance M, Hecht MA. Option or obligation to smile: the effects of power and gender on facial expression. In: Philippot P, Feldman RS, Coats EJ, editors. The social context of nonverbal behavior. Paris: Editions de la Maison des Sciences de l'Homme; 1999. p. 45–70.
5. Gillies H. Experiences with Fascia lata grafts in the operative treatment of facial paralysis: (section of otology and section of laryngology). Proc R Soc Med 1934;27(10):1372–82.
6. Harii K, Ohmori K, Torii S. Free gracilis muscle transplantation, with microneurovascular anastomoses for the treatment of facial paralysis. A preliminary report. Plast Reconstr Surg 1976;57(2):133–43.
7. Klebuc M. Masseter–to-facial nerve transfer: a new technique for facial reanimation. J Reconstr Microsurg 2006;22(03):A101.
8. Wu P, Chawla A, Spinner RJ, et al. Key changes in denervated muscles and their impact on regeneration and reinnervation. Neural Regen Res 2014;9(20): 1796–809.
9. Conley J. Hypoglossal crossover–122 cases. Trans Sect Otolaryngol Am Acad Ophthalmol Otolaryngol 1977;84(4 Pt 1). ORL-763–8.
10. Gavron JP, Clemis JD. Hypoglossal-facial nerve anastomosis: a review of forty cases caused by facial nerve injuries in the posterior fossa. Laryngoscope 1984;94(11 Pt 1):1447–50.
11. Kunihiro T, Kanzaki J, Yoshihara S, et al. Hypoglossal-facial nerve anastomosis after acoustic neuroma resection: influence of the time anastomosis on recovery of facial movement. ORL J Otorhinolaryngol Relat Spec 1996;58(1):32–5.
12. Harii K, Asato H, Yoshimura K, et al. One-stage transfer of the latissimus dorsi muscle for reanimation of a paralyzed face: a new alternative. Plast Reconstr Surg 1998;102(4):941–51.
13. O'Brien BM, Franklin JD, Morrison WA. Cross-facial nerve grafts and microneurovascular free muscle transfer for long established facial palsy. Br J Plast Surg 1980;33(2):202–15.
14. Park SB, Cheshier S, Michaels D, et al. Endoscopic harvesting of the sural nerve graft: technical note. Neurosurgery 2006;58(1 Suppl):ONS-E180 [discussion: ONS-E180].
15. Oliveira MT, Marttos AC Jr, Fallopa F. Endoscopic harvesting of the sural nerve graft: a cadaveric investigation. Orthopedics 2000;23(11):1189–91.
16. Koh KS, Park S. Endoscopic harvest of sural nerve graft with balloon dissection. Plast Reconstr Surg 1998;101(3):810–2.
17. Coert JH, Dellon AL. Clinical implications of the surgical anatomy of the sural nerve. Plast Reconstr Surg 1994;94(6):850–5.
18. Manktelow RT, Zuker RM. Cross-facial nerve graft—the long and short graft: The first stage for microneurovascular muscle transfer. Operat Tech Plast Reconstr Surg 1999;6(3):174–9.

19. Besset M, Penaud A, Quignon R, et al. Donor site morbidity after free gracilis muscle flap. Report of 32 cases. Ann Chir Plast Esthet 2014;59(1):53–60 [in French].
20. Hamra ST. The deep-plane rhytidectomy. Plast Reconstr Surg 1990;86(1):53–61 [discussion: 62–3].
21. Godwin Y, Tomat L, Manktelow R. The use of local anesthetic motor block to demonstrate the potential outcome of depressor labii inferioris resection in patients with facial paralysis. Plast Reconstr Surg 2005;116(4):957–61.
22. Hussain G, Manktelow RT, Tomat LR. Depressor labii inferioris resection: an effective treatment for marginal mandibular nerve paralysis. Br J Plast Surg 2004; 57(6):502–10.

Management of Long-Standing Flaccid Facial Palsy

Static Approaches to the Brow, Midface, and Lower Lip

Marissa Purcelli Lafer, MD[a], Teresa M. O, MD, MArch[b],*

KEYWORDS

- Flaccid facial paralysis • Facial nerve paralysis • Brow ptosis • Static suspension
- External nasal valve collapse • Chemodenervation • Myectomy
- Selective neurectomy

KEY POINTS

- Long-term flaccid facial paralysis is defined as flaccid (no tone) facial paralysis for 2 or more years.
- The face is evaluated in horizontal thirds and contralateral facial symmetry is compared.
- Static techniques can be used alone or as an adjunct to dynamic techniques.
- Browlifting and periocular interventions improve symmetry, visual field defects, protect the cornea and improve patient comfort.
- Contralateral weakening techniques (chemodenervation, myectomy, or neurectomy) are commonly used to improve resting symmetry in the upper and lower face.

INTRODUCTION

Patients who have had flaccid facial paralysis (FFP) for 2 or more years constitute a subset considered to have "long-standing" paralysis. After 2 years of flaccidity, the native facial nerve branches and facial musculature are no longer viable for primary nerve substitution procedures. Successful management of long-standing paralysis can be challenging; afflicted patients suffer psychosocial burden, and surgical interventions are known to improve quality of life.[1] The treatment plan should be individualized and tailored to the individual's deficits, and developed in the context of their overall health.

Disclosure Statement: The authors have nothing to disclose.
[a] Department of Otolaryngology Head and Neck Surgery, New York University, 462 First Avenue, 5th Floor, Suite 5SE5, New York, NY 10016, USA; [b] Facial Nerve Center, Vascular Birthmark Institute of New York, Department of Otolaryngology-Head and Neck Surgery, Manhattan Eye, Ear, and Throat Hospital, Lenox Hill Hospital, 210 East 64th Street, 7th Floor, New York, NY 10065, USA
* Corresponding author.
E-mail address: to@vbiny.org

Otolaryngol Clin N Am 51 (2018) 1141–1150
https://doi.org/10.1016/j.otc.2018.07.010
0030-6665/18/© 2018 Elsevier Inc. All rights reserved.

Physical examination is performed systematically using a horizontal zonal approach to the face. The upper, middle, and lower thirds of the face are each assessed separately comparing the left and right sides. Once the deficits have been identified, a comprehensive plan is developed using dynamic and static techniques to maximize overall symmetry and function.

Although dynamic reanimation should be the gold standard, in a subset of patients, static techniques may be more appropriate. For patients with significant comorbidities, a shortened life span, advanced age, patients who are not good candidates for prolonged general anesthesia, or in whom free muscle transfer may not be appropriate, static correction can still provide improved symmetry and function. Techniques for static reanimation described in this article also can be used as an adjunct to free muscle transfer or nerve transfer.

This article focuses on the management of flaccid paralysis using primarily static approaches to the individual zones of the face to create resting symmetry. In the upper face, brow ptosis and basic periocular considerations are addressed; in the midface, techniques for correction of the nasal valve as well as reestablishment of the nasolabial fold are examined; in the lower face, oral competence is discussed, and finally, considerations for the contralateral hemiface are presented.

UPPER FACE
Unilateral Brow Ptosis

Long-standing frontal branch paralysis leads to atrophy of the frontalis muscle, the primary brow elevator, with resultant brow ptosis. Functionally, patients may complain of visual field deficits, especially with superior gaze.[2] Significant brow ptosis also permits desquamation of epidermal cells onto the cornea, increasing ocular irritation.

The patient is evaluated in the upright position. The degree of ptosis and position of the hairline is noted and compared with the normal side. Manual elevation of the brow to the ideal position will help to determine how much of the visual field deficit is secondary to the brow ptosis alone. Special attention should be paid to any degree of lagophthalmos because exuberant brow lifting may further compromise eye closure.

Solutions for brow ptosis include traditional browlift techniques, direct, midforehead, endoscopic, and indirect, with or without additional fine-tuning procedures, such as contralateral chemodenervation of the frontalis muscle and/or the corrugator complex.[3]

Direct Brow Lift

In patients with deep forehead wrinkling, a direct brow lift may be used and placed just above the brow. An ellipse of tissue is removed, thus lifting the brow. Care must be taken to preserve the supraorbital neurovascular pedicle.

Fixation Device

An in-office procedure may be performed using local anesthetic. A pretrichial or posttrichial incision is used to access the subperiosteal plane. A subperiosteal dissection in a fan-shaped area releases the entire supraorbital rim; care is used to avoid injury to neurovascular bundles. The soft tissue flap is elevated superiorly and secured to a fixation device, either poly lactic co-glycolic acid copolymers, or craniofacial bone screws, which are drilled into the calvarium. The excess soft tissue of the forehead is removed in elliptical fashion and the incision closed (**Fig. 1**).[4] This procedure may also be performed endoscopically.

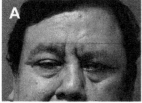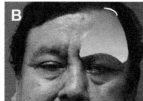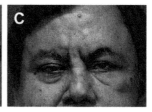

Fig. 1. (A) Left brow ptosis. (B) Pretrichial incision. Area of subperiosteal elevation with fixation device and elliptical excision of redundant skin. (C) After brow lift.

Suture Suspension

Another technique uses a horizontal pretrichial or posttrichial incision and a miniplate fixation to which up to 5 sutures are secured. These sutures are passed along the deep dermis at the level of the superior brow through small stab incisions; sutures are passed up to the trichial incision using long Keith needles and secured to the plate.[1]

In elderly patients with fair skin and excess wrinkling, a direct brow lift also may be used with minimal aesthetic penalty.[4] Bilateral brow ptosis occurs in normal aging. A unilateral brow lift on the paralyzed size may accentuate the contralateral brow ptosis associated with normal aging, thus occasionally bilateral brow lifting is appropriate.[5] Accepted principles for ideal brow positioning can be used (at or slightly above the supraorbital rim with the apex centered between the lateral limbus and the lateral canthus with gender consideration).

Selective chemodenervation

Botulinum toxin is a neurotoxic protein produced by the bacterium *Clostridium botulinum*. The toxin inhibits the release of acetylcholine from presynaptic nerve endings thus inhibiting muscle contraction.[6] In the upper face, injection into the contralateral frontalis muscle may improve symmetry to the brow and forehead zones.

Periocular complex: upper and lower eyelid

Upper eyelid: lagophthalmos and corneal exposure Lagophthalmos in facial paralysis results from paralysis of the orbicularis oculi muscle leading to incomplete eye closure, ectropion, and compromised tear-pumping mechanism. These deficits result in an inability to protect the cornea. Excessive corneal exposure causes rapid evaporation of the tear film, which can lead to ulceration that, if not adequately managed, may lead to visual loss. Patients at increased risk for exposure keratitis can be identified by applying the acronym BAD: absence of *B*ell phenomenon, corneal *A*nesthesia, and history of *D*ry eye.[5]

The levator palpebrae superioris muscle (LPS) is innervated by the oculomotor nerve and serves as a direct antagonist to the orbicularis oculi by raising the upper eyelid. When the orbicularis oculi is paralyzed, the LPS can become foreshortened due to lack of passive opposition from the orbicularis oculi, thereby exacerbating lagophthalmos.[2]

There are both static and dynamic procedures to treat lagophthalmos and corneal exposure. Static procedures include tarsorrhaphy and lid loading while dynamic options include palpebral spring implants and temporalis muscle transfer. Physical therapy with eyelid stretch exercises are useful. The upper lid eyelashes are grasped between 2 fingers. Superior countertraction is placed at the superior orbital rim to stretch and elongate the LPS muscle. These maneuvers mechanically disrupt covalent linkages between adjacent myosin chains, thus, improving eye closure.

All patients benefit from daytime hydrating preservative free eye drops and night-time lubricant. Nighttime taping or eye shield also protects the eye.

Tarsorrhaphy This procedure is especially helpful in the presence of decreased corneal sensation. The lateral upper and lower eyelids are denuded at the lid margin and sutured together. This may be temporary or permanent.

Lid loading/eyelid weight A lid crease incision is made and a thin profile gold or platinum eyelid weight is placed into a precise pocket overlying the tarsal plate. If placed over the tarsus, the profile may be visible in thin-skinned individuals. Moving the weight farther superiorly so that the inferior border of the plate is at the superior border of the tarsus alleviates this problem. However, a slightly heavier weight should be used. Both gold and platinum are well tolerated. Platinum has the advantage of being denser than gold and thus can be smaller and thinner in profile (**Fig. 2**).

Lower eyelid: laxity and ectropion
In the lower eyelid, paralysis of the orbicularis oculi muscle leads to ptosis of the lower eyelid margin. In some cases of excess laxity, the lower eyelid is pulled away from the globe disrupting the tear film and further exposing the eye. Static sling procedures such as lateral tarsal strip elevate the lower lid superolaterally and serve to reestablish contact between the lid margin and the globe. Allografts may also be used in the entire lower eyelid subunit to the orbital rim to lift the lower eyelid margin superiorly.[7]

These procedures are described in detail in "Management of Long-Standing Flaccid Facial Palsy: Periocular Considerations" by Drs Natalie Homer and Aaron Fay, elsewhere in this issue.

MIDFACE

Functional deficits related to midface flaccidity include external nasal valve collapse and nasal obstruction, and lip ptosis with associated drooling and speech difficulty. The entire midface cheek complex also becomes ptotic and displaced inferiorly exacerbating lower eyelid and lip ptosis and appearance of aging.

External Nasal Valve Collapse

Obstructive nasal symptoms are common in patients with long-standing facial paralysis, and result from nasal base rotation, inferomedial alar displacement, and external nasal valve collapse. In addition to collapse of the nasal valve, paralysis of the nasalis muscle prevents dilation of the nostrils during inspiration, which can also contribute to or worsen nasal obstruction.[2] A Cottle maneuver can help identify nasal valve collapse. However, unlike traditional rhinoplasty techniques in which cartilage grafts are used for structural reinforcement in nonparalyzed patients, the obstruction in facial paralysis is compounded by the unopposed pull of the contralateral side with deviation of the philtrum.

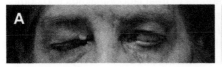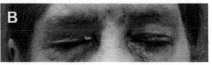

Fig. 2. (*A*) Left upper eyelid lagophthalmos. (*B*) Eye closure after placement of thin profile platinum eyelid weight.

External nasal valve suspension accomplishes lateral displacement of the pyriform aperture region, thereby counterbalancing the unopposed pull of the healthy side. This maneuver will, in most cases, relieve nasal obstruction. Several techniques have been described including suture vector, bone-anchored suture, and static suspension using autologous materials including fascia lata (FL) and palmaris longus tendon. Suture vector techniques or bone-anchored suture techniques (Mitek) are simple office procedures, but have failure rates approaching 25%.[8] Additionally, the presence of a foreign body increases the risk of infection and suture extrusion.

Static suspension of the nasal ala
A thin strip of FL (1–2 cm × 10–15 cm) is harvested from the leg and passed from a preauricular/temporal incision subcutaneously to an alar crease incision, where it is secured to the accessory alar cartilages.[9] This procedure has minimal morbidity and increased long-term benefit with patients reporting improved quality of life.[9] This technique may be combined with static or dynamic reanimation of the midface (**Fig. 3**).

Other sources of tendon or fascia include the palmaris longus tendon or the gracilis or semitendinosus tendons. The palmaris longus tendon is harvested from the forearm with a small incision at the wrist crease and the upper forearm, with minimal morbidity and scarring.[10] The gracilis and semitendinosus tendons may be harvested simultaneously with a gracilis muscle by adding a stab incision at the popliteal fossa. A tendon stripper is used to isolate the tendon, which can then be filleted to become 1 to 2 cm wide and up to 22 cm long (see **Fig. 3**B).

Fascia lata harvest technique
The incision for thigh FL harvest is minimal, and may be performed endoscopically.[11,12] If harvested superiorly, soft tissue bulge can be avoided. Two small incisions are made. The superior incision is 2 cm long and the inferior incision, a stab. The area harvested is 4 cm anterior to the lateral intermuscular septum (preserve iliotibial band), 10 cm superior to the lateral femoral condyle, 15 cm inferior to the anterior superior iliac spine. An area up to 20 × 4 cm can be harvested in this fashion. Saline is used for hydrodissection and an elevator to separate the fascia. The fascia is incised with a blade and the elevator is used to further separate the deep surface. Longitudinal cuts are then made and the fascia is passed from a superior to inferior direction

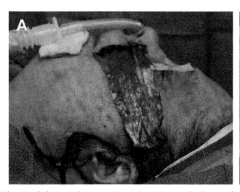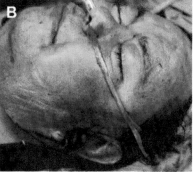

Fig. 3. (*A*) Autologous FL strips at nasal ala, and nasolabial fold. This was combined with a gracilis free muscle at modiolus and lateral upper lip. (*B*) Gracilis tendon to suspend nasal ala combined with gracilis free muscle.

and removed via an inferior skin stab incision.[13] Extending the length of the incisions will allow for the harvest of wider pieces.

Many materials for static suspension have been described. Autologous FL, allografts such as acellular human dermis (AlloDerm), and synthetic grafts such as polytetrafluoroethylene (ie, Gore-Tex) have all been used. Autologous sources are preferred because they eliminate the risk of extrusion and decrease risk of infection.

Nasolabial Fold Asymmetry

The nasolabial fold (NLF), which is effaced in the paralyzed face, is formed by the muscular projections of the upper lip elevators, the fibrous tissue that connects the smiling mechanism to the dermis of the skin in the fold, and striated muscle bundles that originate in the fold fascia.[14,15] Through natural aging, the NLF becomes more prominent. Recreating the NLF can be accomplished through the traditional linear incision at the fold with static suspension toward the temporalis fascia or zygomatic arch. Alternatively, multiple small stab incisions placed medial to the NLF may be used with suture suspension.[1] Multiple anchor points add more strength to the suspension and this gives a more natural appearance. This technique has better aesthetic outcomes when compared with the traditional linear incision. A wider strip of FL with multiple points of insertion gives a more natural, long-lasting effect. Separate strips of FL may be used for the nasal ala, NLF, and the modiolus (oral commissure). In patients undergoing free muscle transfer for smile reanimation, the FL at the modiolus is substituted with free muscle. The widest band of fascia is used to support the NLF.

Nasolabial fold creation

A minimally invasive technique is described by Faris and colleagues.[1] Once the facelift flap is elevated, dissection proceeds superficially over the facial musculature toward the NLF. Several stab incisions or anchor points are placed 2 mm medial to the desired location of the new NLF and are marked and numbered at 5-mm intervals from the commissure to the cephalic portion of the nasofacial isthmus. Approximately 10 nasolabial anchor points are required in adult patients. Stab incisions into the dermis are then made at each marked point with a No. 11 blade. The fascia is then trimmed to the curvature of the desired fold and marked at points corresponding to the nasolabial anchor points. Double-armed 3–0 polypropylene sutures are then passed parallel to the dermis at each of these points and passed to the undersurface of the skin flap and sutured to the inferior end of the FL. The FL is "parachuted" into the wound. The lateral aspect of these FL strips are then secured to the deep temporal fascia. This technique may be used as an adjunct to free muscle transfer (see **Fig. 3**A; **Fig. 4**).

See "Free Gracilis Transfer and Static Facial Suspension for Midfacial Reanimation in Long-Standing Flaccid Facial Palsy" by Drs Nate Jowett and Tessa A. Hadlock, elsewhere in this issue, for further discussion on static suspension of the midface as an adjunct to dynamic reanimation of long-standing facial palsy.

LOWER FACE

Oral incompetence is the most significant functional deficit seen in long-standing paralysis of the lower face. Oral incompetence can lead to difficulties manipulating a food bolus, anterior bolus spillage, sialorrhea, and difficulties with speech articulation.[16] Techniques to correct oral incompetence and improve facial asymmetry include static slings, muscle transfers, wedge resections, and fillers.

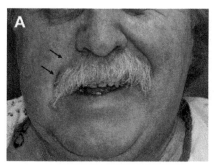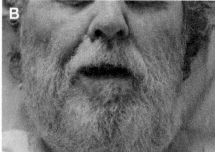

Fig. 4. (*A*) Note partially effaced right nasolabial fold *(black arrows)* with ptosis of oral commissure. (*B*) Recreation of right nasolabial fold after static FL suspension.

Depressor Dysfunction

Lower lip depression is attributed to a combination of actions of the orbicularis oris, depressor labii inferioris, depressor anguli oris, mentalis, and platysma muscles. The main lip depressors are the depressor labii inferioris and the depressor anguli oris, which are innervated by the marginal mandibular branch of the facial nerve. The depressor labii inferioris (DLI) pulls the lower lip downward and laterally while everting the vermillion border. The depressor anguli oris draws the lip downward and laterally, but also depresses the oral commissure. The facial expressions attributed to the lower lip depression are negative emotions such as frown and snarl. However, it is also important in smiling.[16] Although the depressors are not used in a zygomaticus or canine smile, they are used in a full-denture smile. In a full-denture smile, there is equal contraction of lip elevators and depressors, which exposes both the maxillary and mandibular dentition.[2] Symmetry may be created by either inhibiting the opposite lower lip depressors or by reanimating the paralyzed lip.

Contralateral chemodenervation with botulinum toxin

Botulinum toxin is used in the face to weaken contralateral musculature to create a more balanced appearance.[17] It is used in both synkinetic (nonflaccid) facial paralysis and FFP. In a systematic review, Cooper and colleagues[6] concluded that botulinum toxin injections are helpful in restoring overall facial symmetry both at rest and during movement in patients with chronic facial palsy.

Intraoral transection of contralateral depressor labii inferioris muscle The DLI muscle on the contralateral side may be transected and a transverse segment removed via an intraoral incision, which may be performed under local anesthesia.[18,19]

Selective neurectomy of contralateral face If botulinum toxin injections are successful and the patient is pleased with the result, the effect may be made more permanent with highly selective neurectomy. Intraoperative cutaneous nerve stimulation assists in isolating whether the marginal or cervical branch is contributing to the lower lip asymmetry on the contralateral side. The branches that give the most contralateral pull are selectively transected. Preoperative nerve mapping using continuous mapping of the action potential (CMAP) of the lower division of the facial nerve is performed.[20]

A 1 to 2 cm incision over the nerve branch under the mandible permits access to the branch. Once its role is confirmed with stimulation, the isolated branch is transected and ligated, obviating the need for serial injections (**Figs. 5** and **6**).[21]

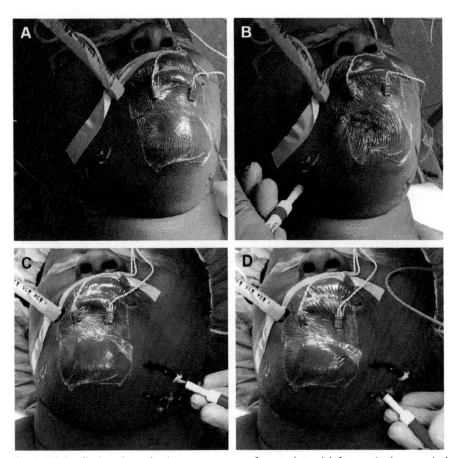

Fig. 5. Minimally invasive selective neurectomy of contralateral left marginal or cervical branches using CMAP (continuous monitoring of the action potential) technology and nerve stimulation. Patient with congenital right lower lip paralysis. (*A*) Stimulation of marginal branch elicits no downward lower lip pull. There is mentalis dimpling. (*B*) There is no downward cervical or platysmal response when area of cervical branches are stimulated. (*C*) Left nonparalyzed side. CMAP nerve monitoring used to initially map the nerve. Direct stimulation of marginal branch elicits no downward lip movement. (*D*) Stimulation of cervical branch elicits strong platysmal downward pull (note eversion of lower lip with pulling of tegaderm downwards). This branch will be transected using a minimally invasive approach.

Dynamic reanimation of the ipsilateral lower lip Digastric muscle transfer and platysma muscle transfer have also been described for lower lip symmetry.[22,23] These techniques require prolonged operative time and the results are not as predictable or reproducible. Given the ease of lower lip weakening techniques, with minimal functional deficits, digastric and platysma muscle transfers are not commonly used.[23,24]

Soft tissue hyaluronic fillers Hyaluronic acid–based fillers can be administered as in-office procedures with low morbidity. The filler can be used to augment thinned areas of the lip thereby improving competence, closure of the lip, and articulation.

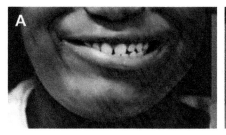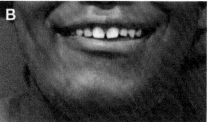

Fig. 6. Minimally invasive selective neurectomy of contralateral lower lip pull. (*A*) Congenital right lower lip paralysis. (*B*) Note symmetric smile after selective neurectomy.

Disadvantages of hyaluronic acid fillers include requirement for repeat injections every 6 to 12 months.[25]

Fat grafting Autologous fat grafting has been used as a more permanent filler to increase lip volume on the paralyzed side, and to improve aesthetic appearance and oral competence. Mobility of this region impacts on graft take, with many patients requiring several staged injections for optimal bulk restoration.[26–28]

TREATING THE CONTRALATERAL FACE

Weakening of select contralateral facial musculature may improve aesthetic facial symmetry. Chemodenervation, myectomy, selective neurectomy, and physical therapy may be used.

SUMMARY

A comprehensive approach to long-standing FFP requires systematic assessment to adequately address facial functional and aesthetic deficits. Static approaches to the brow, midface, and lower lip are important in reestablishing symmetry, and improving function and quality of life.

REFERENCES

1. Faris C, Heiser A, Jowett N, et al. Minimal nasolabial incision technique for nasolabial fold modification in patients with facial paralysis. JAMA Facial Plast Surg 2017;1–6. https://doi.org/10.1001/jamafacial.2017.1425.
2. Bhama PK, Hadlock TA. Management of the paralyzed face. In: Papel ID, Frodel JL, Holt GR, et al, editors. Facial plastic and reconstructive surgery. 4th edition. New York: Thieme Medical Publishers, Inc; 2016. p. 737–44.
3. Moody FP, Losken A, Bostwick J, et al. Endoscopic frontal branch neurectomy, corrugator myectomy, and brow lift for forehead asymmetry after facial nerve palsy. Plast Reconstr Surg 2001;108(1):218–24.
4. Hadlock TA, Greenfield LJ, Wernick-Robinson M, et al. Multimodality approach to management of the paralyzed face. Laryngoscope 2006;116(8):1385–9.
5. Ridgway JM, Crumley RL, Kim JH. Rehabilitation of facial paralysis. In: Flint PW, Haughey BH, Lund VJ, et al, editors. Cummings operative otolaryngology. 6th edition. Philadelphia: Elsevier; 2015. p. 2643–61.
6. Cooper L, Lui M, Nduka C. Botulinum toxin treatment for facial palsy: a systematic review. J Plast Reconstr Aesthet Surg 2017;70(6):833–41.
7. Boahene K. Reanimating the paralyzed face. F1000Prime Rep 2013;5:49.

8. Nuara MJ, Mobley SR. Nasal valve suspension revisited. Laryngoscope 2007; 117(12):2100–6.

9. Lindsay RW, Smitson C, Edwards C, et al. Correction of the nasal base in the flaccidly parayzed face. Plast Reconstr Surg 2010;126:185e–6e.

10. Saeed WR, Kay SP. Harvest of palmaris longus tendon: technique. J Hand Surg Br 1993;18(5):583–4.

11. Tucker JG, Choat D, Zubowicz VN. Videoscopically assisted fascia lata harvest for correction of recurrent ventral hernia. South Med J 1997;90:399–401.

12. Drever JM. A simple method for obtaining fascia lata grafts. Plast Reconstr Surg 1972;50(2):196–7. Available at: http://www.ncbi.nlm.nih.gov/pubmed/5045382.

13. Tay VS-L, Tan KS, Loh ICY. Minimally invasive fascia lata harvest. Plast Reconstr Surg Glob Open 2013;1(1):1–2.

14. Rubin LR, Mishriki Y, Lee G, et al. Anatomy of the nasolabial fold: The keystone of the smiling mechanism. Plast Reconstr Surg 1989;83(1):1–8.

15. Rubin L. The anatomy of the nasolabial fold: the keystone of the smiling mechanism. Plast Reconstr Surg 1999;103(2):687–94.

16. Glenn MG, Goode RL. Surgical treatment of the "marginal mandibular lip " deformity 1987;97:462–8.

17. Stupak HD, Maas CS. New procedures in facial plastic surgery using botulinum toxin A. Facial Plast Surg Clin North Am 2003;11(4):515–20.

18. Hussain G, Manktelow RT, Tomat LR. Depressor labii inferioris resection: an effective treatment for marginal mandibular nerve paralysis. Br J Plast Surg 2004; 57(6):502–10.

19. Lindsay RW, Edwards C, Smitson C, et al. A systematic algorithm for the management of lower lip asymmetry. Am J Otolaryngol 2011;32(1):1–7.

20. Ulkatan S, Waner M, Arranz-Arranz B, et al. New methodology for facial nerve monitoring in extracranial surgeries of vascular malformations. Clin Neurophysiol 2014;125(4):849–55.

21. Klosterman T, Ulkatan S, Romo T, et al. Congenital lower lip facial paralysis: selective neurectomy of the underappreciated cervical branch. Int J Pediatr Otorhinolaryngol 2018;109:144–8.

22. Tan S. Anterior belly of digastric muscle transfer: a useful technique in head and neck surgery. Head Neck 2002;24(10):947–54.

23. Terzis J, Kalantarian B. Microsurgical strategies in 74 patients for restoration of dynamic depressor muscle mechanism: a neglected target in facial reanimation. Plast Reconstr Surg 2000;105(6):1917–31.

24. Manktelow R. Microsurgical strategies in 74 patients for restoration of dynamic depressor muscle mechanism: a neglected target in facial reanimation. No title. Plast Reconstr Surg 2000;105(6):1932–4.

25. Starmer H, Lyford-Pike S, Ishii LE, et al. Quantifying labial strength and function in facial paralysis. JAMA Facial Plast Surg 2015;17(4):274.

26. Biglioli F, Allevi F, Battista V, et al. Lipofilling of the atrophied lip in facial palsy patients. Minerva Stomatol 2014;63(3):69–75.

27. Coleman SR. Facial augmentation with structural fat grafting. Clin Plast Surg 2006;33:567–77.

28. Barret JP, Sarobe N, Grande N, et al. Maximizing results for lipofilling in facial reconstruction. Clin Plast Surg 2009;36(3):487–92.

Facial Rehabilitation
Evaluation and Treatment Strategies for the Patient with Facial Palsy

Mara Wernick Robinson, PT, MS, NCS*, Jennifer Baiungo, PT, MS

KEYWORDS

- Facial rehabilitation • Physical therapy • Neuromuscular retraining • Synkinesis
- Postsurgical facial reanimation

KEY POINTS

- Evaluation of the patient with facial palsy includes the Sunnybrook Facial Grading System, eFACE, FaCE (Facial Clinimetric Evaluation), and the Facial Disability Index.
- Facial rehabilitation treatment strategies are used for adults and children with peripheral unilateral and bilateral facial palsy.
- Neuromuscular retraining, synkinesis management, and chemodenervation are essential in the treatment of postparalysis synkinesis.
- Rehabilitation optimizes facial function after surgical dynamic facial reanimation.
- A multidisciplinary team approach in the management of patients with facial palsy is most effective.

 Video content accompanies this article at http://oto.theclinics.com/.

INTRODUCTION

Rehabilitation of the paralyzed face addresses both the physical and psychological aspects of facial disability. Individuals with facial palsy suffer from lack of facial expression, as well as a host of functional limitations, including oral incompetence, articulation difficulties, and visual impairments. Furthermore, when the ability to express emotions is sacrificed, patients are classified as having a negative affect.[1–3] Quality of life is frequently affected, and anxiety and depression may develop.[1,4] Lack of treatment of the sequelae associated with incomplete or aberrant nerve regeneration can lead to dysfunctional facial movements and devastating psychosocial

Disclosure Statement: No disclosure.
Facial Plastic and Reconstructive Surgery Department, Facial Nerve Center, Massachusetts Eye and Ear Infirmary, Facial Nerve Center, 9th Floor, 243 Charles Street, Boston, MA 02114, USA
* Corresponding author.
E-mail address: mara_robinson@meei.harvard.edu

Otolaryngol Clin N Am 51 (2018) 1151–1167
https://doi.org/10.1016/j.otc.2018.07.011
oto.theclinics.com

consequences. Restoring facial function to the highest degree results in improved self-esteem and quality of life.[5–7] People who experience facial palsy, irrespective of cause, can benefit from facial rehabilitation intervention.[5,6,8–12] Facial rehabilitation is also an essential component of postoperative management following dynamic facial reanimation.[7]

EVALUATION

Initial evaluation of the patient with facial palsy includes review of the medical record, followed by history of the present illness, including timing of onset and degree of facial palsy, and associated symptoms (eg, hearing loss, dizziness). Measurement of impairments, functional limitations, and degree of disability is gathered through clinician-graded outcome measures, still photographs, video, and patient-reported outcome measures.

The most widely used, and objective, clinician-graded outcome measurement among rehabilitation therapists is the Sunnybrook Facial Grading System (FGS). The FGS is a performance-based measure of facial impairment in 3 areas: resting symmetry compared with the unaffected side, symmetry of voluntary movement of 5 facial movements, and associated synkinesis.[13] Reliability and validity,[13,14] as well as intrarater repeatability,[15] have been established. The measurement of synkinesis, however, has been found to be less reliable.[16] An example of the FGS score is shown in **Fig. 1**B. The eFACE is an electronic clinician-graded facial function scale that generates an overall disfigurement score and offers simple graphic output.[17,18] Similar to the Sunnybrook FGS, the eFACE measures static position, dynamic movement, and synkinesis patterns. An example of the eFACE score is shown in **Fig. 1**C. Additional facial movement patterns that are not included in the Sunnybrook FGS and eFACE (eg, lower lip depression, lip approximation, lip rolling, and scowl) should also be examined. It is also useful to analyze facial expression during spontaneous conversation and note the amount of symmetry, movement, and synkinesis when a patient emotes. Gathering personal, professional, and recreational information from the patient while also analyzing spontaneous facial expression helps to formulate individual patient goals. Finally, a set of still photographs and a video of facial expression is a useful adjunct to objective data.

Patient-reported outcome measures provide useful and, perhaps, the most important, data. The FaCE instrument is a disease-specific, self-reported 15-item questionnaire that is widely used in patients with facial nerve disorders.[19] Domains of the questionnaire relate to both impairment and disability categories, and are considered to be quality-of-life measurements for patients with facial palsy. The reliability and validity of the FaCE is strong[19] and a positive correlation between an initial Sunnybrook FGS score and an initial FaCE score has been demonstrated.[20] The Facial Disability Index (FDI) is another widely used self-reporting tool for the assessment of physical disability and psychosocial factors related to facial nerve injury. This 10-item questionnaire has 2 5-item subscales: the physical function subscale, which assesses daily life activities such as tooth brushing, eating, and drinking; and the social wellbeing subscale, which includes items related to psychological and social aspects.[1,21–24] The FDI has been shown to have reliability, as well as construct validity, of the physical function subscale with the clinician's physical examination of facial movement.[24] The Synkinesis Assessment Questionnaire (SAQ) is a simple patient-graded instrument designed to self-rate facial synkinesis associated with facial expression. The SAQ has been demonstrated to have high test-retest reliability, internal consistency, and construct validity.[25]

A   Facial Synkinesis

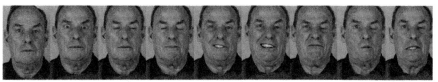

B   Sunnybrook Facial Grading System

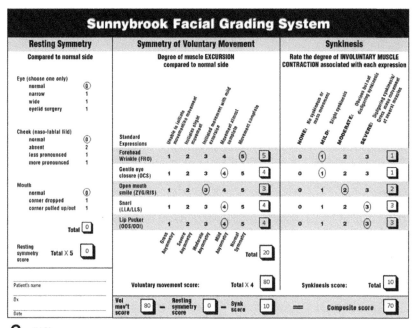

C   eFACE

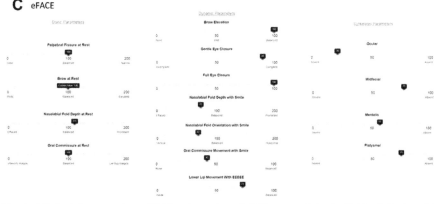

Fig. 1. (*A*) Facial expressions. (*B*) The Sunnybrook FGS score of the individual depicted in the photographic series. (*C*) The eFACE score of the individual depicted in the photographic series. (*Courtesy of* Sunnybrook Health Sciences Centre, Toronto, Ontario, Canada; with permission.)

Given the variability of facial palsy and individual personalities, it is imperative to gain the patient's perspective on their limitations to develop an individualized treatment plan. Inquiring, "What bothers you the most?" is a very useful and direct question that can guide and prioritize treatment intervention. For example, some patients may highlight the inability to smile, or a slight smile asymmetry, whereas others are solely bothered by ocular discomfort or facial tightness.

The remainder of the evaluation of the patient with facial palsy should include testing of sensation to light touch, range of motion of the temporomandibular joint, and screening of the remaining cranial nerves. The latter may prove useful if the referring diagnosis does not support clinical examination findings. Obtaining the patient's past medical history, and screening the patient's neurologic, vestibular, and musculoskeletal systems, is necessary for treatment planning. Finally, and most importantly, the therapist must gain an understanding of the patient's goals and expectations of facial rehabilitation.

Results of the evaluation guide the clinician into thinking globally about the state of the facial muscles. Identifying the specific facial neuromuscular impairments guides the clinician on appropriate treatment strategies. Understanding facial nerve pathologic conditions and the potential for nerve recovery guides the clinician in formulating realistic goals. Generally speaking, patients can be further classified into the acute or subacute stages of facial nerve injury (ie, within 6 months of onset of facial nerve insult) or chronic facial palsy (ie, >6 months), with or without synkinesis (**Fig. 2**).

TREATMENT

Facial rehabilitation for all patients typically includes 5 main components: (1) patient education to explain the pathologic condition and set realistic goals; (2) soft tissue mobilization to address facial muscle tightness and edema; (3) functional retraining to improve oral competence; (4) facial expression retraining, including neuromuscular reeducation; and (5) synkinesis management (when appropriate).

The emphasis of facial rehabilitation is on teaching the patient self-management strategies. Education in the anatomy of the facial nerve, the muscles it innervates, and the role of individual facial muscles during expressions is included. Treatment sessions are designed to identify areas of functional and communicative limitation, and patients are guided on independent soft tissue mobilization techniques and motor control exercises as part of their individualized home program. Patients are taught to identify, develop, and refine appropriate movement patterns and facial expressions through neuromuscular retraining (NMR), a process of facilitating the return of intended facial movement patterns and eliminating or lessening unwanted patterns of facial movement, or synkinesis, due to aberrant nerve regeneration.

VanSwearingen and colleagues initially described 4 basic treatment categories as a guide for therapeutic intervention strategies.[6,11,26,27]

Initiation

Patients who present with complete facial paralysis due to an acute facial nerve injury, or have a delayed recovery following facial nerve damage, begin treatment with initiation strategies because the main goal is to help patients initiate movement from the flaccid or weak muscles. Patients present with lack of muscle activation on the involved side, including incomplete eye closure, and lack synkinesis. Individuals with acute facial palsy typically have impaired articulation, oral incompetence, and inability to express emotions.

Treatment of patients in the initiation category includes education about facial muscle anatomy; expectations for recovery; gentle eyelid stretching; soft tissue

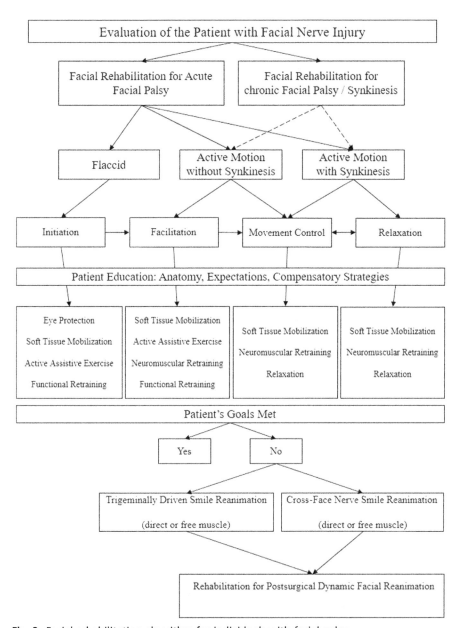

Fig. 2. Facial rehabilitation algorithm for individuals with facial palsy.

mobilization, initiation, or active-assistive movement exercises; and compensatory strategies for functional deficits.

Patients in this category often present with lagophthalmos due to weakness of the orbicularis oculi musculature and unopposed action of the levator palpebrae superioris.[28,29] The lack of active motion of the orbicularis oculi may cause formation of cross-linkages between the myosin and actin filaments in the levator muscle fibers. Patients are taught to stretch the superior eyelid for 30 seconds, to passively lengthen the levator palpebrae superioris, and effectively interrupt the cross-bridges. Immediately following the stretch, patients experience improved eye closure.[28] An example of the eyelid stretch is shown in **Fig. 3**. Soft tissue mobilization techniques are provided to affected facial muscles to improve circulation and muscle health. Some patients complain of tightness and fatigue on the uninvolved side, related to absence of antagonistic activity on the involved side, and can benefit from massage.

Patients are taught exercises to initiate movement of facial expression with manual or passive movement. For example, to improve smile excursion, the patient places the finger at the corner of the mouth and gently assists the oral commissure superiorly to encourage zygomaticus contraction. Importantly, patients are instructed to avoid mass movements of the face and focus on balanced facial expressions. Though symmetry and balance are stressed, education in compensatory strategies may be necessary for issues related to oral incompetence. Education regarding realistic recovery, expectations of rehabilitation, and importance of compliance with a home program is provided. As facial nerve regeneration occurs, the patient transitions to facilitation treatments; when regeneration is unlikely (eg, nerve transection), surgical reanimation is an option (see **Fig. 2**).

Facilitation

Patients with acute facial palsy who present with incomplete flaccid facial palsy without obvious synkinesis begin treatment with facilitation strategies because the main goal is to assist or facilitate motor return. Treatment in this category includes patient education, eyelid stretching, soft tissue mobilization, and NMR. Soft tissue mobilization is included when muscle tightness or tenderness to palpation is present in facial musculature. Active-assistive techniques are used here because minimal contraction is observed. When more obvious movement occurs to form a moderate degree of contraction, neuromuscular reeducation exercises, including mime therapy (ie, emotional expression exercises), are taught.[5,9,11] The importance of slow-controlled symmetric movements and avoidance of mass movement is reinforced.[5,6,11,27] Patients are taught to dampen the uninvolved facial muscles to minimize opposing forces, in an effort to gain movement on the involved side. For example, patients are taught to smile on the unaffected side only to the same degree as possible on the affected side. This permits production of a balanced smile without overpowering the affected side by the opposing force of the unaffected side. Because

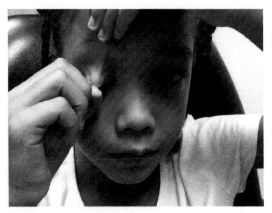

Fig. 3. Eyelid stretch.

the intrinsic muscle and joint receptors that would normally provide proprioceptive feedback are few or absent in the facial muscles, visual feedback, in the form of a mirror[11] or the use of camera technology on hand-held and desktop devices, is used to guide movement. Surface electromyography (EMG) biofeedback can serve as an adjunct to the reeducation process, providing visual or audio feedback to the patient regarding recruitment of motor units during NMR, as well as decreasing muscle activity on the contralateral side for symmetry.[27,30]

Movement Control

Patients who demonstrate active motion in some or all zones of the face but also present with synkinesis due to aberrant nerve regeneration, begin treatment using movement control strategies. Movement control treatment strategies are designed to teach the patient to activate specific facial expressions while also releasing or dampening the synkinesis contractions that are limiting intended movements.

Patient education about the phenomenon of synkinesis and the patient's specific synkinetic patterns are vital components of the treatment plan. NMR teaches patients to mindfully relax or release the tension in the synkinetic musculature while simultaneously performing associated facial movements. For example, the patient is taught to form a small symmetric smile while also controlling periocular synkinesis (**Fig. 4**, Video 1). Controlling synkinesis can be described to the patient as releasing the tension as in slowly draining the air out of an inflated tire. Patients are taught to use the unaffected side as a template for what normal feels like. Conscious control of synkinesis is challenging for most patients and requires utmost concentration. Frequent practice of NMR exercises is required for neural plasticity to permit long-lasting new neural pathways because the ultimate goal is improved spontaneous

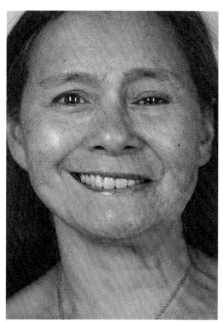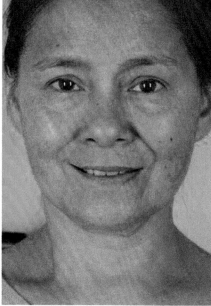

Fig. 4. Smile expression photographs of an individual who presented with chronic left-sided facial palsy and synkinesis at initial evaluation (*left*), followed by facial rehabilitation and chemodenervation (*right*).

facial expression with fewer intense involuntary synkinetic movement patterns. It is important that NMR exercise repetitions are of good quality to avoid reinforcement of the abnormal movement pattern. Recommendations for frequency and duration of the prescribed NMR routine is based on an individual's presentation, motivational level, and specific goals.

As conscious control of synkinesis improves, patients are taught to incorporate NMR concepts into daily facial activities.[11] A patient who experiences periocular synkinesis while eating or drinking is instructed to attempt to control the synkinesis during this activity (Video 2). Although constant attention to automatic movements is unrealistic, some degree of awareness is beneficial. With repetition, neural plasticity may allow for improved facial function over time. Similar to the process in the facilitation category, patients begin learning movement patterns with visual feedback via a mirror or camera, or with EMG biofeedback. As patients develop greater appreciation for synkinetic control with visual feedback, they are encouraged to move away from visual or EMG feedback and rely on kinesthetic awareness. The patient with acute facial palsy who began treatment with initiation or facilitation strategies may transition into needing movement control strategies if synkinesis evolves (see **Fig. 2**).

Relaxation

Patients with chronic facial paralysis who present with severe synkinesis begin treatment with relaxation strategies. Patients present with significant asymmetry related to muscle tightness, and moderate to severe synkinesis. Patients typically complain of facial tension and discomfort on the affected side. Aggressive soft tissue mobilization techniques and synkinesis control through relaxation strategies are taught as a primary intervention. The use of an audio relaxation recording, using guided visual imagery to release facial tension, and using mindfulness to dampen synkinesis, is recommended. With time, patients may learn to spontaneously use relaxation techniques to release facial tension. After muscle tension decreases, the patient can learn movement control strategies.

Instructions for the frequency and intensity of massage and NMR exercises are provided to the patient as an individualized home exercise program encouraging daily practice. Written explanations with illustrations, or video instruction, influence the quality of performance, motivation, and confidence to perform the complex exercises. Subsequent therapy sessions focus on modifying and advancing the home program based on the degree of facial nerve recovery and the patient's degree of motor learning. Reviewing previous exercises and providing new strategies at each session enhances the patient's interest and compliance. Clinician-reported and patient-reported outcomes should be administered every 6 to 8 weeks to gauge progress. The average patient with facial palsy is seen for a total of 6 to 12 months. Yearly reevaluations to ensure maintenance and review the home program are suggested. Given the long-standing nature of facial palsy and synkinesis, long-term commitment to home exercise programs is emphasized.

SPECIAL CONSIDERATIONS

Not all patients belong precisely in a treatment category. The experienced clinician should collaborate with the entire facial nerve team to maximize patient outcomes based on the diagnosis. Additionally, patients with bilateral facial palsy, pediatric cases, or patients with an unclear cause pose a challenge for the rehabilitation therapist.

Bilateral Facial Paralysis

Bilateral facial paralysis, a rare disorder with an incidence of less than 2% of all cases of facial palsy, can stem from various causes.[31] The FGS and eFACE are not reliable scales for this patient population due to lack of an uninvolved side of the face for grading comparison.[14,32] Patients may present with acute onset of bilateral flaccid facial palsy, bilateral chronic facial palsy, or chronic facial palsy on 1 side with the contralateral facial palsy. These scenarios represent a unique management strategy in which elements of each of the different approaches are introduced into the care plan. Compensatory strategies for oral incompetence and impairments in articulation are priority treatments for patients with bilateral facial palsy. Bilateral ocular synkinesis poses a safety concern if there is significant loss of the visual field and is often managed successfully with chemodenervation.

Pediatrics

Facial palsy in the pediatric population is also a rare condition, with an incidence of 21.1 per 100,000 per year for children younger than the age of 15 years.[33] There are many causes of facial palsy in children, including congenital or acquired (eg, inflammatory, neoplastic, traumatic, or iatrogenic causes) facial palsy.[33,34] Classification of a child's facial nerve insult, as well as the basics of the treatment intervention, are similar to that of an adult. However, the strategies and delivery of treatment are altered to be more child-friendly, and to accommodate the specific interest and personality of a child. For example, children are engaged by technology and, therefore, computerized games and applications are successful strategies. Stickers or face paint on the facial muscles can be used in place of surface electrodes to provide feedback about symmetric movements. Lollipops, bubbles, and whistles are used to teach oral motor control. Goals of very young children (and their parents) with facial paralysis typically include improving the ability to drink, eat, and speak clearly, whereas the goals of a teenager are more likely taking photographs for social media, and improving self-confidence in school, recreational activities, and social interactions.

CHEMODENERVATION

Chemodenervation, using botulinum toxin (eg, Botox), is commonly used to eliminate inappropriate movements caused by synkinesis.[35–38] Numerous studies have shown its efficacy, including improvements in Sunnybrook FGS scores,[39] as well as quality-of-life scores.[39,40] Precise botulinum toxin injections decrease the strength of the synkinetic contraction. For example, injection into the superior and inferior oculi will diminish the involuntary eye closure often seen with smiling and puckering in these patients. The pattern and intensity of synkinesis varies among patients, therefore each chemodenervation plan is individualized. To balance facial expression, chemodenervation is also beneficial in treating the contralateral, nonparalyzed side. For example, weakening the contralateral depressor labii inferioris is often used to address lower lip asymmetry during speech and smiling.

The facial rehabilitation therapist plays an integral role in the development and modification of chemodenervation therapy. It is imperative that individuals have a good understanding of the phenomenon of synkinesis and its effect on facial motor control before initiating botulinum toxin injections. Patients seem to gain the most benefit from facial rehabilitation when chemodenervation is initiated after the patient has participated in facial rehabilitation and achieved some degree of conscious control over their synkinesis. **Fig. 5** demonstrates the progress made by a patient with a 4-year history of Bell palsy after participating in facial rehabilitation for 3 months, followed by initial chemodenervation injections. Multiple sessions of skilled facial rehabilitation, including reevaluation with clinician-reported and patient-reported outcome measures, as well

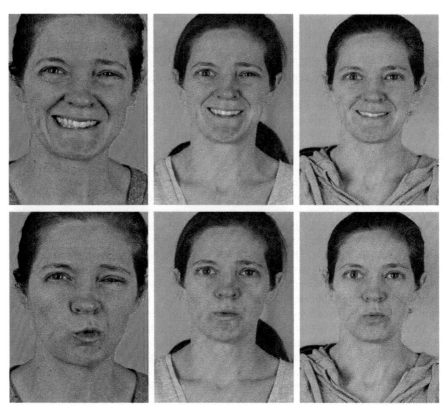

Fig. 5. Smile (*top row*) and pucker (*bottom row*) photographs of an individual who presented with chronic left-side facial palsy and synkinesis, at initial evaluation (*left column*), followed by facial rehabilitation for 3 months (*middle column*), and followed by initial chemodenervation injections (*right column*).

as photographs, enables the therapist and patient to assess the effects of chemodenervation, and to provide feedback to modify injection sites and dosage if needed.

REHABILITATION FOR POSTSURGICAL DYNAMIC FACIAL REANIMATION

For patients with complete facial paralysis, for example, when the facial nerve has been sacrificed during tumor extirpation, or transected secondary to a temporal bone fracture, surgical intervention to restore nerve function may be the only option in hopes of restoration of facial expression. For patients with postparalytic facial palsy who have not regained adequate commissure excursion, facial reanimation surgery is also an option to restore a meaningful smile.[41–43] The decision to advance from facial rehabilitation to dynamic surgical reanimation is made by the patient and the entire treatment team with the primary motivation being patient satisfaction. Facial rehabilitation intervention is then indicated to maximize smile restoration, as well as to maximize function following surgery.

Several surgical procedures have been described for smile restoration.[41,44–46] Common surgical reanimation strategies include nerve transfer to the native facial musculature controlling the smile using the ipsilateral nerve to masseter in isolation or in conjunction with other nerve transfers (eg, cross-facial nerve grafts or hypoglossal nerve transfer), or functional free muscle transfer for smile reanimation using nerve to masseter and/or a cross-facial nerve graft from smile branches of the contralateral facial nerve.

The ipsilateral nerve to masseter provides powerful neuronal input for smile reanimation; however, patients must learn to bite down (ie, clench the jaw) to activate smile. This initially may feel unnatural, necessitating more intense rehabilitation than would otherwise be required when reanimated smile is driven by cross-facial nerve grafting. Though cross-facial nerve graft–driven smile provides spontaneity, axonal density through the graft is far less than that obtained from the nerve to masseter, resulting in higher failure rates.[41,46] The appropriate surgical intervention is based on the location of nerve injury, the degree of facial paralysis, the length of time since onset, and individual patient factors such as age, prognosis, patient choice, and surgeon choice and experience.[41,43] Each approach has advantages and disadvantages and should be individualized for each patient.

For all patients undergoing surgical reanimation, facial rehabilitation includes 4 main components: (1) patient education to review facial anatomy and patient expectations, (2) soft tissue mobilization to manage postoperative edema and muscle tightness, (3) functional retraining to improve oral competence, and (4) smile retraining specific to the facial reanimation surgery performed.

NERVE TO MASSETER–DRIVEN SMILE

Following nerve to masseter transfer to native midfacial musculature, or to free muscle, a smile occurs when the patient bites down as a result of innervation by the trigeminal motor branches. Muscle activity from biting down occurs approximately 2 to 5 months postoperatively, with an average gain in commissure excursion of 8 mm.[47,48] Patients are referred for facial rehabilitation approximately 2 months postoperatively with the goal of educating the patient about movement expectations, soft tissue massage, and identification of any movement from biting down. The goal of soft tissue mobilization is to decrease postsurgical edema that commonly occurs following surgery.

Four rehabilitation stages of motor learning for patients who have undergone nerve to masseter–driven smile reanimation surgery are described in the following sections. The 4 stages are designed to guide therapists and patients with a general framework of progression (**Table 1**).

Stage 1. Biting Down to Engage the Masseter for Commissure Excursion

The patient is instructed to gently bite down on a soft medium placed between the contralateral or unilateral molars. Commonly used mediums include a mouth guard, gauze pad, or chewy soft candy. The patient places the medium between their molars, looks at the affected commissure, and bites down. The goal of this stage is to simply teach the patient that biting down generates movement of the commissure. Next, the patient is taught to grade the amount of tension used to bite down to generate movement, using a visual analog scale from 0 to 10, in which 0 represents no biting and 10 represents maximal bite effort. Therapy involves teaching the patient to bite down with the least amount of effort required to achieve ideal excursion. Initially, patients must often bite down with maximal effort to drive smile, with less effort required over time. Patients are educated that they may experience fatigue in the masseter during practice. In addition to biting down, patients are taught to perform self-guided effleurage massage to the midface. The patient is instructed on range-of-motion exercises to facilitate jaw opening to prevent temporomandibular joint dysfunction that may occur from forceful and repetitive biting.

Table 1
Stages of facial rehabilitation following ipsilateral nerve to masseter–driven smile reanimation surgery

Stage	Key Points of Rehabilitation	Time Frame
1. Commissure excursion: bite down to engage masseter for isolated commissure excursion	Massage the zygomaticus or gracilis Mirror feedback for commissure excursion Bite down on soft medium (eg, candy) Visual analog scale 10–20 repetitions, 2–3/d	Movement begins 2–5 mos after surgery Practice 2–4 wks, depending on the strength of the contraction
2. Voluntary posed smile: bite down to smile symmetrically	Massage the zygomaticus or gracilis Mirror feedback to bite down and smile with goal of • Symmetry • Normal timing between affected and unaffected side 10–20 repetitions, 2–3/d	Smile symmetry practice begins within 2 wks of initial sign of movement Practice 4–12 wks depending on motivation of the patient
3. Voluntary engaging smile: bite down to smile during conversation	Massage the zygomaticus or gracilis Engage frequently in habits of smiling during routine points daily; for example, "good morning" followed by a biting smile	Practice 4–12 wks depending on motivation of the patient
4. Spontaneous smile: smile without biting	Use of smile without biting may eventually become automatic after intense practice	Depends on patient understanding and motivation

Stage 2. Biting Down to Smile Symmetrically: Voluntary Posed Smile

After meaningful commissure excursion (ie, greater than approximately 4 mm of movement) is demonstrated, patients are instructed on integration of bite-effort with concurrent smiling on the contralateral (ie, healthy) side. The patient is instructed to gently bite down, using mirror feedback, while simultaneously forming a small balanced smile. The goal of this stage is to teach the patient that biting down generates a smile. As in stage 1, the patient is taught to grade the amount of tension used to bite down to generate movement, using a visual analog scale. The patient is taught to bite down with the least amount of effort to achieve smile symmetry. Patients are encouraged to envision a happy thought while gently biting down to trigger smile on the healthy side, typically with the lips together to achieve a natural appearing grin (closed-mouth smile). The goal is to form a voluntary posed smile that is balanced and symmetric. This biting smile is considered by patients to be an acceptable posed smile that can be generated in photographs. The patient then progresses to biting down using a thicker structure (eg, thicker gauze) that demands less biting effort.

Stage 3. Biting Down to Smile During Conversation: Voluntary Engaging Smile

The goal of this stage is to voluntarily form a biting smile while engaging in conversation. This smile displays pleasure or demonstrates agreement during conversation. The patient should begin using the biting smile during conversation and to transition into using the biting smile consciously throughout daily interactions. For example, when meeting a friend, coworker, or a family member, the intent is to say a typical pleasant greeting followed by a biting smile. Over time, this type of biting smile should transition from a conscious and voluntary motor plan to an automatic gesture displaying a smile. Video 3 demonstrates a cumulative 4-month process, of stages 1 through

3, of a patient who underwent free gracilis transfer driven by the masseteric branch of the trigeminal nerve.

Stage 4. Smile Without Biting: Spontaneous Smile

The ultimate goal of smile reanimation surgery is a spontaneous smile. The ability for patients who have undergone nerve to masseter reanimation procedures that require biting down to execute a smile to form a spontaneous smile is variable. The percentage of patients who acquire a spontaneous smile following the masseteric nerve surgery has not been well characterized, in part due to the challenge of assessing spontaneous smile.[49] How some patients achieve spontaneous smile following smile reanimation driven by motor branches of the trigeminal nerve is unclear. Coactivation of the masseter muscle with smile is known to occur naturally in some patients and may explain spontaneity seen postopereatively.[50] Alternatively, cortical neuroplasticity might result in spontaneous bite-activated smile in the postoperative state.[49,51]

FACIAL REHABILITATION FOLLOWING FREE MUSCLE TRANSFER DRIVEN BY A CROSS-FACE NERVE GRAFT

Cross-face nerve graft–driven smile reanimation results in spontaneous movement. Patients who have undergone 2-stage free gracilis transfer for smile reanimation by cross-facial nerve grafting are expected to see muscle activity approximately 5 to 9 months following the second stage.[52] Contraction of the free muscle is generated when the patient smiles either voluntarily or spontaneously. Although spontaneous smiling seems straightforward, 2 to 4 rehabilitation sessions are indicated to teach the patient how to facilitate movement and symmetry. Patients are instructed to perform both maximal effort smiles (including exposure to funny videos or situations that facilitate smiling and laughter) followed by symmetric, perhaps even smaller excursion, smiles. The use of a mirror or camera for visual feedback helps the patient appreciate new movement. Surface EMG biofeedback may also be used. Soft tissue mobilization and functional retraining for oral competence is also indicated.

Smile reanimation surgery has become a mainstay in the management of patients with facial palsy. Objective outcomes following free muscle transfer using the gracilis have demonstrated quantifiable improvements in resting symmetry and in the amount of oral commissure excursion.[7,44,47,48] Although outcomes measures from facial rehabilitation following such surgery has yet to be reported in the literature, facial rehabilitation exercises are suggested by most surgeons. Quality-of-life measures have demonstrated improved function following surgical intervention in a clinic where most patients receive facial rehabilitation following surgery.[7,43,44] **Fig. 6** shows preoperative and postoperative photographs of patients who reported excellent patient satisfaction following dynamic facial reanimation surgery and facial rehabilitation.

PSYCHOLOGY OF FACIAL EXPRESSION

The ability to activate facial muscles alone is inadequate to perform the complex interactions involved in facial expression. Facial expression, including functional actions such as communication and personal interactions, are both cortically and subcortically driven. Cortically mediated expressions are voluntary, with an intended facial function, such as protruding the lips to drink from a cup. Subcortical actions are typically driven by a reaction such as surprise or laughter. Although difficult to achieve, the skill of connecting the cortical and subcortical responses is the ultimate goal of facial

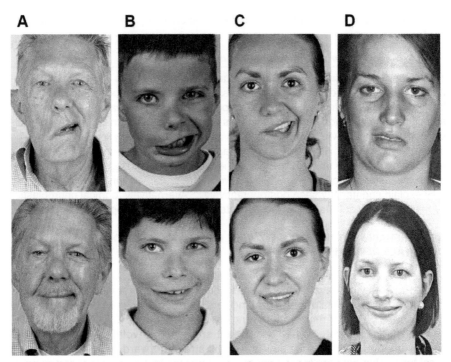

Fig. 6. Smiles of individuals who participated in facial rehabilitation at presentation (*top row*) and after rehabilitation for dynamic reanimation surgery (*bottom row*). (*A*) Functional free muscle (gracilis) transfer using ipsilateral nerve to masseter nerve. (*B*) Functional free muscle (gracilis) driven by a cross-facial nerve graft from smile branches. (*C*) Ipsilateral nerve to masseter nerve to native facial muscles. (*D*) Bilateral free muscle (gracilis) driven by ipsilateral nerves to masseter nerves.

rehabilitation. Because emotions elicit a set of stereotypical facial muscle contractions of an expression, the alternative may also be true. Facial muscle activity may elicit or reinforce emotions (facial feedback hypothesis); for example, the inability to smile and psychological distress.[8,53] Little is actually known about the contribution of deficient facial feedback to the psychosocial problems of individuals with facial palsy; however, limited social interactions and depression are commonly reported. Therapists should guide treatment in specific facial expressions connected to emotions for optimal recovery.[8,9,11,54]

Additionally, individuals with facial palsy are taught to alter their verbal tone and body language to improve self-expression and nonverbal communication. Hairstyle modifications can help to minimize appearances of facial asymmetries, especially in the brow region. The use of accessories, such as eye glasses, earrings, necklaces, scarves, and make-up, may draw attention away from facial asymmetry. Patients are encouraged to participate in physical exercise to alleviate stress and improve health and overall wellbeing. When emotional distress interferes with rehabilitation, referral for psychological support is indicated.

SUMMARY

Although facial rehabilitation cannot restore perfect premorbid appearance and function, appropriate intervention can make a substantial difference in facial muscle motor control with the ultimate goal of improved physical function, enhanced appearance, and increased patient self-confidence. Patient education, including management of expectations, is crucial. Rehabilitation goals must be tailored to the individual on a functional, cosmetic, and emotional level. Realistic functional outcomes include improved ability to smile, eat, drink, speak clearly, and blink on the affected side. Additionally, reduction of facial pain and tension in the affected musculature is achieved. At the interpersonal level, willingness to participate in social activities and improved self-confidence are realistic goals. Patients who possess the motivation necessary to commit to a consistent and thorough home program are most successful.

SUPPLEMENTARY DATA

Supplementary data related to this article can be found online at https://doi.org/10.1016/j.otc.2018.07.011.

REFERENCES

1. Coulson SE, O'dwyer NJ, Adams RD, et al. Expression of emotion and quality of life after facial nerve paralysis. Otol Neurotol 2004;25(6):1014–9.
2. Ishii LE, Godoy A, Encarnacion CO, et al. What faces reveal: impaired affect display in facial paralysis. Laryngoscope 2011;121(6):1138–43.
3. Bogart KR, Tickle-Degnen L, Ambady N. Communicating without the face: holistic perception of emotions of people with facial paralysis. Basic Appl Soc Psych 2014;36(4):309–20.
4. Fu L, Bundy C, Sadiq SA. Psychological distress in people with disfigurement from facial palsy. Eye 2011;25(10):1322–6.
5. Diels HJ, Combs D. Neuromuscular retraining for facial paralysis. Otolaryngol Clin North Am 1997;30(5):727–43.
6. Lindsay RW, Robinson M, Hadlock TA. Comprehensive facial rehabilitation improves function in people with facial paralysis: a 5-year experience at the Massachusetts Eye and Ear Infirmary. Phys Ther 2010;90(3):391–7.
7. Lindsay RW, Bhama P, Hadlock TA. Quality-of-life improvement after free gracilis muscle transfer for smile restoration in patients with facial paralysis. JAMA Facial Plast Surg 2014;16(6):419.
8. Byrne PJ. Importance of facial expression in facial nerve rehabilitation. Curr Opin Otolaryngol Head Neck Surg 2004;12:332–5.
9. Beurskens CHG, Heymans PG. Mime therapy improves facial symmetry in people with long-term facial nerve paresis: a randomised controlled trial. Aust J Physiother 2006;52(3):177–83.
10. Manikandan N. Effect of facial neuromuscular re-education on facial symmetry in patients with Bell's palsy: a randomized controlled trial. Clin Rehabil 2007;21(4):338–43.
11. VanSwearingen J. Facial rehabilitation: a neuromuscular reeducation, patient-centered approach. Facial Plast Surg 2008;24(2):250–9.
12. Teixeira LJ, Valbuza J, Prado GF. Physical therapy for Bell s palsy (idiopathic facial paralysis). Cochrane Database Syst Rev 2008;(3):CD006283.
13. Ross BG, Fradet G, Nedzelski JM. Development of a sensitive clinical facial grading system. Otolaryngol Head Neck Surg 1996;114(3):380–6.
14. Neely JG, Cherian NG, Dickerson CB, et al. Sunnybrook facial grading system: Reliability and criteria for grading. Laryngoscope 2010;120(5):1038–45.

15. Kanerva M, Poussa T, Pitkäranta A. Sunnybrook and House-Brackmann facial grading systems: intrarater repeatability and interrater agreement. Otolaryngol - Head Neck Surg 2006;135(6):865–71.

16. Coulson SE, Croxson GR, Adams RD, et al. Reliability of the "Sydney," "Sunnybrook," and "House Brackmann" facial grading systems to assess voluntary movement and synkinesis after facial nerve paralysis. Otolaryngol - Head Neck Surg 2005;132(4):543–9.

17. Banks CA, Bhama PK, Park J, et al. Clinician-graded electronic facial paralysis assessment: the eFACE. Plast Reconstr Surg 2015;136(2):223e–30e.

18. Banks CA, Jowett N, Azizzadeh B, et al. Worldwide testing of the eFACE facial nerve clinician-graded scale. Plast Reconstr Surg 2017;139(2):491e–8e.

19. Kahn JB, Gliklich RE, Boyev KP, et al. Validation of a patient-graded instrument for facial nerve paralysis: the FaCE scale. Laryngoscope 2001;111(3):387–98.

20. Ng JH, Ngo RYS. The use of the facial clinimetric evaluation scale as a patient-based grading system in Bell's palsy. Laryngoscope 2013;123(5):1256–60.

21. Brach JS, VanSwearingen J, Delitto A, et al. Impairment and disability in patients with facial neuromuscular dysfunction. Otolaryngol Head Neck Surg 1997;117(4):315–21.

22. Ho AL, Scott AM, Klassen AF, et al. Measuring quality of life and patient satisfaction in facial paralysis patients: a systematic review of patient-reported outcome measures. Plast Reconstr Surg 2012;130(1):91–9.

23. Samsudin WSW, Sundaraj K. Evaluation and grading systems of facial paralysis for facial rehabilitation. J Phys Ther Sci 2013;25(4):515–9.

24. VanSwearingen JM, Brach JS. The Facial Disability Index: reliability and validity of a disability assessment instrument for disorders of the facial neuromuscular system. Phys Ther 1996;76(12):1288–98, 300.

25. Mehta RP, Wernickrobinson M, Hadlock TA. Validation of the Synkinesis Assessment Questionnaire. Laryngoscope 2007;117(5):923–6.

26. Brach JS, VanSwearingen J. Physical therapy for facial paralysis: a tailored treatment approach. Phys Ther 1999;79:397–404.

27. Wernick Robinson M, Baiungo J, Hohman M, et al. Facial rehabilitation. Oper Tech Otolaryngol - Head Neck Surg 2012;23(4):288–96.

28. Aramideh M, Koelman JHTM, Devriese PP, et al. Thixotropy of levator palpebrae as the cause of lagophthalmos after peripheral facial nerve palsy. J Neurol Neurosurg Psychiatry 2002;72(5):665–7.

29. Cronin GW, Steenerson RL. The effectiveness of neuromuscular facial retraining combined with electromyography in facial paralysis rehabilitation. Otolaryngol Head Neck Surg 2003;128(4):534–8.

30. Nakamura K, Toda N, Sakamaki K, et al. Biofeedback rehabilitation for prevention of synkinesis after facial palsy. Otolaryngol Head Neck Surg 2003;128(4):539–43.

31. Gaudin RA, Jowett N, Banks CA, et al. Bilateral facial paralysis: a 13-year experience. Plast Reconstr Surg 2016;138(4):879–87.

32. Gaudin RA, Robinson M, Banks CA, et al. Emerging vs time-tested methods of facial grading among patients with facial paralysis. JAMA Facial Plast Surg 2016;18(4):251–7.

33. Banks CA, Hadlock TA. Pediatric facial nerve rehabilitation. Facial Plast Surg Clin North Am 2014;22(4):487–502.

34. Ciorba A, Corazzi V, Conz V, et al. Facial nerve paralysis in children. World J Clin Cases 2015;3(12):973–9.

35. Husseman J, Mehta RP. Management of synkinesis. Facial Plast Surg 2008;24(2):242–9.

36. Filipo R, Spahiu I, Covelli E, et al. Botulinum toxin in the treatment of facial synkinesis and hyperkinesis. Laryngoscope 2012;122(2):266–70.
37. Cabin JA, Massry GG, Azizzadeh B. Botulinum toxin in the management of facial paralysis. Curr Opin Otolaryngol Head Neck Surg 2015;23(4):272–80.
38. Mehdizadeh OB, Diels J, White WM. Botulinum toxin in the treatment of facial paralysis. Facial Plast Surg Clin North Am 2016;24(1):11–20.
39. Couch SM, Chundury RV, Holds JB. Subjective and objective outcome measures in the treatment of facial nerve synkinesis with onabotulinumtoxinA (Botox). Ophthal Plast Reconstr Surg 2014;30(3):246–50.
40. Mehta RP, Hadlock TA. Botulinum toxin and quality of life in patients with facial paralysis. Arch Facial Plast Surg 2008;10(2):84–7.
41. Henstrom DK. Masseteric nerve use in facial reanimation. Curr Opin Otolaryngol Head Neck Surg 2014;22(4):284–90.
42. Bhama PK, Hadlock TA. Contemporary facial reanimation. Facial Plast Surg 2014;30(2):145–51.
43. Jowett N, Hadlock TA. A contemporary approach to facial reanimation. JAMA Facial Plast Surg 2015;17(4):293–300.
44. Bhama PK, Weinberg JS, Lindsay RW, et al. Objective outcomes analysis following microvascular gracilis transfer for facial reanimation: a review of 10 years' experience. JAMA Facial Plast Surg 2014;16(2):85–92.
45. Garcia RM, Hadlock TA, Klebuc MJ, et al. Contemporary solutions for the treatment of facial nerve paralysis. Plast Reconstr Surg 2015;135(6):1025e–46e.
46. Sforza C, Frigerio A, Mapelli A, et al. Double-powered free gracilis muscle transfer for smile reanimation: a longitudinal optoelectronic study. J Plast Reconstr Aesthet Surg 2015;68(7):930–9.
47. Hontanilla B, Marre D, Cabello Á. Masseteric nerve for reanimation of the smile in short-term facial paralysis. Br J Oral Maxillofac Surg 2014;52(2):118–23.
48. Klebuc MJA. Facial reanimation using the masseter-to-facial nerve transfer. Plast Reconstr Surg 2011;127(5):1909–15.
49. Hontanilla B, Cabello A. Spontaneity of smile after facial paralysis rehabilitation when using a non-facial donor nerve. J Craniomaxillofac Surg 2016;44(9):1305–9.
50. Schaverien M, Moran G, Stewart K, et al. Activation of the masseter muscle during normal smile production and the implications for dynamic reanimation surgery for facial paralysis. J Plast Reconstr Aesthet Surg 2011;64(12):1585–9.
51. Buendia J, Loayza FR, Luis EO, et al. Functional and anatomical basis for brain plasticity in facial palsy rehabilitation using the masseteric nerve. J Plast Reconstr Aesthet Surg 2016;69(3):417–26.
52. Lindsay RW, Bhama P, Weinberg J, et al. The success of free Gracilis muscle transfer to restore smile in patients with nonflaccid facial paralysis. Ann Plast Surg 2014;73(2):177–82.
53. VanSwearingen JM, Cohn JF, Bajaj-Luthra A. Specific impairment of smiling increases the severity of depressive symptoms in patients with facial neuromuscular disorders. Aesthetic Plast Surg 1999;23(6):416–23.
54. Merkel KE, Schmidt KL, Levenstein RM, et al. Positive affect predicts improved lip movement in facial movement disorder. Otolaryngol Head Neck Surg 2007;137(1):100–4.

Surgical Management of Postparalysis Facial Palsy and Synkinesis

Babak Azizzadeh, MD[a,b,]*, Julia L. Frisenda, MD[b]

KEYWORDS

- Synkinesis • Facial paralysis • Smile dysfunction • Neurectomy
- Platysma myotomy • Spontaneous smile

KEY POINTS

- The treatment goals for patients with postfacial paralysis synkinesis are to improve resting oral commissure position, oral competence, facial and cervical tightness, and smile symmetry and spontaneity.
- Modified selective neurectomy of the facial nerve with platysma myotomy improves the spontaneous smile mechanism and overall function in patients with postfacial paralysis synkinesis.
- Modified selective neurectomy provides long-term results and can be performed in an outpatient setting with a short recovery period.
- This technique should be considered a stand-alone treatment of incomplete facial palsy and an alternative or adjunct to more invasive surgical options, such as free functional muscle transfer and temporalis myoplasty.

 Video content accompanies this article at http://www.oto.theclinics.com/.

INTRODUCTION

Synkinetic facial movement develops following facial nerve injury. It manifests as involuntary movement in the presence of voluntary movement. Any form of facial nerve repair, regeneration, or cranial nerve substitution after nerve insult can lead to synkinesis. Oral and smile dysfunction are among the most distressing

Disclosure Statement: Dr B. Azizzadeh receives royalties from Wiley, Thieme, Elsevier, and Springer. J.L. Frisenda has no financial or conflicts of interest to disclose. No funding was received for this article.
[a] Division of Head and Neck Surgery, David Geffen School of Medicine at the University of California, Los Angeles, Los Angeles, CA 90024, USA; [b] Department of Facial Plastic & Reconstructive Surgery, Center for Advanced Facial Plastic Surgery, 9401 Wilshire Boulevard, Suite 650, Beverly Hills, CA 90212, USA
* Corresponding author. Center for Advanced Facial Plastic Surgery, 9401 Wilshire Boulevard, Suite 650, Beverly Hills, CA 90212.
E-mail address: Drazizzadeh@gmail.com

Otolaryngol Clin N Am 51 (2018) 1169–1178
https://doi.org/10.1016/j.otc.2018.07.012
0030-6665/18/© 2018 Elsevier Inc. All rights reserved.

consequences of facial palsy because of the psychosocial impact and negative effect on quality of life.[1] Components of a natural smile include symmetric dental show, a superolateral oral commissure excursion, and appropriate orientation of the nasolabial fold. Spontaneity and symmetry are critical elements of an emotional and authentic smile.[2]

Synkinesis may begin as early as 3 to 4 months after the onset of facial paralysis and affects a significant percentage of patients after reversible facial nerve injury.[3-5] There are several theories to explain the mechanism of synkinesis. The most widely accepted theory is that of aberrant regeneration.[5-10] This theory hypothesizes that after nerve injury, proximal axons reroute, sprout, and/or degenerate leading to aberrant reinnervation of both correct and inappropriate muscles (**Fig. 1**). This phenomenon leads to opposing contraction of facial muscles and resulting deformity. Most patients with moderate to severe synkinesis have significant aesthetic consequences as well as functional deficits, such as narrowing of the eyelid aperture, facial asymmetry, platysmal tension, poor manipulation of the food bolus, and oral incompetence. Dysfunctional synkinetic movement of the orbicularis oris, platysma, depressor anguli oris, and buccinator muscles produce an inferior and lateral vector of pull on the oral commissure that is antagonistic to the key smile muscles (zygomatic major/minor, levator labii superioris, levator labii alaeque nasi, and depressor labii inferioris). Patients are left with a frozen or frowning smile and decreased upper and lower teeth show. The psychosocial sequelae of synkinesis can significantly impact patients' well-being.[11]

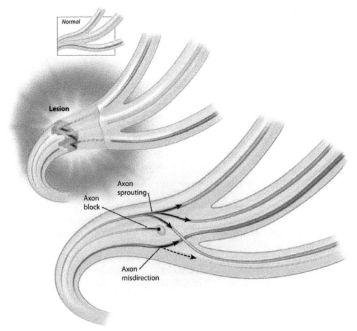

Fig. 1. Aberrant regeneration theory of synkinesis. After nerve injury, proximal axons reroute, sprout along multiple distal pathways, and/or degenerate, leading to reinnervation of both correct and incorrect muscles. (*Courtesy of* The Facial Paralysis Institute, Beverly Hills, CA; with permission.)

Treatment goals for patients with postfacial paralysis synkinesis are to improve oral competence, facial and cervical tightness, resting oral commissure position, and smile symmetry and spontaneity.[12–27] (Azizzadeh B, Irvine LE, Diels J, et al: Modified selective neurectomy for the treatment of post-facial paralysis synkinesis. Submitted for publication.) Very few, if any, previously described reanimation techniques achieve the components of a natural, spontaneous smile. This article details the authors' novel surgical approach for treating smile dysfunction in postfacial paralysis synkinesis with modified selective neurectomy.

SURGICAL PROCEDURE: MODIFIED SELECTIVE NEURECTOMY

All procedures are performed on an outpatient basis under general anesthesia. A standard rhytidectomy incision is used. The incision and the subcutaneous plane of the face is injected with 1:100,000 epinephrine. Lidocaine hydrochloride is not used in order to prevent inadvertent paresis of the facial nerve.

Facial nerve monitoring electrodes are placed in the periorbital and perioral regions. The skin flap is elevated anteriorly toward the nasolabial fold and toward the midline neck for approximately 5 cm. An incision is made in the superficial muscular aponeurotic system (SMAS) and the platysma and in an oblique vector from the lateral zygomatic arch to the cervical region passing through the angle of the mandible (**Fig. 2**). The SMAS and platysma are undermined for 3 to 5 cm. Blunt dissection is carried out deep to the masseteric and subplatysmal fascia in order to identify the branches of the facial nerve as they exit the parotid capsule.

All the visible branches of zygomatic, buccal, marginal mandibular, and cervical divisions of the facial nerve are identified and carefully dissected (**Fig. 3**). The connections between the zygomatic and buccal branches are isolated as well as side branches of the cervical branches, as they enter the underbelly of the platysma.[28] The nerve branches are then stimulated at 0.5 to 2.0 mA to evaluate the elicited movement. Video documentation is performed at this point to document the muscular activity (Video 1).

The nerves to be transected are branches that cause platysmal tightening or downward and lateral excursion of the oral commissure. Vascular clips are placed on the most proximal and distal portion of the dissected nerve, and 0.5 to 4.0 cm of intervening nerve is resected (**Fig. 4**). The zygomatic branches that purely elevate the oral commissure and the marginal mandibular branch that stimulates the depressor labii inferioris are carefully preserved.

The platysmal myotomy is performed below the identified marginal mandibular nerve.

After the modified selective neurectomy and platysmal myotomy are completed, the SMAS is returned to its native position. A drain is placed in the subcutaneous plane before closure. If patients are undergoing a simultaneous symmetrizing rhytidectomy, the SMAS is suspended in a superolateral vector. Deep plane rhytidectomy is often performed on the contralateral side to improve symmetry between the two sides.

Patients are discharged the same day. Patients usually return to work and routine social function in 7 to 10 days and start neuromuscular retraining in 1 month. Patients obtain fillers and/or botulinum toxin-A (BTX-A) for the periorbital region and contralateral face 1 week postoperatively as needed.

There have been no serious complications during or following the procedure. The most common side effects are hematoma formation and temporary oral incompetence. Seventeen percent of patients require a second procedure in which additional nerve branches are resected in order to obtain ideal results.

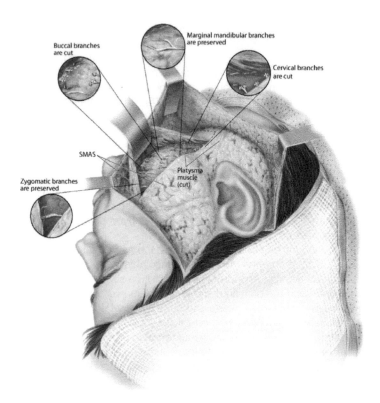

Fig. 2. Modified selective neurectomy surgery. After entering the plane deep to the SMAS and platysma muscle, multiple distal nerves are identified and tagged. Stimulation of each nerve is performed with video documentation, and cervical and buccal branches that cause downward or lateral excursion of the oral commissure and upper lip are transected. The marginal mandibular branches are identified and preserved along with zygomatic branches. (*Courtesy of* The Facial Paralysis Institute, Beverly Hills, CA; with permission.)

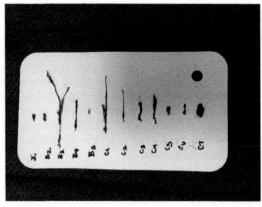

Fig. 3. Transected buccal and cervical nerve branches.

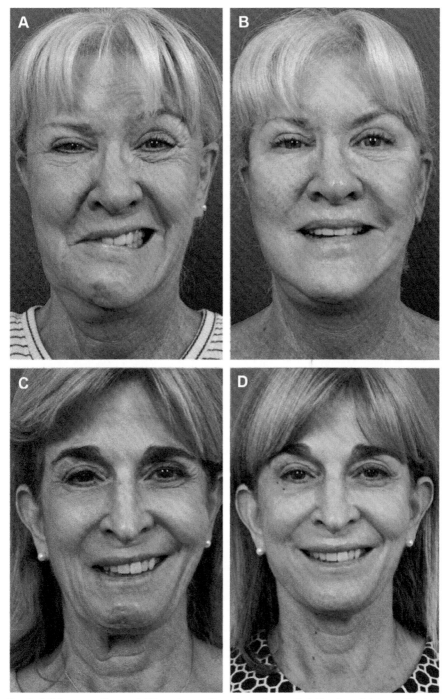

Fig. 4. (*A*) Preoperative and (*B*) postoperative photo 1 month following right modified selective neurectomy, platysma myotomy, revision bilateral rhytidectomy, autologous fat grafting, and periorbital botulinum toxin A. (*C*) Preoperative and (*D*) postoperative photos 10 months following right modified selective neurectomy, platysma myotomy, bilateral rhytidectomy, autologous fat grafting, and fractionated carbon dioxide laser resurfacing.

OUTCOMES

The electronic clinician-graded facial function scale (eFACE) has been shown by a cohort of facial nerve experts to be a useful cross-platform digital instrument for facial function assessment.[29,30] The eFACE application creates static, dynamic, and synkinesis scores as well as periocular, lower face and neck, midface, and smile scores. Using the eFACE, the authors' institution has previously reported that patients undergoing modified selective neurectomy with platysma myotomy have statistically significant improvement in oral commissure movement with smile, nasolabial fold depth at rest, nasolabial fold orientation with smile, lower lip movement with making the sound, "EEEE," midfacial synkinesis, mentalis synkinesis, platysmal synkinesis, static score, dynamic score, synkinesis score, lower face and neck score, midface and smile score, and total score. (Azizzadeh B, Irvine LE, Diels J, et al: Modified selective neurectomy for the treatment of post-facial paralysis synkinesis. Submitted for publication.) Patients had significant smile restoration by 4 months with the expected final outcome by 1 year.

PREVIOUSLY DESCRIBED TECHNIQUES IN SURGICAL MANAGEMENT

Coleman[31] first proposed total neurectomy of the main trunk of the facial nerve for hemifacial spasm in 1937. Complete facial nerve paralysis that was rehabilitated with a hypoglossal-facial or spinal accessory-facial nerve anastomoses was considered better than hemifacial spasm.[31] In 1946, Greenwood[32] reported partial neurectomy of the intraparotid or postparotid branches of the facial nerve for hemifacial spasm. In 1950, Marino and Alurralde[33] advocated peripheral selective neurectomy for spastic facial palsy. Multiple reports of selective neurectomy for blepharospasm have been described.[34,35] Smile analysis was not performed in any of these studies.

In the midface, myectomy of the zygomaticus major and levator labii superioris has been described for oculofacial synkinesis.[36] For the lower face and neck, neurectomy of the cervical branches of the facial nerve has been described to specifically improve platysmal banding associated with synkinesis.[17,37] Henstrom and colleagues[38] also described the use of platysmectomy for the treatment of platysmal hypertonicity and synkinesis. Comprehensive myectomy of synkinetic facial muscles along with transection of peripheral branches of the facial nerve followed by reconstruction with gracilis muscle flap innervated by masseteric or spinal accessory nerve was described by Chuang and colleagues[24] for patients with synkinesis. Smile change with neurectomy and muscle resection was not evaluated, as patients underwent simultaneous reconstruction, precluding this measure. In 2012, Terzis and Karypidis[39] discussed selective neurectomy as one of many strategies for postfacial paralysis synkinesis; but selective neurectomy was performed on only 6 patients with minor synkinesis, and the surgical details were not outlined.

Historically, surgical treatment of facial synkinesis has paralleled that of flaccid paralysis and centered around augmenting and increasing power to the elevators of the lip and oral commissure.[24] Modified selective neurectomy of the facial nerve focuses on reducing the counterproductive activity of the depressor muscles while preserving smile elevators and enhancing the overall smile mechanism. The traditional treatment of increasing power of the elevators may not be necessary. The senior author (B.A.) thinks that patients with synkinesis have functional mimetic facial muscles. Smile dysfunction in patients with postparalysis synkinesis is due to cocontraction of muscles that oppose desired muscle actions. Modified selective neurectomy reestablishes the patients' own natural smile mechanism by reducing the activity of antagonistic muscles (buccinator, platysma, depressor anguli oris, and orbicularis oris) while preserving the neural input into the key smile muscles (zygomatic major/minor, levator labii superioris, levator labii superioris alaeque nasi, and depressor labii inferioris). All elements of the smile mechanism are maintained, as the native facial musculature is motorized by the ipsilateral facial nucleus via an uninterrupted facial nerve.

The key differentiating factors in the modified selective neurectomy versus other neurectomy procedures described in the literature include identification of a significant number of peripheral branches, preservation of the marginal mandibular nerve, ablation of multiple buccal as well as cervical branches that cause lateral and inferior excursion of the oral commissure, and transection of connections between buccal and zygomatic branches that may lead to oculofacial synkinesis. This procedure leads to objective improvement in synkinesis as well as the smile mechanism. There is no improvement of ocular synkinesis, which is expected given the nerves to the orbital region are not modified.

Modified selective neurectomy achieves results rarely seen in traditional facial reanimation procedures by producing a perfectly timed, natural, spontaneous, and symmetric smile (**Fig. 5**A). Furthermore, patients with apparent marginal mandibular dysfunction due to synkinetic activity may also have improvement in depressor labii inferioris motion and lower teeth show (**Fig. 5**B). Marginal mandibular rehabilitation has significant relevance because the asymmetry of lower teeth show has been found to be one of the main factors influencing disfigurement after facial paralysis.[40]

Although patients demonstrate significant improvement in smile after modified selective neurectomy, their natural lip movement during normal conversation and articulation does not change significantly with this procedure. Despite reduction of neural input into various muscles of facial expression, no patients reported long-term worsening of their oral competence, articulation, or lip pursing function.

The authors have noted better outcomes and a decreased revision rate as the senior author has performed more procedures. Initially, there is a natural tendency toward conservative nerve transection given the potential consequences of over-resection. With increased experience, the surgeon may more readily identify nerves that can be sacrificed without complications to yield optimal results. The most common finding

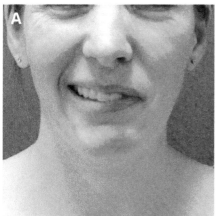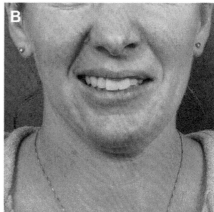

Fig. 5. (A) Preoperative and (B) postoperative photos 5 months after revision left modified selective neurectomy with improvement in left lower teeth show and left lower lip inferior excursion.

in revision cases was identification of nerve branches that were not transected in the primary surgery. Revision cases rarely require repeat platysma myotomy.

SUMMARY

Modified selective neurectomy of the facial nerve is a safe and effective outpatient facial reanimation procedure that reduces facial synkinesis, thus, significantly improving a spontaneous, emotional, and dynamic smile. This technique should be considered an alternative to more invasive surgical options as a stand-alone treatment of incomplete facial palsy.

SUPPLEMENTARY DATA

Supplementary data related to this article can be found online at https://doi.org/10.1016/j.otc.2018.07.012.

REFERENCES

1. Neely JG, Neufeld PS. Defining functional limitation, disability, and societal limitations in patients with facial paresis: initial pilot questionnaire. Am J Otol 1996; 17(2):340–2.
2. Helwig NE, Sohre NE, Ruprecht MR, et al. Dynamic properties of successful smiles. PLoS One 2017;12(6):e0179708.
3. Beurskens CH, Oosterhof J, Nijhuis-van der Sanden MW. Frequency and location of synkineses in patients with peripheral facial nerve paresis. Otol Neurotol 2010; 31(4):671–5.
4. Yamamoto E, Nishimura H, Hirono Y. Occurrence of sequelae in Bell's palsy. Acta Otolaryngol Suppl 1988;446:93–6.
5. Celik M, Forta H, Vural C. The development of synkinesis after facial nerve paralysis. Eur Neurol 2000;43(3):147–51.
6. Takeda T, Takeda S, Okada T, et al. Experimental studies on the recovery processes from severe facial palsy and the development of its sequelae. Otol Neurotol 2015;36(5):896–903.
7. Moran CJ, Neely JG. Patterns of facial nerve synkinesis. Laryngoscope 1996; 106(12 Pt 1):1491–6.
8. Guntinas-Lichius O, Irintchev A, Streppel M, et al. Factors limiting motor recovery after facial nerve transection in the rat: combined structural and functional analyses. Eur J Neurosci 2005;21(2):391–402.
9. Eekhof JL, Aramideh M, Speelman JD, et al. Blink reflexes and lateral spreading in patients with synkinesis after Bell's palsy and in hemifacial spasm. Eur Neurol 2000;43(3):141–6.
10. Bratzlavsky M, vander Eecken H. Altered synaptic organization in facial nucleus following facial nerve regeneration: an electrophysiological study in man. Ann Neurol 1977;2(1):71–3.
11. Brach JS, VanSwearingen J, Delitto A, et al. Impairment and disability in patients with facial neuromuscular dysfunction. Otolaryngol Head Neck Surg 1997;117(4):315–21.
12. Armstrong MW, Mountain RE, Murray JA. Treatment of facial synkinesis and facial asymmetry with botulinum toxin type A following facial nerve palsy. Clin Otolaryngol Allied Sci 1996;21(1):15–20.
13. Beurskens CH, Heymans PG. Positive effects of mime therapy on sequelae of facial paralysis: stiffness, lip mobility, and social and physical aspects of facial disability. Otol Neurotol 2003;24(4):677–81.

14. Bran GM, Lohuis PJ. Selective neurolysis in post-paralytic facial nerve syndrome (PFS). Aesthetic Plast Surg 2014;38(4):742–4.
15. Dall'Angelo A, Mandrini S, Sala V, et al. Platysma synkinesis in facial palsy and botulinum toxin type A. Laryngoscope 2014;124(11):2513–7.
16. Hadlock TA, Greenfield LJ, Wernick-Robinson M, et al. Multimodality approach to management of the paralyzed face. Laryngoscope 2006;116(8):1385–9.
17. Laskawi R, Rohrbach S, Rödel R. Surgical and nonsurgical treatment options in patients with movement disorders of the platysma. J Oral Maxillofac Surg 2002; 60(2):157–62.
18. Naumann M, Carruthers A, Carruthers J, et al. Meta-analysis of neutralizing antibody conversion with onabotulinumtoxinA (BOTOX(R)) across multiple indications. Mov Disord 2010;25(13):2211–8.
19. Rogers CR, Schmidt KL, VanSwearingen JM, et al. Automated facial image analysis: detecting improvement in abnormal facial movement after treatment with botulinum toxin A. Ann Plast Surg 2007;58(1):39–47.
20. Toffola ED, Furini F, Redaelli C, et al. Evaluation and treatment of synkinesis with botulinum toxin following facial nerve palsy. Disabil Rehabil 2010;32(17): 1414–8.
21. Cabin JA, Massry GG, Azizzadeh B. Botulinum toxin in the management of facial paralysis. Curr Opin Otolaryngol Head Neck Surg 2015;23(4):272–80.
22. Mehdizadeh OB, Diels J, White WM. Botulinum toxin in the treatment of facial paralysis. Facial Plast Surg Clin North Am 2016;24(1):11–20.
23. Lindsay RW, Bhama P, Weinberg J, et al. The success of free gracilis muscle transfer to restore smile in patients with nonflaccid facial paralysis. Ann Plast Surg 2014;73(2):177–82.
24. Chuang DC, Chang TN, Lu JC. Postparalysis facial synkinesis: clinical classification and surgical strategies. Plast Reconstr Surg Glob Open 2015;3(3):e320.
25. Byrne PJ, Kim M, Boahene K, et al. Temporalis tendon transfer as part of a comprehensive approach to facial reanimation. Arch Facial Plast Surg 2007; 9(4):234–41.
26. Terzis JK, Olivares FS. Mini-temporalis transfer as an adjunct procedure for smile restoration. Plast Reconstr Surg 2009;123(2):533–42.
27. Yoleri L, Songür E, Yoleri O, et al. Reanimation of early facial paralysis with hypoglossal/facial end-to-side neurorrhaphy: a new approach. J Reconstr Microsurg 2000;16(5):347–55 [discussion: 355–6].
28. Tzafetta K, Terzis JK. Essays on the facial nerve: part I. microanatomy. Plast Reconstr Surg 2010;125(3):879–89.
29. Banks CA, Bhama PK, Park J, et al. Clinician-graded electronic facial paralysis assessment: the eFACE. Plast Reconstr Surg 2015;136(2):223e–30e.
30. Banks CA, Jowett N, Hadlock TA. Test-retest reliability and agreement between in-person and video assessment of facial mimetic function using the eFACE facial grading system. JAMA Facial Plast Surg 2017;19(3):206–11.
31. Coleman CC. Surgical treatment of facial spasm. Ann Surg 1937;105(5):647–57.
32. Greenwood J Jr. The surgical treatment of hemifacial spasm. J Neurosurg 1946; 3(6):506–10.
33. Marino H, Alurralde A. Spastic facial palsy; peripheral selective neurotomy. Br J Plast Surg 1950;3(1):56–9.
34. Hohman MH, Lee LN, Hadlock TA. Two-step highly selective neurectomy for refractory periocular synkinesis. Laryngoscope 2013;123(6):1385–8.
35. Fisch U, Esslen E. The surgical treatment of facial hyperkinesia. Arch Otolaryngol 1972;95(5):400–5.

36. Guerrissi JO. Selective myectomy for postparetic facial synkinesis. Plast Reconstr Surg 1991;87(3):459–66.

37. Nakamura K, Murakami S, Kozawa T, et al. Surgical treatment of synkinesis. Eur Arch Otorhinolaryngol 1994;251(1):S380–2.

38. Henstrom DK, Malo JS, Cheney ML, et al. Platysmectomy: an effective intervention for facial synkinesis and hypertonicity. Arch Facial Plast Surg 2011;13(4): 239–43.

39. Terzis JK, Karypidis D. Therapeutic strategies in post-facial paralysis synkinesis in adult patients. Plast Reconstr Surg 2012;129(6):925e–39e.

40. Banks CA, Jowett N, Hadlock CR, et al. Weighting of facial grading variables to disfigurement in facial palsy. JAMA Facial Plast Surg 2016;18(4):292–8.

Evaluation and Management of Facial Nerve Schwannoma

Alicia M. Quesnel, MD*, Felipe Santos, MD

KEYWORDS

- Facial nerve schwannoma • Facial paresis
- Management of facial nerve schwannoma

KEY POINTS

- Facial nerve schwannomas are benign peripheral nerve sheath tumors that arise from Schwann cells, and most commonly present with facial paresis and/or hearing loss.
- Management decisions are primarily based on facial function, tumor size, and hearing status.
- Observation is favored for small to medium tumors with good facial function.
- For patients with poor facial function (House-Brackmann score of IV or greater), the authors favor surgical resection with facial reanimation.
- There is growing evidence to support radiation treatment in patients with progressively worsening moderate facial paresis and growing tumors.

BACKGROUND

Introduction

Facial nerve schwannomas (FNSs) are rare, benign tumors arising from the Schwann cells that ensheath the facial nerve at any point along the nerve. The most common symptom is facial paresis but these tumors may also affect hearing and balance. Imaging with a combination of computed tomography (CT) and MRI is critical to the initial diagnosis. Management options include observation, facial nerve decompression, facial nerve resection with or without the fascicle-sparing technique, and stereotactic radiation therapy. This article reviews tumor biology, natural history, and diagnostic imaging, and highlights recent management trends for FNSs.

Definition and Genetics

The 3 major types of benign peripheral nerve sheath tumors (PNSTs) are schwannomas, neurofibromas, and perineuriomas. When tumors include a combination of

Disclosure Statement: The authors have no relationships to disclose or conflicts of interest.
Department of Otolaryngology, Otology, Neurotology, and Skull Base Surgery, Harvard Medical School, Massachusetts Eye and Ear, 243 Charles Street, Boston, MA 02114, USA
* Corresponding author.
E-mail address: alicia_quesnel@meei.harvard.edu

Otolaryngol Clin N Am 51 (2018) 1179–1192
https://doi.org/10.1016/j.otc.2018.07.013
0030-6665/18/© 2018 Elsevier Inc. All rights reserved.

oto.theclinics.com

schwannoma, neurofibroma, and/or perineurioma, they are considered to be a distinct tumor type based on the World Health Organization classification and are called hybrid PNSTs.[1] The Schwann cell is the principal neoplastic cell in both schwannomas and neurofibromas; however, neurofibromas are pathologically distinct from schwannomas. Neurofibroma tumors include a mixture of nonneoplastic fibroblasts, lymphocytes, perineurial cells, and degenerated axons.[2] Perineuriomas are derived from perineurial cells that form the perineurium, a connective tissue layer that surrounds endoneurial bundles and lies deep in the epineurial layer.[3]

In schwannomas, the primary neoplastic cell and dominant cell type in the tumor is the Schwann cell. Schwann cells are the principal glial cell of the peripheral nervous system (PNS). They provide trophic support to neurons; play a role in development and, potentially, regeneration of the PNS; and conduct action potentials along axons.[4] These cells develop from neural crest stem cells, and may develop into either myelinating or nonmyelinating Schwann cells. Schwannomas may occur anywhere in the body along the PNS, which includes cranial nerves (except cranial nerve II, which represents a tract of the diencephalon), spinal nerve rootlets, and all other peripheral nerves. Schwann cells do not exist in the central nervous system and, therefore, do not occur in the brain and spinal cord. Common locations for schwannomas include the spine (from spinal nerve rootlets)[5]; gastrointestinal system, including stomach, small and large intestine[6]; the head and neck, including vestibular nerves,[7] oral cavity,[8] carotid sympathetic plexus[9]; and (rarely) other cranial nerves, such as the facial nerve (**Fig. 1**).

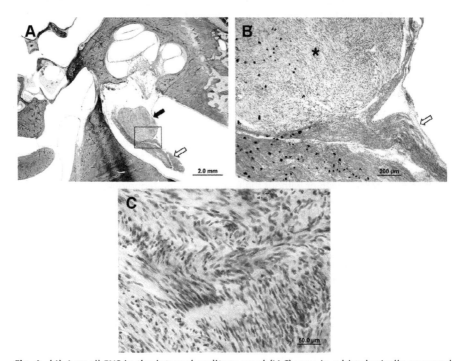

Fig. 1. (*A*) A small FNS in the internal auditory canal (IAC) seen in a histologically prepared temporal bone specimen photographed at 1.25 × magnification. The solid arrow indicates the tumor and the open arrow indicates the facial nerve. (*B*) At 10 × magnification, the relationship of the FNS (*asterisk*) to the facial nerve (*open arrow*) is seen. (*C*) At 40 × magnification, features of Antoni A patterns with Verocay bodies can be seen.

Although there is a paucity of genetic studies specific to sporadic FNSs, multiple large genetic and genomic studies of vestibular schwannomas and mixed types of schwannomas exist. Loss of function of a tumor suppressor gene, the neurofibromatosis type 2 (NF2) gene on chromosome 22, is associated with development of vestibular schwannomas. The NF2 gene was mutated in 62% of 61 vestibular schwannoma specimens from a combination of 29 unilateral sporadic tumors and 32 bilateral tumors in NF2 subjects.[10] In a study of 126 schwannomas, including both vestibular schwannomas and spinal schwannomas, 76% of the tumors had loss of NF2 function either by mutation or chromosome 22q deletion identified by whole exome sequencing.[11] In a separate study, whole exome sequencing on 46 sporadic vestibular schwannoma specimens also identified an NF2 mutation in 76% of cases and found that all other cases had mutations in genes related to or linked to the function of NF2.[12] In a single case report of a subject with bilateral FNSs, genetic screening of the subject's blood sample identified a germline mutation in the NF2 gene.[13]

Pathologic Findings

Macroscopically, schwannomas are pink or tan, appear encapsulated, and have a smooth rounded surface. On a cut surface, the tumor appears tan or yellow with occasional areas of microhemorrhage.[14] Microscopically, the tumor may be composed of several different juxtaposed cellular arrangements. In Antoni A areas, oval or spindle shaped cells are arranged in whorls, and there may be areas of aligned or palisading nuclei termed Verocay bodies (**Fig. 2**A). In Antoni B subgroup 1, cystic areas with fatty degeneration and polymorphic cells with a honeycombed appearance dominate (**Fig. 2**B). In Antoni B subgroup 2, hyalin deposition is seen between cells, disrupting the honeycomb or orderly appearance, resulting in lower cell density.[15]

Areas of necrosis due to microvascular infarcts, calcification, and a chronic inflammatory cell infiltrate may also be present.[14] In a study comparing rapidly growing versus slowly growing vestibular schwannomas, an increased density of M2-type macrophages identified by CD163 immunostaining and an increased microvessel density was found in the rapidly growing tumor specimens.[16] This observation suggests a potential role of inflammation and angiogenesis in tumor growth in schwannomas.

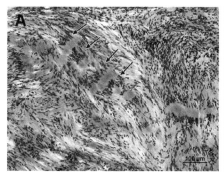 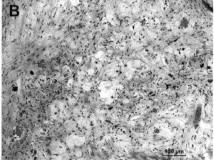

Fig. 2. Schwannoma microscopic pathologic features. A vestibular schwannoma in the IAC from a cadaveric temporal bone specimen photographed in high-power (40 ×) magnification to demonstrate Antoni A (*A*) pattern and Antoni B patterns (*A*) in schwannomas. (*A*) Note the elongated oval shaped cells, arranged in whorls. Arrows indicate Verocay bodies created by the alignment of tumor nuclei. (*B*) Note the loose but orderly architecture of large polymorphic cells.

Schwannomas almost universally demonstrate robust nuclear and cytoplasmic S100 expression and have significant amounts of pericellular type IV collagen that can been demonstrated by immunostaining. Glial fibrillary acid protein is expressed in most schwannomas.[2] Classically, neurofilament staining is present only on the surface of the tumor in residual axons, which stands in contradistinction to neurofibromas, which are another type of benign tumor that arises from the Schwann cell. More recently, however, disrupted and entangled axons have been noted throughout schwannomas.[17] Pathologic variants of schwannomas include plexiform, cellular, and melanotic schwannomas[2]; however, these are particularly uncommon in FNSs. In FNSs from patients with NF2, fusion tumors with schwannomas and meningiomas may be seen.

Epidemiology

FNSs are so rare that estimation of the clinical incidence is problematic. In clinical practice, FNSs are far more rare than vestibular schwannomas, which have an incidence reported to range from 15.5 to 22.1 per million per year.[18–20] Among 2000 subjects presenting to a facial nerve center with facial paralysis, benign facial nerve tumors (ie, schwannomas, meningiomas, and hemangiomas, which were not reported separately) accounted for the cause of facial paralysis in 103 subjects; the most common causes of facial paralysis were Bell palsy, vestibular schwannoma treatment, and head and neck cancer.[21] In a review of a temporal bone collection consisting of 600 specimens, 5 FNSs were identified and only 1 out of the 5 specimens had a clinical history indicating facial paresis during life.[22] This incidence of 0.83% cannot be extrapolated to the general population because the temporal bone specimens collected in a temporal bone bank do not represent the typical otologic disease distribution among the population.

The average age of presentation with FNSs ranges from 43 to 51 years among multiple large series of subjects.[23–33] Men and women are equally affected, and the tumors are evenly distributed between the right and left sides.[26,30] Sporadic FNSs represent almost all cases (see **Fig. 1**); however, FNSs may also occur in the NF2 syndrome (**Fig. 3**). In a series that included 88 subjects with FNSs seen at a single institution, 8 (9%) of the FNSs occurred in subjects with NF2, whereas the other 91% were considered sporadic FNSs.

EVALUATION
Clinical Presentation: Symptoms and Signs

Facial paresis is the most common presenting symptom in patients with FNSs in most series, though it is not uniformly present at the time of diagnosis. Among multiple large series of FNSs, 41% to 82% of subjects presented with a facial paresis.[23,24,26,27,31] In a single-institution series of 79 subjects with FNSs, the percentage of subjects presenting with House-Brackmann (HB) facial nerve scores of I, II, III, IV, V, and VI out of VI before any treatment was 40.5% (normal facial function), 22.8%, 16.5%, 6.3%, 10.1%, and 3.8% (no facial movement), respectively.[30] Facial twitching or spasms were reported in 26% of a series of 80 subjects with FNSs with or without facial paresis.[31] Although rare and self-resolving periocular or perioral twitching is fairly common and benign, persistent or progressive hemifacial twitching or spasms suggests an ongoing degenerative or denervating process of the facial nerve, and should increase suspicion for a facial nerve tumor. A facial nerve examination that demonstrates elements of both weakness and hypertonicity or synkinesis in different zones of the face highly suggests an FNS or other primary facial nerve tumor. Patients who

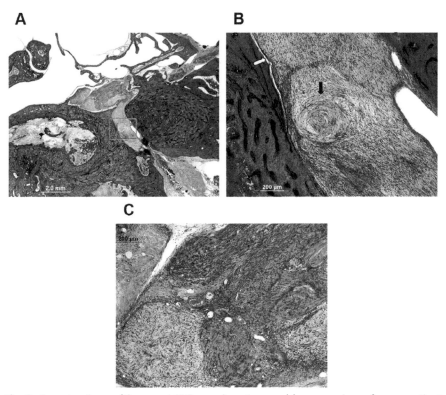

Fig. 3. An extensive multisegment FNS seen in a temporal bone specimen from a patient with NF2. (A) At 1.25 × magnification, the IAC, labyrinthine, and geniculate portions of the facial nerve are seen. On the left, the vestibule and lateral semicircular canal are seen filled with fibrous tissue and new bone growth. The box in (A) is depicted at 10 × magnification in (B). (B) The labyrinthine portion of the facial nerve shows (*open arrow*) a whorl pattern of neoplastic spindle cells (solid black arrow). (C) The geniculate portion of the facial nerve, shown at 10 × magnification, is also involved with schwannoma.

have normal facial nerve function on the initial examination may also report a history of transient facial paresis. Out of 56 subjects with an FNS, McRackan and colleagues[26] reported that 9% had a history of transient facial paresis. Additional symptoms, such as dysgeusia or dry eye, may occur when an intratemporal facial schwannoma is located medial to the entry point of the chorda tympani nerve or greater superficial petrosal nerve, respectively.

Hearing loss is common at the time of presentation with an FNS. One series reported it as more common than facial paresis at the time of presentation.[31] Thus, an audiogram is recommended as part of the initial evaluation whether or not the patient reports hearing loss. Most commonly, sensorineural hearing loss (rather than conductive hearing loss) occurs, which can range from mild hearing loss to anacusis. In a series with a higher percentage of internal auditory canal (IAC) tumor extension than most other series, 43% of subjects presented with American Academy of Otolaryngology–Head and Neck Surgery (AAO-HNS) class D hearing (ie, nonserviceable hearing). Profound sensorineural hearing loss or anacusis may occur in cases in which the facial schwannoma involves the IAC, or in which there has been significant expansion of the labyrinthine segment with a fistula into the basal turn of the cochlea, or in patients with NF2 who commonly have concurrent schwannomas in the IAC or labyrinth. Sensorineural hearing loss has been noted, however, even in cases in which the FNS does not involve the IAC or cause a cochlear fistula. Remenschneider and colleagues[33] reported that 5 out of 20 (25%) subjects with tympanic segment FNSs that did not extend into the IAC had sensorineural hearing loss. There may be intracochlear disease that occurs in response to an FNS even when the schwannoma is not directly in contact with the cochlea or IAC, analogous to the intracochlear protein deposition and hair cell losses that have been noted in patients with vestibular schwannoma.[34] Conductive hearing loss may occur in geniculate ganglion, tympanic, or mastoid segment schwannomas that directly contact the ossicular chain or the undersurface of the tympanic membrane.[33]

Vestibular symptoms may occur in patients with facial nerve tumors but have not been routinely reported in series of FNSs. In a series of 80 subjects with 49% of tumors involving the IAC, 39% of subjects reported dizziness.[31] Vestibular function loss may occur when the schwannoma extends into or lies entirely within the IAC, presumably due to the juxtaposition of the vestibular nerve and possibly due to direct compression, cytotoxic, or immune mechanisms affecting the vestibular nerves or the labyrinth. The exact pathophysiologic mechanism is not well understood in FNS.

Rarely, an incidentally found middle ear mass may be the only presenting history for a tympanic FNS.[35] If an FNS is suspected, complete imaging of the temporal bone and brain should be performed to evaluate the radiologic characteristics of the tumor and to evaluate for additional tumors that would establish a diagnosis of NF2, such as vestibular schwannomas or meningiomas. Clarifying the radiologic diagnosis of a middle ear mass is important to avoid a biopsy, which may lead to complete facial paralysis.[36]

FNSs may also be diagnosed incidentally on MRIs obtained for evaluation of unrelated symptoms. In a series of 80 FNSs, 6% were identified incidentally.[31]

Imaging

When the clinical history is concerning for a possible facial nerve tumor, imaging should be obtained. Key features about the facial paresis that should increase the index of suspicion for a facial nerve tumor include a subacute onset (ie, occurring over weeks); a slowly progressive course (ie, occurring over months)[37]; an acute paralysis (ie, presumed Bell palsy) that fails to show any recovery after 4 months[38]; and a mixed picture of weakness, hypertonicity, and synkinesis. The radiologic differential diagnosis of a mass that involves the facial nerve includes schwannoma, hemangioma (also called lymphovascular malformation), meningioma, and epidermoid (also called cholesteatoma), as well as other benign or malignant tumors. Both MRI and CT may be needed to help narrow the differential diagnosis for facial nerve tumors.

MRI with high-resolution images through the IAC and temporal bone with and without gadolinium contrast is the primary mode of imaging for evaluation of facial schwannomas. Facial schwannomas, like vestibular schwannomas, are avidly enhancing, generally well-circumscribed lesions that are most commonly T1 isointense and T2 hypointense (**Fig. 4**). T1-enhanced images may be used to identify enhancement along the intratemporal course of the facial nerve and pathologic enlargement of the nerve. Radiologically, tumors may be classified into 4 general types based on the location of involvement of the tumor: (1) tumors primarily involving the geniculate ganglion with or without extension into the labyrinthine segment, (2) tumors involving both the geniculate ganglion and the IAC creating a dumbbell shape, (3) tumors primarily involving the tympani and/or mastoid segments, and (4) tumors in the IAC with or without extension into the cerebellopontine angle (CPA).[27] Facial

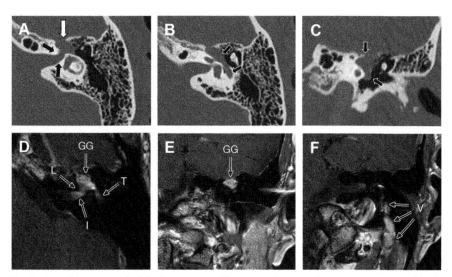

Fig. 4. A multisegment facial schwannoma illustrates the complementary nature of high-resolution temporal bone CT and gadolinium-enhanced IAC protocol MRI for diagnosis. (*A*, *B*) Axial left ear CT images through the facial nerve tumor. (*A*) Widening the labyrinthine segment of the facial nerve (*black arrows*) and enlargement of geniculate ganglion (*white arrow*). (*B*) Enlargement of the tympanic and mastoid segments of the facial nerve (*black arrows*). (*C*) A coronal CT image shows smooth bony expansion of adjacent temporal bone in the enlarged geniculate ganglion and tympanic segments without calcifications (*black arrows*), as are more commonly seen in geniculate ganglion vascular malformations. (*D*) Axial MRI T1 with gadolinium image shows enhancing tumor involving the IAC (I), labyrinthine (L), geniculate ganglion (GG), and tympanic (T) portions of the facial nerve. (*E*) The rounded and significantly enlarged geniculate ganglion portion of the tumor is avidly enhancing and measured 6.1 mm (GG) in the superior-inferior dimension shown in a coronal T1 with gadolinium image. (*F*) A coronal T1 with gadolinium demonstrates the nodular, bulbous expansion of the vertical segment of the facial nerve (V).

schwannomas often involve multiple adjacent segments of the facial nerve, with a median of 4 segments (average of 3.83) involved based on high-resolution contrasted enhanced MRI imaging in 30 cases.[24] The most common involved segment based on MRI is the geniculate ganglion, followed by the labyrinthine segment. In a series of 44 MRIs for facial schwannomas, the geniculate ganglion was involved in 68.2% and the labyrinthine segment in 52.3%.[28] Facial schwannomas can usually be distinguished from vestibular schwannomas by the location of enhancement along the facial nerve and this multisegment involvement. Facial schwannomas that are isolated to the IAC (type IV) may be more difficult to radiologically distinguish from the much more common vestibular schwannoma. However, a clinical presentation with facial paresis in a patient with an isolated IAC mass should increase suspicion for a facial schwannoma because facial paresis is exceedingly rare in patients with vestibular schwannoma before treatment. An FNS at the geniculate ganglion may be distinguished from a geniculate ganglion meningioma on MRI by lack of an enhancing adjacent meninges (ie, dural tail). Heavily T2-weighted images (eg, CISS [constructive interference in steady state] sequence) may be used to determine whether the enhancement is associated with a mass when the enhancement extends into the IAC.[39] Diffusion-weighted imaging may be used to evaluate for epidermoid tumor but, generally, the location within the temporal bone and lack of clear predilection for the course of the facial nerve can distinguish an epidermoid from a facial schwannoma.

High-resolution CT of the temporal bone with fine collimation (≤0.6 mm) is complementary to the MRI for the radiologic diagnosis of intratemporal facial schwannomas. At the authors' institution, we regularly obtain both an MRI and a CT to best determine the diagnosis of a facial nerve mass. On CT, schwannomas create smooth remodeling of the surrounding bony Fallopian canal due to expansion of the tumor,[39] as compared with hemangiomas, which usually create a more irregular bony erosion and often contain spicules of bone within the tumor mass itself (see **Fig. 4**). When the FNS involves the mastoid segment, however, expansion can lead to loss of mastoid air cell septations and may create some irregularity in the bony contour.[40]

Electrophysiology

Tumors that are confined to the CPA may be clinically and radiographically indistinguishable from vestibular schwannomas. This is particularly true when preoperative facial function is normal. Intraoperative electrophysiological measures of facial nerve function can help to differentiate tumors of facial nerve origin misdiagnosed preoperatively as being of vestibular nerve origin. Electrophysiological measures can assist with intraoperative clarification of the nerve of tumor origin. This allows the surgeon to follow the best clinical course of action to preserve normal facial function. This course may include termination of surgery in favor of observation in the appropriate clinical setting. Although the use of preoperative testing of facial function has been reported in the assessment of vestibular schwannomas,[41] in the absence of facial weakness this is not routinely used in the authors' practice.

There is no natural history data for facial schwannomas that longitudinally tracks facial function with electrophysiological measures using electroneuronography (ENoG) or electromyography (EMG). Wilkinson and colleagues[30] reported on the pretreatment and posttreatment ENoG data of 27 subjects with FNSs. Although there was a correlation between ENoG and facial function at diagnosis there were not enough data to assess the effect of decline in ENoG on facial nerve outcome. To date, the authors have relied on clinical assessment of function over electrophysiological measures when selecting appropriate candidates for surgical resection. Anecdotally, we have used ENoG and EMG for the prognostic value in assessing the likelihood of recovery in a patient with an FNS who had recurrent episodes of facial paresis when surgical decompression was under consideration in the recurrent acute setting. Collective longitudinal data using standardized electrophysiological measures are still needed to better define the role of testing in the surveillance of FNS.

MANAGEMENT
Observation

As a function of improved and more readily accessible MRI imaging, the number of diagnosed asymptomatic vestibular schwannomas has increased.[42] Although fewer, the same may be extrapolated for schwannomas arising from the facial nerve. Increasingly, FNSs are diagnosed when facial function is good. Unlike vestibular schwannomas in which physiologic adaptation can occur following resection of the tumor, there is no compensatory adaptation for loss of facial function. Moreover, complete recovery of facial function is not yet feasible with reanimation. Observation of an FNS in which facial function is good has, therefore, become the mainstay of management.

The threshold for what constitutes good facial function is prone to subjective interpretation. Complete surgical resection of the tumor unambiguously leaves no remaining function. Therefore, the authors rely on the best outcomes that can be achieved with static and dynamic reanimation in the decision-making process. Most clinicians agree that slight to moderate movement of forehead function cannot be achieved with current reanimation protocols and, thereby, the authors have used HB grade IV or worse as a relative indication for surgical resection. This is not an absolute indication because not all patients with this degree of facial dysfunction are good surgical candidates and there are patients with better facial nerve function who may be candidates for surgery, for example, in the setting of clinically significant compression of the brainstem.

When considering observation as a management choice, the likelihood of tumor growth must be considered. The reported average rate of annual growth of facial schwannomas is 2.0 mm per year; this rate is comparable to the growth rate of vestibular schwannomas. Patients with larger tumors at diagnosis may be more likely to grow than tumors smaller than 1 cm in their largest dimension.[31] Collective natural history data point to a trend observed in the natural history of vestibular schwannomas[43]; after diagnosis, most FNSs remain clinically stable without measurable progression over years. Of 14 subjects observed in 1 series with HB grade III function or better, 12 of 14 remained in observation (range 6 months to 13 years) without clinical or radiographic progression.[44] In a second series, 20 of 53 subjects were observed for as long as 8 years and maintained good facial nerve function.[41]

Although contemporary series do not achieve statistical significance, they suggest that growing tumors are likely to be associated with worse function. In a series of 21 subjects observed with annual imaging surveillance, 18 of 21 maintained HB grade III or better function. Nine of the 21 subjects did show evidence of growth and 8 of the 9 that grew had worsening facial function. Three of these subjects progressed to HB grade IV or worse. The average length of follow-up was 6.4 years (range 4–9 years).[45]

Hearing loss is reported in up to 78.6% of subjects with FNSs.[26] The average reported rate of hearing loss over an average observation period of 35.7 months was an increase in 5.9 dB of the pure tone average.[30] The effect of tumor size and growth on hearing remains uncertain.

Finally, whether or not duration of observation adversely affects reanimation outcomes in patients who ultimately undergo treatment is not known. It is likely that with time there is an increased risk of loss of cell bodies in the facial motor nucleus and motor end plates of the facial musculature. Serial electrophysiological measures could be used to monitor this risk over time.

Surgical Management

Surgical resection

Large tumors with poor facial function (HB ≤IV) that are within the CPA can be approached by a translabyrinthine, transotic, or suboccipital craniotomy. The likelihood of preservation of residual hearing and vestibular function with tumor resection by suboccipital craniotomy must be assessed by the surgeon and/or team. Translabyrinthine and transotic approaches offer a more favorable exposure for cable grafting to distal intratemporal segments of the facial nerve.

For tumors involving the IAC, geniculate ganglion, tympanic, and mastoid segments, the authors favor a combined middle fossa and transmastoid approach. This approach permits preservation of residual hearing and vestibular function. When the tympanic segment of the facial nerve is resected or mobilized, the incus is often disarticulated from the stapes to decompress a nondehiscent segment. The ossicular chain can be left intact by reapproximating the ossicles; however, placement of a partial ossicular reconstruction prosthesis should be considered a possibility in the preoperative planning and counseling. All approaches to the CPA and intratemporal segments of the nerve can be combined with transfacial approaches to the intraparotid facial nerve. It has been the authors' practice to perform concurrent reanimation (most frequently reinnervation using the masseteric nerve to a distal branch of the facial nerve) with surgical resection. Dynamic and static reanimation procedures are increasingly becoming integrated into the primary surgical management of FNSs, occasionally requiring careful incision planning to permit both preauricular and postauricular cutaneous incisions.

Unanticipated surgical decision-making

An FNS in the CPA or parotid that does not involve the intratemporal segments of the nerve may be misdiagnosed preoperatively. The surgeon may make the diagnosis with intraoperative facial nerve monitoring when the tumor is exposed. If facial function is good to normal, the surgeon must decide how to proceed. Resection is likely to result in facial paresis or paralysis.

Bacciu and colleagues[29] described their experience with intraoperative decision-making in 23 subjects with CPA FNSs who underwent surgery with a preoperative diagnosis of vestibular schwannoma. Subjects with facial nerve function of greater than HB grade III underwent total resection with grafting and those with better function had subtotal and total resections described as fascicle preservation surgery resections. Eight of 9 subjects undergoing fascicle preservation surgery were reported as having HB grade I or II postoperatively. Decompression was performed in 4 subjects with small tumors preoperatively considered candidates for hearing preservation. This experience highlights intraoperative options for management favoring preservation of facial function and raises important questions about the surgical management of FNSs: (1) what is the role of nerve-sparring resection, (2) can biopsy of a facial schwannoma be safely performed, and (3) what is the role of facial nerve decompression?

Fascicle preservation surgery

The role of fascicle or nerve-sparing surgery and biopsy assume that the tumor is histologically eccentric to sufficient nerve fibers such that resection would not compromise existing function of the nerve. Reported clinical experience supports that this approach is (sometimes) possible, beginning with Pulec[46] in 1972. Subsequently, multiple groups have reported cases of both stable and improved function, often using monopolar stimulation to distinguish between tumor and viable nerve, with follow-up periods as long as 19 years.[47–50] Hajjaj and Linthicum[36] reviewed the histopathology of 23 facial schwannomas and found nerve fibers widely disseminated within 8 tumors, which would argue against the universal safety of this strategy. As management has shifted to observation, the authors have not recommended fascicle preservation surgery or routine biopsy in light of the risk of loss of function. If improved preoperative imaging, intraoperative imaging, or visualization can distinguish between functional nerve fibers and tumor, this strategy may gain more traction.

Decompression

Decompression refers to the removal of bone surrounding the intratemporal facial nerve. This maneuver can be performed from the porus acusticus to the stylomastoid foramen. The rationale for decompression is that an enlarging tumor can cause direct compression or indirect compression by edema of viable axons, thereby leading to facial weakness. The facial paresis of an FNS is typically not acute in onset as seen in Bell palsy. In the setting of an FNS, decompression is directed at preventing further degeneration, in addition to reversing the less frequently observed acute changes more frequently seen in Bell Palsy. One study to date has compared the effect of decompression to observation.[30] There was no observed difference in facial nerve function outcomes, though the investigators reported improved function in 3 subjects. When patients present with good function, the authors have favored observation over decompression. Decompression may play a role in patients with worsening but still good function. In this setting, CT of the temporal bone can be helpful to look for evidence of bone expansion as a radiological correlate to neural compression.

Radiation

The goal of radiation therapy is to prevent further tumor growth and preserve residual facial function without a need for surgical intervention. The risks of radiation include failure to control tumor growth, further deterioration of facial function, hearing loss, and malignant transformation. Understanding of the effects of radiation on preventing further growth and preserving facial function are limited by the low incidence of these tumors.

Radiation for an FNS has gained traction as a treatment option in part because of the accumulation of longitudinal data for radiation of vestibular schwannomas in which the facial nerve is in the radiation field. The incidence of new facial nerve weakness following radiation for a vestibular schwannoma with a marginal dose less than 14 Gy is less than 5%.[51]

Overall, short-term tumor-control rates for facial schwannomas with stereotactic radiosurgery (SRS) are good. In a meta-analysis of 45 cases with a minimum of 2 years of follow-up, tumor control was achieved in 93% of subjects.[52] Sheehan and colleagues[25] reviewed the results of 42 subjects treated at 8 separate centers of the North American Gamma Knife Consortium. The mean marginal dose in this cohort was 12.5 Gy and the mean follow-up was 42 months. Actuarial 5-year tumor control was 90%. This was similar to the findings of Hasegawa and colleagues[27] who reviewed 42 cases of FNSs from 10 Gamma Knife centers in Japan. The actuarial 5-year progression-free survival rate was 92%. The long-term risk of tumor progression remains unknown.

In the aforementioned studies, the rates of worsening facial nerve ranged from 10.5% to 12.8%. McRackan and colleagues identified 30 subjects with available hearing data pretreatment and posttreatment and found that of those with serviceable hearing (AAO-HNS class A to B) before SRS (n = 14), 9 (64.3%) remained stable and 5 (36.7%) deteriorated after SRS. The mean posttreatment follow-up period was 42.1 months.[26] To date, few cases of malignant transformation of cranial nerve schwannoma have been reported in the literature; however, patients should be counseled on this small risk. The mean latency period to malignant transformation in a recent review of 26 cases was 5.8 years.[53]

In summary, radiation is a viable option for older patients with good facial function with enlarging tumors or showing early signs of decline in facial function. Patients must be counseled on the unknown long-term risks of radiation, the short-term risk of deterioration of facial function despite or as a consequence of treatment in 10% of cases, and limited data suggesting that as many as a third of patients may incur hearing loss.

SUMMARY

FNSs are rare tumors that often present with minimal to no facial paresis. The combination of CT and MRI is critical in establishing the diagnosis. In the setting of good facial nerve function, observation has become the primary choice of management. Surgical resection and reanimation still play an important role in patients with poor facial function (HB >IV) and large tumors compressing the brainstem. The roles of decompression and fascicle preservation surgery are not well defined but can be considered when the diagnosis is made intraoperatively or in large tumors with good facial function, respectively. There are limited longitudinal data on radiation therapy but it is a compelling option in patients with enlarging tumors and good or declining function (HB <IV). The patient's age, risk of loss of facial function, hearing loss, and continued growth remain important considerations in the decision-making process.

REFERENCES

1. Ud Din N, Ahmad Z, Abdul-Ghafar J, et al. Hybrid peripheral nerve sheath tumors: report of five cases and detailed review of literature. BMC Cancer 2017; 17(1):349.
2. Rodriguez FJ, Folpe AL, Giannini C, et al. Pathology of peripheral nerve sheath tumors: diagnostic overview and update on selected diagnostic problems. Acta Neuropathol 2012;123(3):295–319.
3. Markovchick V. Suture materials and mechanical after care. Emerg Med Clin North Am 1992;10(4):673–89.
4. Castelnovo LF, Bonalume V, Melfi S, et al. Schwann cell development, maturation and regeneration: a focus on classic and emerging intracellular signaling pathways. Neural Regen Res 2017;12(7):1013–23.
5. Ottenhausen M, Ntoulias G, Bodhinayake I, et al. Intradural spinal tumors in adults-update on management and outcome. Neurosurg Rev 2018. [Epub ahead of print].
6. Lin YM, Chiu NC, Li AF, et al. Unusual gastric tumors and tumor-like lesions: Radiological with pathological correlation and literature review. World J Gastroenterol 2017;23(14):2493–504.
7. Kshettry VR, Hsieh JK, Ostrom QT, et al. Incidence of vestibular schwannomas in the United States. J Neurooncol 2015;124(2):223–8.
8. Santos PP, Freitas VS, Pinto LP, et al. Clinicopathologic analysis of 7 cases of oral schwannoma and review of the literature. Ann Diagn Pathol 2010;14(4):235–9.
9. Navaie M, Sharghi LH, Cho-Reyes S, et al. Diagnostic approach, treatment, and outcomes of cervical sympathetic chain schwannomas: a global narrative review. Otolaryngol Head Neck Surg 2014;151(6):899–908.
10. Welling DB. Clinical manifestations of mutations in the neurofibromatosis type 2 gene in vestibular schwannomas (acoustic neuromas). Laryngoscope 1998; 108(2):178–89.
11. Agnihotri S, Jalali S, Wilson MR, et al. The genomic landscape of schwannoma. Nat Genet 2016;48(11):1339–48.
12. Havik AL, Bruland O, Myrseth E, et al. Genetic landscape of sporadic vestibular schwannoma. J Neurosurg 2017;128(3):911–22.
13. Fenton JE, Morrin MM, Smail M, et al. Bilateral facial nerve schwannomas. Eur Arch Otorhinolaryngol 1999;256(3):133–5.
14. Hilton DA, Hanemann CO. Schwannomas and their pathogenesis. Brain Pathol 2014;24(3):205–20.
15. Merchant SN, McKenna MJ. Neoplastic growth. In: Merchant SN, Nadol JB, editors. Schuknecht's pathology of the ear. 3rd edition. Shelton (CT): People's Medical Publishing House; 2010. p. 492–510.

16. de Vries M, Briaire-de Bruijn I, Malessy MJ, et al. Tumor-associated macrophages are related to volumetric growth of vestibular schwannomas. Otol Neurotol 2013; 34(2):347–52.

17. Nascimento AF, Fletcher CD. The controversial nosology of benign nerve sheath tumors: neurofilament protein staining demonstrates intratumoral axons in many sporadic schwannomas. Am J Surg Pathol 2007;31(9):1363–70.

18. Kleijwegt M, Ho V, Visser O, et al. Real incidence of vestibular schwannoma? Estimations from a national registry. Otol Neurotol 2016;37(9):1411–7.

19. Stepanidis K, Kessel M, Caye-Thomasen P, et al. Socio-demographic distribution of vestibular schwannomas in Denmark. Acta Otolaryngol 2014;134(6):551–6.

20. Stangerup SE, Caye-Thomasen P. Epidemiology and natural history of vestibular schwannomas. Otolaryngol Clin North Am 2012;45(2):257–68, vii.

21. Hohman MH, Hadlock TA. Etiology, diagnosis, and management of facial palsy: 2000 patients at a facial nerve center. Laryngoscope 2014;124(7):E283–93.

22. Saito H, Baxter A. Undiagnosed intratemporal facial nerve neurilemomas. Arch Otolaryngol 1972;95(5):415–9.

23. Shirazi MA, Leonetti JP, Marzo SJ, et al. Surgical management of facial neuromas: lessons learned. Otol Neurotol 2007;28(7):958–63.

24. Thompson AL, Aviv RI, Chen JM, et al. Magnetic resonance imaging of facial nerve schwannoma. Laryngoscope 2009;119(12):2428–36.

25. Sheehan JP, Kano H, Xu Z, et al. Gamma Knife radiosurgery for facial nerve schwannomas: a multicenter study. J Neurosurg 2015;123(2):387–94.

26. McRackan TR, Rivas A, Wanna GB, et al. Facial nerve outcomes in facial nerve schwannomas. Otol Neurotol 2012;33(1):78–82.

27. Hasegawa T, Kato T, Kida Y, et al. Gamma Knife surgery for patients with facial nerve schwannomas: a multiinstitutional retrospective study in Japan. J Neurosurg 2016;124(2):403–10.

28. Kertesz TR, Shelton C, Wiggins RH, et al. Intratemporal facial nerve neuroma: anatomical location and radiological features. Laryngoscope 2001;111(7):1250–6.

29. Bacciu A, Nusier A, Lauda L, et al. Are the current treatment strategies for facial nerve schwannoma appropriate also for complex cases? Audiol Neurootol 2013; 18(3):184–91.

30. Wilkinson EP, Hoa M, Slattery WH 3rd, et al. Evolution in the management of facial nerve schwannoma. Laryngoscope 2011;121(10):2065–74.

31. Carlson ML, Deep NL, Patel NS, et al. Facial nerve schwannomas: review of 80 cases over 25 years at Mayo clinic. Mayo Clin Proc 2016;91(11):1563–76.

32. Prasad SC, Laus M, Dandinarasaiah M, et al. Surgical management of intrinsic tumors of the facial nerve. Neurosurgery 2017. [Epub ahead of print].

33. Remenschneider AK, Gaudin R, Kozin ED, et al. Is the cause of sensorineural hearing loss in patients with facial schwannomas multifactorial? Laryngoscope 2017;127(7):1676–82.

34. Roosli C, Linthicum FH Jr, Cureoglu S, et al. Dysfunction of the cochlea contributing to hearing loss in acoustic neuromas: an underappreciated entity. Otol Neurotol 2012;33(3):473–80.

35. Sarolia SP, Danner CJ, Erdem E. Facial nerve schwannoma presenting as a tympanic mass. Ear Nose Throat J 2006;85(6):366–8.

36. Hajjaj M, Linthicum FH Jr. Facial nerve schwannoma: nerve fibre dissemination. J Laryngol Otol 1996;110(7):632–3.

37. Chen WJ, Ye JY, Li X, et al. Case analysis of temporal bone lesions with facial paralysis as main manifestation and literature review. Cancer Biomark 2017;20(2): 199–205.

38. Quesnel AM, Lindsay RW, Hadlock TA. When the bell tolls on Bell's palsy: finding occult malignancy in acute-onset facial paralysis. Am J Otolaryngol 2010;31(5): 339–42.

39. Veillon F, Taboada LR, Eid MA, et al. Pathology of the facial nerve. Neuroimaging Clin N Am 2008;18(2):309–20, x.

40. Wiggins RH 3rd, Harnsberger HR, Salzman KL, et al. The many faces of facial nerve schwannoma. AJNR Am J Neuroradiol 2006;27(3):694–9.

41. McMonagle B, Al-Sanosi A, Croxson G, et al. Facial schwannoma: results of a large case series and review. J Laryngol Otol 2008;122(11):1139–50.

42. Sughrue ME, Yang I, Aranda D, et al. The natural history of untreated sporadic vestibular schwannomas: a comprehensive review of hearing outcomes. J Neurosurg 2010;112(1):163–7.

43. Stangerup SE, Caye-Thomasen P, Tos M, et al. The natural history of vestibular schwannoma. Otol Neurotol 2006;27(4):547–52.

44. Doshi J, Heyes R, Freeman SR, et al. Clinical and radiological guidance in managing facial nerve schwannomas. Otol Neurotol 2015;36(5):892–5.

45. Yang W, Zhao J, Han Y, et al. Long-term outcomes of facial nerve schwannomas with favorable facial nerve function: tumor growth rate is correlated with initial tumor size. Am J Otolaryngol 2015;36(2):163–5.

46. Pulec JL. Facial nerve neuroma. Laryngoscope 1972;82(7):1160–76.

47. Lu R, Li S, Zhang L, et al. Stripping surgery in intratemporal facial nerve schwannomas with poor facial nerve function. Am J Otolaryngol 2015;36(3):338–41.

48. Mowry S, Hansen M, Gantz B. Surgical management of internal auditory canal and cerebellopontine angle facial nerve schwannoma. Otol Neurotol 2012; 33(6):1071–6.

49. Lee JD, Kim SH, Song MH, et al. Management of facial nerve schwannoma in patients with favorable facial function. Laryngoscope 2007;117(6):1063–8.

50. Perez R, Chen JM, Nedzelski JM. Intratemporal facial nerve schwannoma: a management dilemma. Otol Neurotol 2005;26(1):121–6.

51. Kondziolka D, Mousavi SH, Kano H, et al. The newly diagnosed vestibular schwannoma: radiosurgery, resection, or observation? Neurosurg Focus 2012; 33(3):E8.

52. Moon JH, Chang WS, Jung HH, et al. Gamma knife surgery for facial nerve schwannomas. J Neurosurg 2014;121(Suppl):116–22.

53. Husseini ST, Piccirillo E, Sanna M. On "malignant transformation of acoustic neuroma/vestibular schwannoma 10 years after gamma knife stereotactic radiosurgery" (skull base 2010;20:381-388). Skull Base 2011;21(2):135–8.

Management of Vestibular Schwannoma (Including NF2)
Facial Nerve Considerations

Vivian Kaul, MD, Maura K. Cosetti, MD*

KEYWORDS

- Management • Vestibular schwannoma • Facial nerve • Facial paralysis
- Intraoperative monitoring

KEY POINTS

- Vestibular schwannomas (VS) may be treated with observation, microsurgical resection, stereotactic radiotherapy, or a combination of these, with the goal of achieving maximal tumor control with minimal functional deficit.
- Stereotactic radiosurgery has low rates of facial nerve injury and high rates of long-term tumor control.
- Careful preoperative assessment and planning, interdisciplinary surgical team, and judicious use of intraoperative monitoring can facilitate intraoperative decision-making and improve facial nerve outcomes.
- Large intracranial tumor burden, tumor biology, limited reconstructive options, and bilateral disease make VS management and facial nerve considerations in neurofibromatosis type 2 (NF2) patients uniquely challenging.

INTRODUCTION TO VESTIBULAR SCHWANNOMA

Vestibular schwannomas (VS) are benign tumors derived from Schwann cells of the vestibular portion of cranial nerve (CN) VIII and can occur in the internal auditory canal (IAC) or cerebellopontine angle (CPA). The two primary types of VS, which are physiologically distinct, are sporadic VS and neurofibromatosis type 2 (NF2). Most VS are sporadic with a combined lifetime risk of 1:1000 for developing a unilateral tumor.[1] There is a higher incidence of VS diagnosis secondary to incidental findings from more frequent MRI.[2,3] Because of their anatomic location, these tumors often present with progressive hearing loss (90%) and tinnitus (>60%), with facial paresthesia (12%) and facial nerve (FN) palsy (6%) occurring almost exclusively among larger tumors.[1] For sporadic VS, mean age at presentation is 50 to 55 years old, without gender

Disclosure Statement: None.
Department of Otolaryngology–Head and Neck Surgery, Icahn School of Medicine at Mount Sinai, New York Eye and Ear of Mount Sinai, Floor 6, 310 East 14th Street, New York, NY 10003, USA
* Corresponding author.
E-mail address: Maura.Cosetti@mountsinai.org

predilection, and can occur on either side. Presentation of NF2 is typically earlier and less often incidental and is discussed later. A history of radiation exposure is a risk factor for VS development; however, other environmental factors have not been identified. Mobile cellphone use has not shown to increase the risk for developing VS according to the Interphone study.[4] Because sporadic, unilateral VS are benign, slow-growing tumors with only a 0.2% to 1% mortality rate, management options are predominately focused on minimizing morbidity and maximizing outcomes of hearing, balance, and FN function.[5,6]

Because a vast amount of data is available on nearly all aspects of VS, this article focuses on FN considerations related to the presentation, diagnosis, and management of VS.

CLINICAL PRESENTATION

As with most slow-growing intracranial tumors, symptom presentation (**Table 1**) is a factor of tumor biology and anatomic location. Unsurprisingly, when symptomatic, VSs most commonly presents with vestibulocochlear symptoms linked to their location in the IAC/CPA (**Fig. 1**).

Hearing Loss

VS develops slowly, typically resulting in progressive, unilateral sensorineural hearing loss (SNHL) followed by high-pitched tinnitus, likely from ischemic compression of the cochlear nerve.[3] Sudden SNHL may also occur, although more rarely, ranging from 5% to 22% of patients.[7] Asymmetrical hearing loss is the primary symptom leading to a diagnosis of VS.

Vestibular Symptoms

Imbalance, falls, vertigo, disequilibrium, and ataxia are less common presenting symptoms, presumably caused by effective compensation from a slow unilateral vestibulopathy caused by indolent tumor growth. Some data suggesting that tumors

Table 1 Symptoms of VS by presenting frequency	
Symptom	**Percentage**
Asymmetrical hearing loss	80
Progressive	72
Sudden	8
Tinnitus	6
Ataxis	4
Vertigo	3
Asymptomatic/incidental	2
Headache	2
Facial numbness	2
Otalgia	<1
Facial pain	<1
Seizure	<1
Syncope	<1

From Foley RW, Shirazi S, Maweni RM, et al. Signs and symptoms of acoustic neuroma at initial presentation: an exploratory analysis. Cureus 2017;9(11):e1846; with permission.

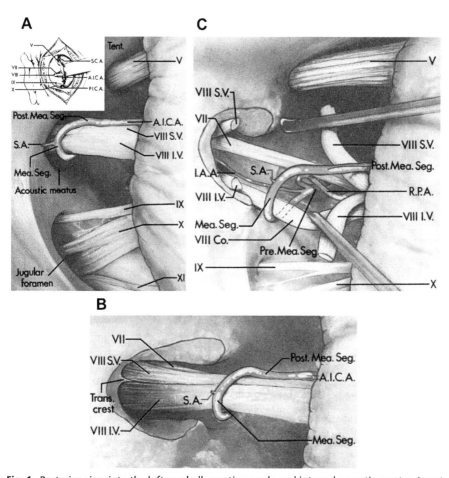

Fig. 1. Posterior view into the left cerebellopontine angle and internal acoustic meatus. Insert shows the orientation. (*A*) The tentorium (Tent.) is above the trigeminal nerve (V). The facial and vestibulocochlear nerves enter the internal acoustic meatus. The posterior surface of the vestibulocochlear nerve is formed by the inferior (VIII I.V.) and superior vestibular (VIII S.V.) nerves. The glossopharyngeal (IX), vagus (X), and spinal accessory nerves (XI) enter the jugular foramen. The premeatal segment of the anterior inferior cerebellar artery (A.I.C.A.) is not visible because it is anterior to the nerves. The meatal segment (Mea. Seg.) passes posterior to the nerves and gives rise to the subarcuate artery (S.A.). The postmeatal segment (Post. Mea. Seg.) passes above the nerves. The insert shows the superior cerebellar artery (S.C.A.) above the trigeminal nerve, and the posterior inferior cerebellar artery (P.I.C.A.) below the glossopharyngeal nerve. (*B*) The posterior wall of the internal acoustic canal has been removed. The facial nerve (VII) is anterior to the superior vestibular nerve. The subarcuate artery had to be divided to gain access to the posterior wall of the acoustic canal. The transverse crest (Trans. Crest) separates the superior and inferior vestibular nerves at the lateral end of the canal. (*C*) The superior and inferior vestibular nerves have been divided to expose the facial and cochlear nerves (VIII Co.). The premeatal segment (Pre. Mea. Seg.) gives origin to the internal auditory (I.A.A.) and recurrent perforating (R.P.A.) arteries. The initial segment of the recurrent perforating artery loops toward the meatus before turning medially to reach the side of the brainstem. (*From* Martin RG, Grant JL, Peace D, et al. Microsurgical relationships of the anterior inferior cerebellar artery and the facial-vestibulocochlear nerve complex. Neurosurgery 1980;6:490; with permission.)

associated with vestibular symptoms are typically larger (>2.5 cm) support this theory[3] Overall, however, as with audiometric data, prior studies have not shown a clear relationship between tumor size and vestibular symptoms.

Facial Nerve Paresis/Paralysis

Facial paralysis is a rare presentation of VS and when encountered, may raise concerns for other non-VS CPA or temporal bone pathology, including primary FN tumors, such as facial schwannoma or facial paraganglioma. Primary FN tumors of the IAC and CPA are difficult, or impossible, to distinguish from other more common pathology on imaging or by clinical presentation. Symptoms of facial schwannomas can mimic VS, more frequently presenting with facial twitching with progressive paresis, in conjunction with hearing loss, tinnitus, and vestibular symptoms.[8] Radiographically, primary FN tumors often have characteristic findings in the region of the geniculate ganglion or tympanic segment of the FN or have skip lesions. All of these findings should raise concern for non-VS pathology. For tumors treated surgically, intraoperative use of FN electromyography (EMG) (discussed later) and pathology analysis is the final confirmation.

DIAGNOSIS OF VESTIBULAR SCHWANNOMA

VS may be diagnosed incidentally from radiologic imaging obtained for unrelated complaints or as a consequence of asymmetrical hearing loss and/or other unilateral otologic complaints (**Table 2**). Although routinely (and appropriately) used for all hearing-related complaints, behavioral audiometry (including pure-tones, speech discrimination testing) and auditory brainstem response testing cannot reliably predict CPA pathology.[9–12] The literature is replete with studies examining the predictive value of various audiometric and electrophysiologic tests (including vestibular nystagmography) to predict retrocochlear pathology and none approach the sensitivity and specificity of radiographic imaging; data suggest that auditory brainstem response testing may be normal in 25% of CPA tumors (**Table 3**).

Gold Standard for Diagnosis of Internal Auditory Canal or Cerebellopontine Angle Pathology: MRI with and Without Gadolinium, Fine Cuts of the Internal Auditory Canal

Many CPA tumors present with a similar constellation of symptoms and audiometric findings and, therefore, the diagnosis relies heavily on radiographic imaging. MRI with gadolinium is gold standard for diagnosis of CPA pathology and should include fluid attenuated inversion recovery, T1- and T2-weighted and diffusion-weighted sequences. VS are classically hypo-to-isointense on MRI T1-weighted images, show variable

Table 2
MRI guidelines

Guideline	Amount of Asymmetry	Across How Many Frequencies	Accounts for Unilateral Tinnitus
Oxford	15 dB	Mean of all frequencies tested	Yes
Northern	20 dB	Two contiguous frequencies	Yes
Charing	20 dB/or 15 dB if one ear is normal hearing	Two contiguous frequencies/one frequency if other ear is normal hearing	No
Nashville	15 dB	One frequency	Yes

From Obholzer RJ, Rea PA, Harcourt JP. Magnetic resonance imaging screening for vestibular schwannoma: analysis of published protocols. J Laryngol Otol 2004;118(5):330; with permission.

Table 3
AAO-HNS class A-D hearing classification

Class	PTA (dB)	WRS (%)
A	<30	>70
B	<50	>50
C	Any	>50
D	Any	Any

Abbreviations: AAO-HNS, American Academy of Otolaryngology-Head and Neck Surgery; PTA, pure tone average; WRS, word recognition score.

From Brackmann DE, Fayad JN, Slattery WH 3rd, et al. Early proactive management of vestibular schwannomas in neurofibromatosis type 2. Neurosurgery 2001;49(2):278. [discussion: 280–3]; with permission.

intensity on T2-weighted images, and enhance with gadolinium contrast (**Fig. 2**).[13] These tumors may be solid or cystic, the latter showing hyperintensity on T2-weighted imaging (**Fig. 3**).[14] Thin-slice, T2-weighted three-dimensional sequences can assess tumor volume, an important measurement when following tumors over time.

Facial schwannomas are difficult to differentiate from VS preoperatively because their clinical and radiographic presentation may mimic VS. FN paresis/paralysis (as detailed previously) combined with enhancement in the geniculate (or perigeniculate) ganglion should raise suspicion for a facial schwannoma.[15,16] When treated surgically, confirmation of diagnosis can occur intraoperatively using FN EMG or by pathologic analysis.

VESTIBULAR SCHWANNOMA MANAGEMENT

Unilateral VS may be treated with clinical observation and serial imaging, microsurgical resection, stereotactic radiotherapy, or a combination of these. Medical therapy, especially as part of a clinical trial, is also an emerging option.[17] Optimal management of VS is topic of significant research and ongoing debate. Although there is an extraordinary amount of published literature on each treatment modality, expert consensus

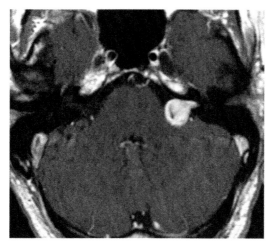

Fig. 2. Axial T1-weighted gadolinium-enhanced MRI of a unilateral left vestibular schwannoma involving of the internal auditory canal and cerebellopontine angle.

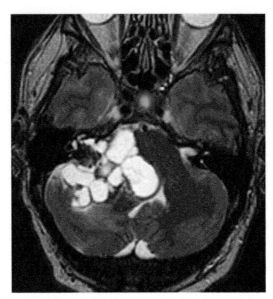

Fig. 3. Axial T2-weighted MRI of a unilateral right, cystic vestibular schwannoma involving the internal auditory canal and cerebellopontine angle.

has not been achieved. Treatment decision-making is individualized, typically incorporating several patient-, tumor-, and provider-specific factors, including age, hearing and CN status, neurologic function, tumor size, tumor location, provider training and experience, and patient preference. Overall, the primary goals of VS management are focused on balancing tumor control with functional outcomes related to hearing, balance, and facial function.

Observation

For patients with small- to medium-sized asymptomatic tumors or those with mild hearing loss, advanced age, or comorbidities precluding surgical intervention, observation with serial imaging to assess for tumor growth may be appropriate. This conservative strategy, also known as "watch and wait," is based on data documenting the natural history of these tumors. Longitudinal studies suggest that most tumors grow slowly, approximately 0 mm to 4 mm per year, although this growth may be nonlinear, sporadic, and unpredictable.[14] Cystic VS demonstrate greater variability in growth rates, likely caused by more rapid enlargement of the cystic portions (see **Fig. 3**).[15] Despite significant research in this area, there are no tumor characteristics that can reliably predict tumor growth, including patient age, gender, tumor size at diagnosis, or location.[18,19] One management algorithm for VS observation recommends imaging at first presentation, 6 months later, and then annual scans for the next 3 years, then increasing to every 2 years for a minimal surveillance of 10 years.[1]

The predominant reason for failure of "watch and wait" was progressive growth of the tumor (88%), vertigo (12%), patient preference (6.7%), FN palsy (0.7%), and midline shift (0.7%).[19] Most of the failures were within the first 2 years of surveillance (70%). Prasad and colleagues[20] compared postsurgical FN outcomes in patients who failed conservative observation against patients treated with initial surgery; after controlling for tumor size, there was no statistical difference in risk of injury of FN caused by "watch and wait" compared with initial surgery.

Radiotherapy

Primary radiotherapy

Stereotactic radiation (SRS) may be used as a primary treatment modality or as an adjunct to microsurgery in cases of tumor recurrence or growth of residual tumor following subtotal resection. SRS is effective at controlling tumor growth with greater than 95% tumor control after more than 10 years of follow-up.[21–26] Rates of hearing preservation range from 50% to 75% in the initial years to approximately 50% at long-term (>10 year) follow-up.[22–26] For patients with hearing that is available to preserve, these rates meet or surpass microsurgical resection. Notably, when compared with microsurgical resection, SRS has superior FN function outcomes.[23,25–27] Although there is significant debate on size criteria for SRS, some data caution against SRS for tumors greater than 3 cm because of post-SRS intratumoral edema that can cause further intracranial compromise. Attributed to cellular swelling following SRS-induced apoptosis, these known sequelae can influence treatment options; for this reason, many large tumors are treated with microsurgical resection (partial, subtotal, or total, as discussed later).[28,29]

Among SRS, there are three main types used: (1) Gamma knife (GK), (2) linear accelerator, and (3) fractionated stereotactic radiotherapy (FSRT). Proton beam therapy has also been used for VS, although rarely, because of its high cost and limited availability.

GK uses 192 fixed Cobalt-60 sources to deliver focused gamma rays onto the tumor during a single treatment. Linear accelerator delivers focused X rays rotated around the target in radiating arcs, also in a single dose. GK delivers a marginal dose at 50% isodense line, whereas the linear accelerator delivers 90% at the isodense line. The dose at which SRS is delivered has in recent years reduced to 12 Gy to 13 Gy with a local tumor control of up to 91% to 100% in 10 years with minimal CN V and VII morbidity.[21] In 2018, The Congress of Neurosurgeons published a statement guideline indicating that there are no differences between tumor control using either GK or linear accelerator–based therapy. Radiographically, the tumor control rates had no statistical difference.[29]

Unlike the single dosing of GK or linear accelerator, FSRT gives the radiation in focused doses over many sessions. Suggested benefits of this modality include better targeting of irregular tumor shapes to achieve a more homogenous treatment along the entirety of the tumor instead of a heterogeneous concentrated dose. A recent systematic review demonstrates similar regional control and hearing outcomes between FSRT and SRS, with a slightly higher incidence of facial and trigeminal nerve paresis with FSRT.[30,31] Other studies on FSRT suggest rates of FN damage are rare and equivalent to other forms of SRS (**Table 4**).[31,32]

Compared with surgical intervention, risks of SRS include lack of pathologic diagnosis, delayed cyst formation, vertigo and imbalance, malignant transformation, and failure of tumor control requiring salvage surgery (discussed later). Incidence of malignant transformation or malignant peripheral nerve sheath tumor is low, but nearly universally fatal.[33]

Salvage radiotherapy

SRS may also be used in cases of tumor growth after planned subtotal resection. Tumor may be intentionally left behind during microsurgical resection in an attempt to minimize risk of hearing loss or FN damage and maximize postoperative outcomes (discussed later). Residual tumor may be followed radiographically and SRS performed in cases of tumor growth, often referred to as "salvage SRS." Salvage SRS has shown minimal complications while providing high tumor control rates of up to 82% to 93% at the 5-year follow-up.[29,34] Although somewhat lower than seen in primary SRS, rates of FN function are high with salvage SRS. Jeltema and colleagues[35] found 85% of patients had either no FN deficit or transient mild deficit after salvage SRS (**Table 5**).

Table 4
Different primary modalities of management and the FN outcomes and local tumor control

	Specific Modality	FN Status Immediately After Management	FN Status at Next Follow-up	Requiring Further Treatment
Primary radiotherapy	SRS (including GK)	73% had HB I–II,[37] 19.4%–27% had new-onset FN palsy (HB IV–VI)[32,37]	96.2% had HB I–II at mean of 54 follow-up[24]	1.7%–9.5%[14,34,66]
	FSRT	9% with new-onset palsy (HB IV–VI)[32]	88% had HB I–II[67]	20%–22.2%[32,67]
Primary surgery	Retrosigmoid	17%–75% had HB I–II (Torres, Hong), 3%–21.1% with new-onset palsy (HB IV–VI)[32,66,68]	7%–74.4% had HB I–II (Torres, Hong), 8% had HB III–IV at 1 y out[35,68]	8% of patients after all types of microsurgical resection required radiosurgery[69]
	Translabyranthine	55% had HB I–II, 23% had HB III–IV at postoperative day 8[68]	37%–62.5% had HB I–II, 48% had HB III–IV at 1 y[35,68]	1.2% required revision surgery[37]
	Middle cranial fossa	1% had HB I–II, 1% had HB III–IV at postoperative day 8[68]	7% had HB I–II, 8% had HB III–IV at postoperative day 8[68]	

Abbreviations: FN, facial nerve; FSRT, fractionated stereotactic radiotherapy; GK, Gamma Knife; HB, House-Brackmann; SRS, stereotactic radiosurgery.

Salvage microsurgical resection

Alternatively, patients treated with primary SRS with incomplete control may require surgical excision, termed "salvage surgery." Herein lies the primary downside to SRS: rates of complications, including unilateral profound hearing loss and temporary and permanent facial paralysis are higher when surgery follows prior radiation.[36,37] Data suggest that radiation-induced changes may be responsible for loss of native

Table 5
Different secondary modalities of management and the facial nerve outcomes and local tumor control

	Specific Modality	Facial Nerve Status Immediately After Management	Facial Nerve Status at Next Follow up
Secondary radiotherapy after microsurgery	SRS	23% of HB I–III developed worsened FN function[70]	No data
Secondary radiotherapy after radiotherapy		No worsening facial nerve function[71]	
Secondary surgery after radiotherapy	Retrosigmoid	20%–80% range, mean is 19.4% develop HB IV–VI[68]	73%–82% had HB I–II at long-term follow-up[37,45]
	Translabrynthine	40.4% developed worsening function from HB I–IV[25]	73%–79.3% had HB I–II at 1-y follow-up[11]

Abbreviations: FN, facial nerve; HB, House-Brackmann; SRS, stereotactic radiosurgery.

tumor planes and decreased ability to maintain anatomic integrity of the cochlear or FNs during tumor resection. More recent data suggest that postoperative FN function following salvage and primary surgical treatment may be similar (see **Table 5**).[37]

Microsurgical Resection

For large tumors, those with brainstem compression or neurologic compromise, tumors with demonstrable growth on prior imaging, and/or patients who prefer tumor excision, craniotomy with microsurgical resection is the modality of choice. Historically and before the introduction of SRS, surgery was the primary treatment modality for VS. There are several routes to the IAC/CPA and choice of approach is based on various tumor- and patient-specific characteristics. The approaches include translabrynthine (TL), transotic, middle cranial fossa (MCF), or retrosigmoid approach (RS). Two of these approaches offer the possibility of hearing preservation (MCF and RS), whereas the others intentionally breach the vestibular or cochlear apparatus of the inner ear leading to profound hearing loss. Additionally, the anatomic relationship between the FN and the tumor in each approach has implications for postoperative FN outcomes.

- Middle cranial fossa: The MCF approach is commonly used for intracanalicular tumors limited to the IAC or with minimal (up to 1 cm) CPA extension.[38] This surgical route requires a temporal craniotomy, retraction of the temporal lobe, and has the option of hearing preservation. The dissection is extradural and IAC is drilled from the middle fossa using a variety of techniques to identify and uncover the superior roof of the IAC. Because of the anatomic configuration of the IAC, the FN typically lies beneath the bony roof of the IAC and thus, between the surgeon and the VS, which arises from the superior or inferior vestibular nerve. Tumor access and resection requires retraction of CN VII (**Fig. 4**). Despite this, rates of normal FN function (House-Brackmann [HB] I or HB II) range from 72% to 100%.[38–40] Because tumor dissection is extradural and the temporal lobe sits on the roof of the temporal bone, rates of cerebrospinal fluid leak are low with this approach. Hearing preservation is possible in this approach; however, rates are variable and range from 64% to 82.7%.[38] Because this approach requires retraction of the temporal lobe, there is an increased risk of temporal lobe injury, seizures, or rarely, postoperative hemiparesis.[40]
- Retrosigmoid/suboccipital: This commonly used approach requires a posterior fossa craniotomy and allows access to the CPA, petrous apex, clivus, and the IAC. For tumors with significant residual hearing that are not impacted against the fundus of the IAC, this approach has the potential for hearing preservation. Drilling of the IAC is performed from the posterior, petrous face of the temporal bone with care not to violate the endolymphatic sac or cochleovestibular structures of the inner ear. Typical tumor position within the IAC and CPA place the FN on the underside of the tumor allowing tumor dissection without having to first displace the FN (as with MCF approach.) Identification of the FN may occur in the lateral most aspect of the IAC and followed proximally into the IAC and ultimately into the fundus and cisternal segment in the CPA.[40] Cerebrospinal fluid leak is a known complication of this approach, occurring in approximately 5% to 10% of patients.[41,42]
- Translabyrinthine/transotic: This transtemporal approach accesses the IAC and CPA through the labyrinth, leading to intentional and profound SNHL. As with the RS approach, the FN anatomy is typically favorable with the nerve on the underside of the tumor, away from the surgeon.[38] TL and transotic approaches allow access to the entirety of the temporal course of the FN and the option of distal FN identification, such as in the labyrinthine segment beyond the IAC.

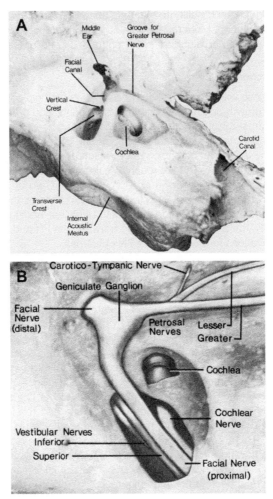

Fig. 4. Middle fossa approach to internal acoustic meatus. (*A*) Cochlea exposed in angle between the groove for the greater petrosal nerve and labyrinthine part of the facial canal. (*B*) Specimen with nerves intact. Dura and bone above facial canal and internal acoustic meatus removed. Cochlear nerve exposed medial to geniculate ganglion. (*From* Pait TG, Harris FS, Paullus WS, et al. Microsurgical anatomy and dissection of the temporal bone. Surg Neurol 1977;8:374; with permission.)

When controlling for other critical factors, such as tumor size (discussed later), TL and RS approaches have similar FN outcomes.[40,43]

Extent of resection: total versus subtotal versus partial

Treatment options for VS management are individualized, incorporating patient- and tumor-specific factors and may not include total tumor resection in all cases. In fact, significant data suggest that subtotal resection in favor of preservation of CN function is a frequent and reasonable goal in current VS management.[44] Residual tumor is intentionally left on the FN and followed postoperatively with MRI. Tumor growth seen radiographically is then commonly treated with "salvage SRS" (discussed previously). Recurrence following gross total resection is uncommon and estimated to be less than 10% in long-term (15 year) follow-up.[44] However, recurrence rates for subtotal resection can vary from 18% to 55% at 15 years.[44,45] This was supported by Monfared and colleagues[46] who found that there was a three times higher likelihood of tumor regrowth following subtotal resections compared with gross total resection.

Intraoperative Facial Nerve Monitoring

Introduced in 1979, FN electromyogram (colloquially referred to as FN monitoring) is the cornerstone of intraoperative monitoring.[13,47] This monitoring is routinely used in VS tumor resection regardless of approach. Successful use requires general anesthesia without (or with limited, short-acting) neuromuscular blockade. Before commencing surgery, needle recording electrodes are inserted into the lateral aspect of the orbicularis oculi and orbicularis oris, and ground electrodes are placed elsewhere in the head and neck according to surgeon preference.

Continuous EMG identifies neurotonic discharges generated by mechanical or metabolic stimuli and can alert the surgeon to possible FN injury from surgical manipulation, whereas direct stimulation allows confirmation of neural integrity from the site of stimulation to the motor end plates of the patient's facial muscles. Modern EMG technology allows for continuous loud-speaker monitoring and intermittent handheld stimulation using a FN probe. The continuous loudspeaker monitoring provides surgeons with real-time audible information about the functional status of the nerve. The most sensitive type of train activity for FN paresis is type A. This produces a sinusoidal, high-frequency pattern that is highly correlated with FN dysfunction.[48] Direct stimulation creates a compound muscle action potential (CMAP) and is generated by a variety of handheld probes, including specifically designed microsurgical instruments with integrated FN monitoring capabilities.

Once the tumor is encountered, the universal first step involves direct stimulation of the tumor capsule to confirm the diagnosis (ie, that it is *not* an FN schwannoma) and also to ensure the FN is not in an unexpected position. Direct electrical stimulation is used throughout the procedure to allow identification and mapping of the FN location relative to the tumor. Several EMG parameters have been found to predict postoperative FN function, including train time, amplitude, and threshold stimulation intensity (milliampere) of the CMAP.

Prell and colleagues[49] showed that train time of up to 10 seconds correlated with a postoperative deterioration of one HB grade. Other authors showed successful CMAP generation with stimulation thresholds of less than or equal to 0.1 mA predicted normal facial function with 98% probability.[50,51] Response amplitude can also have implications for postoperative function with amplitudes of greater than or equal to 200 μV portending good FN outcome. Amplitude ratios (constructed from lateral and distal stimulation points) of greater than or equal to 0.3 suggested the potential for long-term recovery, whereas those less than or equal to 0.1 suggested lack of anatomic integrity necessitating grafting or neural anastomosis surgery.[51]

Often, especially at the start of surgical resection, direct stimulation is of limited utility because the nerve is inaccessible or obscured by tumor bulk. Additionally, if the FN has been significantly thinned and/or stretched by a large tumor, localized direct stimulation may not contact enough nerve fibers to allow action potential generation, thereby yielding inconsistent information about the location and integrity of the FN.

To address this problem, another option for intraoperative FN monitoring is transcranial stimulation of the motor cortex (TCMEP). This modality is an alternative to the triggered CMAP of continuous EMG in that it allows evaluation of the entire FN without direct stimulation. Stimulating corkscrew electrodes are placed into the scalp along the homunculus of the motor cortex and recording occurs (as with direct stimulation) at the needle electrodes in the facial muscles. Stimulation occurs at routine intervals throughout the procedure, at the discretion of the surgical team, and is typically performed by an experienced neuroelectrophysiologist. Data suggest that TCMEP is useful to predict short- and long-term FN function after VS resection.[52–54]

Factors Affecting Facial Nerve Outcome

Although facial paresis or paralysis can occur with any treatment modality (including watchful waiting), it is typically discussed in the context of microsurgical resection. Despite significant advances in nearly all aspects of VS treatment, FN injury remains a central concern with an overall 8% to 20% incidence of permanent FN paresis/paralysis following surgery.[55] Although myriad factors are known to affect FN function, including tumor location, surgical approach, prior SRS, and the use and type of intraoperative monitoring, the most consistent predictor of FN outcome is tumor size.[5,40,56,57] Simply put, larger tumors have greater risk of postoperative facial paresis or paralysis, irrespective of other variables. In addition, it is often the largest tumors that demand surgical resection (SRS and watchful waiting are often inappropriate for large tumors).

Preoperative considerations

Preoperative imaging should be carefully reviewed, preferably with an experienced neuroradiologist. Tumor diameter (>3 cm), volume (>10 cm^3), and location (anterior extension beyond the fundus) predict statistically significant FN disruption (20% vs 5%) compared with smaller tumors.[57] Intratumor characteristics, specifically tumor structure (solid vs cystic) or histologic type (Antoni A vs Antoni B), have not been found to be predictive of FN injury.[57] Importantly, many of these characteristics are interrelated and difficult to analyze in isolation.[15] For example, surgeons may perform a less radical removal of cystic tumors, allowing a thin tumor capsule to be retained onto the FN resulting in improved outcomes.[15] Preoperative use of intravenous steroids (at the start of the procedure) is routine in VS resection; however, no data exist to specifically assess their independent benefit on postoperative function.

Intraoperative technique

Intraoperative technique is highly surgeon-dependent and heavily informed by surgical team experience and intraoperative monitoring technology. Familiarity with facial EMG (and TCMEP, if available) is crucial for intraoperative decision making and input from a neuroelectrophysiologist can assist in synthesizing real-time recording with surgical decision-making.

Preservation of FN function is a well-recognized goal of CPA/IAC tumor surgery, often surpassing complete tumor resection. Of the 1000 VS resections Samii and colleagues[56] performed in 15 years, 93% achieved FN preservation. Review of current trends suggests that modern surgical technique is biased toward near total or subtotal resection, with surgeons opting for leaving a thin rind of tumor on the FN instead of risking nerve injury and compromised postoperative function. Although conceptually simple, this can lead to a myriad of challenging intraoperative scenarios. First, large tumors frequently cause extensive thinning and stretching of the nerve, creating a "veil" often at the porus; in these cases, it is difficult to ascertain anatomic continuity, either visually or with direct EMG, especially in the presence of residual tumor. Occasionally, TCMEP is helpful to indicate neural integrity. Another scenario includes loss of facial EMG in the setting of anatomic continuity. Despite significant advances in lateral skull-base surgery, this persists one of the most vexing intraoperative conundrums in VS surgery: anatomic continuity with loss of electrophysiologic function. The cause of immediate paresis/paralysis is incompletely understood, but may include a conduction block, neuropraxia or axonotmesis caused by intraoperative mechanical/iatrogenic manipulation, edema, vasoconstriction/spasm of neuronal blood supply, herpes virus reactivation, or some combination of these. A temporary conduction block may recover rapidly over a period of days, whereas neuropraxia or axonotmesis may require months to improve and may not reach preoperative function.[58] Optimal intraoperative decision-making in this setting remains elusive and surgeon specific and more data and guidance in this area are needed. For some, to have residual tumor burden and poor facial outcome would seem to have achieved the "worst of both worlds" with failure in functional outcome and tumor control. However, because of the real possibility of delayed recovery of FN function, deference to anatomic continuity (vs total tumor resection compromising the FN) is common.

Some data exist to suggest medical therapies may be helpful intraoperatively, especially to address FN compromise caused by vasospasm/construction. Nimodipine, a dihydropyridine calcium antagonist commonly used as an antihypertensive, has been investigated in VS surgery to improve facial function and hearing preservation. Patients who received perioperative dosing of nimodipine (combined with hydroxyethyl starch, an intravascular volume expander) showed some improved rates of FN function and significant improvement in hearing preservation rates compared with a control group.[59–61]

Gelfoam soaked in papavarine, a vasoactive agent, has also been used anecdotally as a topical agent placed directly onto the facial or cochlear nerve during surgery to improve blood supply. This maneuver is supported by some animal data showing improved hearing function in rabbits; however, no human trials have been reported.

In cases of obvious FN transection identified intraoperatively, options for reanimation include immediate or delayed FN primary coaptation; interposition grafting; and static procedures, such as eyelid weight and tarsorrhaphy. Unlike other locations along the FN course, transection within the CPA or IAC can lead to faster central degeneration than injury farther from the FN nucleus. The closer the transection is to the brainstem, the faster the degeneration and loss of neural plasticity occurs.[56] When possible, immediate reconstruction with an interposition graft can offer the best long-term outcome. Neurorrhaphy in the CPA can range from technically challenging to frequently impossible, especially if the remaining neural elements or stumps are insufficient for grafting. Data suggest that when achieved, immediate nerve reconstruction at the CPA site can achieve HB I to HB III in up to three-quarters of patients.[56]

Postoperatively

Preserved anatomic continuity does not guarantee postoperative outcome. In cases of complete, immediate postoperative FN paralysis with surgical confidence in neural integrity, observation for 6 to 12 months is recommended. Temporary conduction blocks may improve rapidly, whereas neurapraxia and axonotmesis may take months and follow typical regeneration rates of 1 mm per day. Serial EMGs at each surveillance visit can follow this recovery and guide management options. Specifically, polyphasic potentials suggest motor end plates are intact and regenerating, supporting additional observation for management, whereas fibrillation or lack of signal portend less hope for functional recovery and reconstruction options should be pursued.

Perioperative intravenous steroids with transition to an oral taper is commonly used following intracranial tumor resection and may improve FN function.

Meticulous eye care is required to prevent exposure keratopathy. Adjunctive static procedures, such as lid loading with gold or platinum weight implants and/or tarsorrhaphy, canthopexy, or canthoplasty, should be used judiciously to prevent ocular complications of impaired eye closure.[49]

Facial Nerve Reconstruction and Rehabilitation

Dynamic surgical procedures are used when functional recovery is not expected; options include cross-FN grafting, reanimation using hypoglossal or facial to facial reinnervation, muscle transposition, tendon transfer, and free muscle transfer. Static procedures include facial sling and multivector suture techniques and are often reserved for patients who have failed prior dynamic options, or cannot tolerate other options secondary to comorbidities, or as adjunct procedures to dynamic reanimation.[55]

Physical rehabilitation with a therapist skilled in FN paresis/paralysis is an important adjunctive treatment. Soft tissue mobilization, active assistive exercises, relaxation, and meditation have all been shown to improve FN function.[62] Use of laser therapy, EMG for neuromuscular retraining, and physical and biofeedback may also be used as part of a comprehensive rehabilitation program.[55]

Facial Nerve Considerations in Neurofibromatosis Type 2

NF2 is an autosomal-dominant syndrome caused by the loss of tumor suppressor gene Merlin on chromosome 22q12 leading to bilateral VS, which occurs exclusively among this population, and other concurrent intracranial and spinal tumors (**Table 6**).[19] Large intracranial tumor burden, specific tumor biology, limited options for reconstruction, and potential for bilateral CN dysfunction make VS management and FN considerations in these patients uniquely challenging (**Figs. 5** and **6**). Options for VS treatment mimic those for sporadic VS and include observation/watchful waiting, SRS and microsurgical resection, plus targeted chemotherapy/immunotherapy.

Because much is known about Merlin and related signaling pathways, use of targeted chemotherapy and immunotherapy to reduce disease burden, improve hearing and CN function, and improve quality of life is being actively studied. The current drugs in development are lapatinib (epidermal growth factor receptor inhibitor), everolimus (mTOR inhibitor), bevacizumab (vascular endothelial growth factor inhibitor), and AR-42 (histone deacetylase inhibitor). These drugs are all currently in clinical trials phase 0 to 2, but the initial results are promising to inhibit cell proliferation and VS growth.[63]

Table 6 NF2 diagnostic criteria	
Primary Finding	**Additional Details Needed for Diagnosis**
Bilateral VS	Before 70 years old, because after 70 years old there is a higher rate of spontaneous bilateral VS, or unilateral VS before 70 years old, and first-degree relative with NF2
Unilateral VS	AND any two: meningioma, non-VS, neurofibroma, glioma, posterior subcapsular lenticular opacities
Multiple meningiomas	AND unilateral VS or any two: neurofibroma, glioma, nonvestibular schwannoma, cataract
First-degree relative with NF2	AND unilateral vestibular schwannoma, or any two: meningioma, nonvestibular schwannoma, glioma, neurofibroma, posterior subcapsular lenticular opacities

Data from Baser ME, Friedman JM, Wallace AJ, et al. Evaluation of clinical diagnostic criteria for neurofibromatosis 2. Neurology 2002;59(11):1759–65 and Halliday J, Rutherford SA, McCabe MG, et al. An update on the diagnosis and treatment of vestibular schwannoma. Expert Rev Neurother 2018;18(1):29–39.

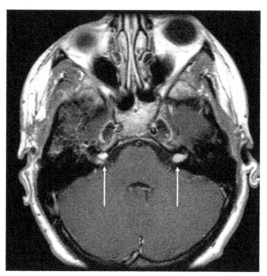

Fig. 5. Axial T1-weighted gadolinium-enhanced MRI of bilateral VS in NF2. *White arrows* indicate the location of the VS in the internal auditory canals bilaterally.

Unlike sporadic VS, surgical excision is favored over SRS in NF2 for a variety of reasons. The more rapid tumor growth and aggressive course of disease in NF2 combined with a younger age at presentation make single modality treatment less effective.[64,65] Only 50% of NF2 patients treated with SRS have tumor control and most require "salvage surgery," typically with worse functional outcomes compared with those treated with primary surgery.[64] Facial dysfunction in NF2 often heralds greater morbidity because of other, concurrent skull base tumors leading to CN

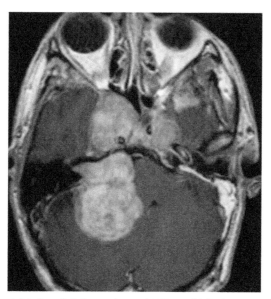

Fig. 6. Axial, T1-weighted gadolinium-enhanced MRI multiple intracranial tumors in NF2. Demonstrated are a large right vestibular schwannoma and bilateral trigeminal schwannomas.

dysfunction. Specifically, NF2 patients with facial paralysis are at greater risk of blindness from exposure keratitis, lagophthalmic keratopathy, and corneal ulcers because of decreased sensation from trigeminal nerve injury. Aggressive eye precautions and early lid loading should be considered in cases of CN V and VII compromise. Facial reanimation options of free muscle transfer or hypoglossal-facial should take into consideration the tumor burden and function of other CNs.

Current NF2 management is centered on maximizing functional outcomes, including facial, hearing, and lower CN functions of voice and swallowing. These patients are best cared for in tertiary care centers with significant multidisciplinary experience in managing this complex and debilitating disease.

SUMMARY

Consensus on optimal treatment of VS remains elusive and includes observation, SRS, microsurgical resection, or a combination. Treatment decision-making should be individualized and incorporate the multitude of patient- and tumor-specific characteristics known to affect outcome. In all cases, treatment should aim to achieve maximum tumor control with minimal functional deficit. When surgical resection is appropriate, the surgical team may use many resources and techniques to guide intraoperative surgical strategy and decision-making, including patient age, preoperative function, tumor size, location, and characteristics and intraoperative monitoring, such as facial EMG and TCMEP. On the horizon, other adjunctive treatments include various chemotherapy and immunotherapeutic agents for NF2 and sporadic VS, and laser and vasoactive drugs for the improvement of FN rehabilitation. It is hoped that clinicians will arrive at a better understanding of single-modality treatment failures so as to better counsel patients and guide therapy.

REFERENCES

1. Schmidt RF, Boghani Z, Choudhry OJ, et al. Incidental vestibular schwannomas: a review of prevalence, growth rate, and management challenges. Neurosurg Focus 2012;33(3):e4.
2. Foley RW, Shirazi S, Maweni RM, et al. Signs and symptoms of acoustic neuroma at initial presentation: an exploratory analysis. Cureus 2017;9(11):e1846.
3. Halliday J, Rutherford SA, McCabe MG, et al. An update on the diagnosis and treatment of vestibular schwannoma. Expert Rev Neurother 2018;18(1):29–39.
4. Group IS. Acoustic neuroma risk in relation to mobile telephone use: results of the INTERPHONE international case-control study. Cancer Epidemiol 2011;35(5): 453–64.
5. Sughrue ME, Yang I, Aranda D, et al. Beyond audiofacial morbidity after vestibular schwannoma surgery. J Neurosurg 2011;114(2):367–74.
6. Sughrue ME, Yang I, Rutkowski MJ, et al. Preservation of facial nerve function after resection of vestibular schwannoma. Br J Neurosurg 2010;24(6):666–71.
7. Moffat DA, Baguley DM, von Blumenthal H, et al. Sudden deafness in vestibular schwannoma. J Laryngol Otol 1994;108(2):116–9.
8. Wilkinson EP, Hoa M, Slattery WH 3rd, et al. Evolution in the management of facial nerve schwannoma. Laryngoscope 2011;121(10):2065–74.
9. Neary WJ, Newton VE, Laoide-Kemp SN, et al. A clinical, genetic and audiological study of patients and families with unilateral vestibular schwannomas. II. Audiological findings in 93 patients with unilateral vestibular schwannomas. J Laryngol Otol 1996;110(12):1120–8.

10. Kanzaki J, Ogawa K, Ogawa S, et al. Audiological findings in acoustic neuroma. Acta Otolaryngol Suppl 1991;487:125–32.

11. Nadol JB Jr, Diamond PF, Thornton AR. Correlation of hearing loss and radiologic dimensions of vestibular schwannomas (acoustic Neuromas). Am J Otol 1996; 17(2):312–6.

12. Tutar H, Duzlu M, Goksu N, et al. Audiological correlates of tumor parameters in acoustic neuromas. Eur Arch Otorhinolaryngol 2013;270(2):437–41.

13. Vivas EX, Carlson ML, Neff BA, et al. Congress of neurological surgeons systematic review and evidence-based guidelines on intraoperative cranial nerve monitoring in vestibular Schwannoma surgery. Neurosurgery 2018;82(2):e44–6.

14. Kirchmann M, Karnov K, Hansen S, et al. Ten-year follow-up on tumor growth and hearing in patients observed with an intracanalicular vestibular Schwannoma. Neurosurgery 2017;80(1):49–56.

15. Piccirillo E, Wiet MR, Flanagan S, et al. Cystic vestibular Schwannoma: classification, management, and facial nerve outcomes. Otol Neurotol 2009;30(6):826–34.

16. Calzada AP, Go JL, Tschirhart DL, et al. Cerebellopontine angle and intracanalicular masses mimicking vestibular schwannomas. Otol Neurotol 2015;36(3): 491–7.

17. Van Gompel JJ, Agazzi S, Carlson ML, et al. Congress of neurological surgeons systematic review and evidence-based guidelines on emerging therapies for the treatment of patients with vestibular Schwannomas. Neurosurgery 2018;82(2): e52–4.

18. Fayad JN, Semaan MT, Lin J, et al. Conservative management of vestibular schwannoma: expectations based on the length of the observation period. Otol Neurotol 2014;35(7):1258–65.

19. Olshan M, Srinivasan VM, Landrum T, et al. Acoustic neuroma: an investigation of associations between tumor size and diagnostic delays, facial weakness, and surgical complications. Ear Nose Throat J 2014;93(8):304–16.

20. Prasad SC, Patnaik U, Grinblat G, et al. Decision making in the wait-and-scan approach for vestibular Schwannomas: is there a price to pay in terms of hearing, facial nerve, and overall outcomes? Neurosurgery 2017. [Epub ahead of print].

21. Murphy ES, Suh JH. Radiotherapy for vestibular Schwannomas: a critical review. Int J Radiat Oncol Biol Phys 2011;79(4):985–7.

22. Meijer OW, Vandertop WP, Baayen JC, et al. Single-fraction vs. fractionated linac-based stereotactic radiosurgery for vestibular Schwannoma: a single-institution study. Int J Radiat Oncol Biol Phys 2003;56(5):1390–6.

23. Kondziolka D, Mousavi SH, Kano H, et al. The newly diagnosed vestibular schwannoma: radiosurgery, resection, or observation? Neurosurg Focus 2012; 33(3):e8.

24. Yang I, Sughrue ME, Han SJ, et al. A comprehensive analysis of hearing preservation after radiosurgery for vestibular schwannoma. J Neurosurg 2010;112(4): 851–9.

25. Hasegawa T, Kida Y, Kato T, et al. Long-term safety and efficacy of stereotactic radiosurgery for vestibular schwannomas: evaluation of 440 patients more than 10 years after treatment with Gamma Knife surgery. J Neurosurg 2013;118(3): 557–65.

26. Wolbers JG, Dallenga AH, Mendez Romero A, et al. What intervention is best practice for vestibular schwannomas? A systematic review of controlled studies. BMJ Open 2013;3(2):e001345.

27. Putz F, Muller J, Wimmer C, et al. Stereotactic radiotherapy of vestibular schwannoma: Hearing preservation, vestibular function, and local control following primary and salvage radiotherapy. Strahlenther Onkol 2017;193(3):200–12.

28. Regis J, Pellet W, Delsanti C, et al. Functional outcome after gamma knife surgery or microsurgery for vestibular Schwannomas. J Neurosurg 2002;97(5):1091–100.

29. Germano IM, Sheehan J, Parish J, et al. Congress of neurological surgeons systematic review and evidence-based guidelines on the role of radiosurgery and radiation therapy in the management of patients with vestibular Schwannomas. Neurosurgery 2018;82(2):e49–51.

30. Noren G. Long-term complications following gamma knife radiosurgery of vestibular schwannomas. Stereotact Funct Neurosurg 1998;70(Suppl 1):65–73.

31. Persson O, Bartek J Jr, Shalom NB, et al. Stereotactic radiosurgery vs. fractionated radiotherapy for tumor control in vestibular schwannoma patients: a systematic review. Acta Neurochir (Wien) 2017;159(6):1013–21.

32. Patel MA, Marciscano AE, Hu C, et al. Long-term treatment response and patient outcomes for vestibular Schwannoma patients treated with hypofractionated stereotactic radiotherapy. Front Oncol 2017;7:200.

33. King AT, Rutherford SA, Hammerbeck-Ward C, et al. Malignant peripheral nerve sheath tumors are not a feature of neurofibromatosis type 2 in the unirradiated patient. Neurosurgery 2018;83(1):38–42.

34. Chung WY, Pan DH, Lee CC, et al. Large vestibular Schwannomas treated by Gamma Knife surgery: long-term outcomes. J Neurosurg 2010;113(Suppl): 112–21.

35. Jeltema HR, Bakker NA, Bijl HP, et al. Near total extirpation of vestibular schwannoma with salvage radiosurgery. Laryngoscope 2015;125(7):1703–7.

36. Pollock BE, Lunsford LD, Kondziolka D, et al. Vestibular Schwannoma management. Part II. Failed radiosurgery and the role of delayed microsurgery. J Neurosurg 1998;89(6):949–55.

37. Wise SC, Carlson ML, Tveiten OV, et al. Surgical salvage of recurrent vestibular schwannoma following prior stereotactic radiosurgery. Laryngoscope 2016; 126(11):2580–6.

38. Ginzkey C, Scheich M, Harnisch W, et al. Outcome on hearing and facial nerve function in microsurgical treatment of small vestibular Schwannoma via the middle cranial fossa approach. Eur Arch Otorhinolaryngol 2013;270(4):1209–16.

39. Meyer TA, Canty PA, Wilkinson EP, et al. Small acoustic neuromas: surgical outcomes versus observation or radiation. Otol Neurotol 2006;27(3):380–92.

40. Colletti V, Fiorino F. Middle fossa versus retrosigmoid-transmeatal approach in vestibular Schwannoma surgery: a prospective study. Otol Neurotol 2003;24(6): 927–34.

41. Ansari SF, Terry C, Cohen-Gadol AA. Surgery for vestibular Schwannomas: a systematic review of complications by approach. Neurosurg Focus 2012;33(3):e14.

42. Mangus BD, Rivas A, Yoo MJ, et al. Management of cerebrospinal fluid leaks after vestibular schwannoma surgery. Otol Neurotol 2011;32(9):1525–9.

43. Gurgel RK, Dogru S, Amdur RL, et al. Facial nerve outcomes after surgery for large vestibular schwannomas: do surgical approach and extent of resection matter? Neurosurg Focus 2012;33(3):e16.

44. Nakatomi H, Jacob JT, Carlson ML, et al. Long-term risk of recurrence and regrowth after gross-total and subtotal resection of sporadic vestibular Schwannoma. J Neurosurg 2017;1–7.

45. Fukuda M, Oishi M, Hiraishi T, et al. Clinicopathological factors related to re-growth of vestibular Schwannoma after incomplete resection. J Neurosurg 2011;114(5):1224–31.
46. Monfared A, Corrales CE, Theodosopoulos PV, et al. Facial nerve outcome and tumor control rate as a function of degree of resection in treatment of large acoustic neuromas: preliminary report of the acoustic neuroma subtotal resection study (ANSRS). Neurosurgery 2016;79(2):194–203.
47. Prass RL, Luders H. Acoustic (loudspeaker) facial electromyographic monitoring: Part 1. Evoked electromyographic activity during acoustic neuroma resection. Neurosurgery 1986;19:392–400.
48. Youssef AS, Downes AE. Intraoperative neurophysiological monitoring in vestibular schwannoma surgery: advances and clinical implications. Neurosurg Focus 2009;27(4):e9.
49. Prell J, Rampp S, Romstock J, et al. Train time as a quantitative electromyographic parameter for facial nerve function in patients undergoing surgery for vestibular schwannoma. J Neurosurg 2007;106(5):826–32.
50. Neff BA, Ting J, Dickinson SL, et al. Facial nerve monitoring parameters as a predictor of postoperative facial nerve outcomes after vestibular schwannoma resection. Otol Neurotol 2005;26(4):728–32.
51. Goldbrunner RH, Schlake HP, Milewski C, et al. Quantitative parameters of intraoperative electromyography predict facial nerve outcomes for vestibular schwannoma surgery. Neurosurgery 2000;46(5):1140–6 [discussion: 1146–8].
52. Cosetti MK, Xu M, Rivera A, et al. Intraoperative transcranial motor-evoked potential monitoring of the facial nerve during cerebellopontine angle tumor resection. J Neurol Surg B Skull Base 2012;73(5):308–15.
53. Liu BY, Tian YJ, Liu W, et al. Intraoperative facial motor evoked potentials monitoring with transcranial electrical stimulation for preservation of facial nerve function in patients with large acoustic neuroma. Chin Med J (Engl) 2007;120(4):323–5.
54. Bhimrao SK, Le TN, Dong CC, et al. Role of facial nerve motor-evoked potential ratio in predicting facial nerve function in vestibular Schwannoma surgery both immediate and at 1 Year. Otol Neurotol 2016;37(8):1162–7.
55. Rudman KL, Rhee JS. Habilitation of facial nerve dysfunction after resection of a vestibular schwannoma. Otolaryngol Clin North Am 2012;45(2):513–30.
56. Samii M, Matthies C. Management of 1000 vestibular schwannomas (acoustic neuromas): the facial nerve–preservation and restitution of function. Neurosurgery 1997;40(4):684–94 [discussion: 694–5].
57. Grahnke K, Garst JR, Martin B. Prognostic indices for predicting facial nerve outcome following the resection of large acoustic neuromas. J Neurol Surg B Skull Base 2017;78(6):454–60.
58. Bernat I, Grayeli AB, Esquia G, et al. Intraoperative electromyography and surgical observations as predictive factors of facial nerve outcome in vestibular Schwannoma surgery. Otol Neurotol 2010;31:306–12.
59. Strauss C, Romstock J, Fahlbusch R, et al. Preservation of facial nerve function after postoperative vasoactive treatment in vestibular schwannoma surgery. Neurosurgery 2006;59(3):577–84 [discussion: 577–84].
60. Scheller C, Wienke A, Tatagiba M, et al. Prophylactic nimodipine treatment for cochlear and facial nerve preservation after vestibular schwannoma surgery: a randomized multicenter Phase III trial. J Neurosurg 2016;124(3):657–64.
61. Scheller C, Wienke A, Tatagiba M, et al. Prophylactic nimodipine treatment and improvement in hearing outcome after vestibular schwannoma surgery: a

combined analysis of a randomized, multicenter, Phase III trial and its pilot study. J Neurosurg 2017;127(6):1376–83.

62. Kumral TL, Uyar Y, Berkiten G, et al. How to rehabilitate long-term facial paralysis. J Craniofac Surg 2015;26(3):831–5.

63. Blakeley J. Development of drug treatments for neurofibromatosis type 2-associated vestibular schwannoma. Curr Opin Otolaryngol Head Neck Surg 2012;20(5): 372–9.

64. Tysome JR, Macfarlane R, Durie-Gair J, et al. Surgical management of vestibular schwannomas and hearing rehabilitation in neurofibromatosis type 2. Otol Neurotol 2012;33(3):466–72.

65. Maniakas A, Saliba I. Neurofibromatosis type 2 vestibular schwannoma treatment: a review of the literature, trends, and outcomes. Otol Neurotol 2014; 35(5):889–94.

66. Nonaka Y, Fukushima T, Watanabe K. Surgical management of vestibular Schwannomas after failed radiation treatment. Neurosurg Rev 2016;39(2): 303–12 [discussion: 312].

67. Teo M, Zhang M, Li A, et al. The outcome of hypofractionated stereotactic radiosurgery for large vestibular Schwannomas. World Neurosurg 2016;93:398–409.

68. Torres R, Nguyen Y, Vanier A, et al. Multivariate analysis of factors influencing facial nerve outcome following microsurgical resection of vestibular Schwannoma. Otolaryngol Head Neck Surg 2017;156(3):525–33.

69. Breshears JD, Osorio JA, Cheung SW, et al. Surgery after primary radiation treatment for sporadic vestibular Schwannomas: case series. Oper Neurosurg (Hagerstown) 2017;13(4):441–7.

70. Yomo S, Arkha Y, Delsanti C, et al. Repeat gamma knife surgery for regrowth of vestibular Schwannomas. Neurosurgery 2009;64(1):48–54 [discussion: 54–5].

71. Hahn CH, Stangerup SE, Caye-Thomasen P. Residual tumour after vestibular schwannoma surgery. J Laryngol Otol 2013;127(6):568–73.

Management of Bilateral Facial Palsy

Leahthan F. Domeshek, MD, Ronald M. Zuker, MD, FRCS, Gregory H. Borschel, MD*

KEYWORDS

- Facial paralysis • Facial reanimation • Facial nerve • Mobius syndrome • Gracilis

KEY POINTS

- Treatment of bilateral facial paralysis is best accomplished via a multidisciplinary approach.
- Reanimation in bilateral facial paralysis cannot typically be performed using a standard cross-facial nerve graft from the contralateral facial nerve; free functional muscle transfer will be innervated by an alternate source, commonly the nerve to masseter.
- Bilateral facial paralysis is uncommon.

INTRODUCTION

Bilateral facial paralysis is uncommon. With an incidence of approximately 1 in 5,000,000 annually, the condition accounts for only 0.3% to 3%[1–3] of all facial paralysis cases. It is seen in both the pediatric and adult populations, and the cause can be congenital or acquired.

There are multiple potential causes of bilateral facial paralysis, many of which are similar to those in unilateral facial paralysis. The source may be infectious, autoimmune, traumatic, iatrogenic, metabolic, idiopathic, or congenital.

Bilateral facial paralysis can have a variety of functional and psychosocial effects depending on involved anatomic distributions and circumstances of paralysis. Upper facial dysfunction can threaten ocular integrity through lagophthalmos and resulting corneal exposure. Lower facial paralysis not only affects the ability to smile but can also impair speech and ability to eat. The decreased ability to emote inhibits nonverbal communication and can be a significant psychosocial detriment.[4] In the pediatric population with congenital palsy, this can hinder social integration, becoming especially problematic.

Depending on the cause, bilateral facial nerve palsy may be self-limited or amenable to medical management. However, when conservative or medical treatment fails or

Disclosures: The authors have nothing to disclose.
Division of Plastic and Reconstructive Surgery, The Hospital for Sick Children, 555 University Avenue, Toronto, Ontario M5G 1X8, Canada
* Corresponding author.
E-mail address: Gregory.borschel@sickkids.ca

Otolaryngol Clin N Am 51 (2018) 1213–1226
https://doi.org/10.1016/j.otc.2018.07.014
0030-6665/18/© 2018 Elsevier Inc. All rights reserved.
oto.theclinics.com

the cause dictates a natural history of permanent paralysis, surgical intervention is required to restore cosmetic resting tone or facial animation.

Determining the cause and time course of paralysis is paramount in devising a treatment approach. This article reviews the differential diagnosis of bilateral facial paralysis and discusses evaluation and management of these patients. Surgical treatment options, with focus on the authors' technique for free functional muscle transfer for smile restoration in the congenital population, are reviewed.

CAUSES OF BILATERAL FACIAL PARALYSIS

Unlike unilateral facial paralysis, which is most often attributed to Bell palsy, bilateral facial nerve paralysis most commonly has an identifiable cause.[1]

In a recent study by Gaudin and colleagues,[1] although Bell palsy remained the single most common diagnosis, it accounted for only approximately one-third of bilateral facial paralysis cases seen in their unit. Among the remaining patients, the more common diagnoses were Lyme disease, Mobius syndrome, Guillain-Barré syndrome, benign neoplastic processes (ie, neurofibromatosis type 2), vascular malformations, and trauma.

Mobius syndrome is the most common congenital cause of bilateral facial paralysis. This syndrome, which involves variable cranial nerve palsies, as well as limb and chest wall anomalies, occurs in only approximately 1 in every 50,000 live births. The cause is unclear, though it may be related to ischemic or hypoxic events affecting the distribution of the developing subclavian artery. Bilateral cranial nerves VI (abducens) and VII (facial) are the most commonly affected, though others, including the twelfth (hypoglossal, the third most commonly affected nerve), third, fourth, fifth, ninth, and tenth, can be involved. There are known genetic, as well as acquired, causes[5] particularly causes related to misoprostol exposure in utero.[6] Facial paralysis in affected patients is variable and most commonly bilateral.

ASSESSMENT OF THE PATIENT WITH BILATERAL FACIAL PARALYSIS

The cause and time course of paralysis inform the patient's potential for spontaneous functional recovery and the role of medical versus surgical management. These factors, in addition to the specific functions affected and patient goals, influence the course of treatment.

A thorough history (**Table 1**) and physical examination (**Table 2**) are crucial in the workup of the patient with bilateral facial paralysis.

Adjunctive Studies

The need for adjunctive studies, imaging or laboratory, depends on the level of suspicion for a given diagnosis. A gamut of laboratory tests may be required to rule in or rule out infectious or autoimmune causes. MRI will be obtained in diagnosing disorders of the central nervous system. When trauma is suspected, adequate imaging of the skull base, in the form of a fine-cut computed tomography (CT) scan, is used to evaluate for the presence of skull base fractures. Electrodiagnostic studies may be obtained in select patients with acquired palsies to predict the likelihood of spontaneous recovery (they have no role in congenital causes).

MANAGEMENT OF BILATERAL FACIAL PARALYSIS

Management depends on affected functions and patient desires. Both function and cosmesis are addressed. Many aspects of treatment are similar to those used in unilateral facial paralysis.

Table 1 Patient history	

Circumstances of onset	• Recent viral illnesses, otitis media
	• Potential exposure to ticks (Lyme disease)
	• Oncologic history (space occupying lesions or neural tumors)
	• Trauma
	  ○ Blunt force trauma (concern for base of skull fractures)
	  ○ Sharp trauma (concern for direct laceration of the facial nerve)
	• Iatrogenic injury or resection (ie, resection of bilateral acoustic neuroma in neurofibromatosis type 2)
	• Congenital
	  ○ Birth history (potential for trauma due to use of forceps)
	  ○ Associated anomalies (concern for syndromic cause)

Progression and duration of symptoms	• Timing of onset
	  ○ Sudden (more suggestive of trauma or iatrogenic, cerebrovascular incident, or infection)
	  ○ Gradual onset (oncologic concern)
	  ○ Congenital
	• Duration of symptoms
	• Synchronous vs asynchronous palsy
	• Waxing or waning of symptoms
	• Improvement or plateau of recovery and time over which symptoms changed (even in the setting of self-limited processes, improvement is often slow, occurring over several months)

Specific functional deficits	• Eye
	  ○ Changes in ability to blink or close eyes
	  ○ Change in lower lid position
	  ○ History of corneal exposure or degradation of vision or dry eyes
	  ○ Double vision
	• Nasal airway: difficulty breathing through nose
	• Lower face
	  ○ Change in smile
	  ○ Change in speech, particularly with bilabial consonants, such as p and b sounds
	  ○ Drooling
	  ○ Difficulty eating or cheek biting with chewing
	• Other: hyperacusis, loss of taste, dry mouth (may indicate more proximal lesion of the facial nerve)
	• Dysfunction of other cranial nerves (ie, deviation of tongue to 1 side with protrusion)

Psychosocial concerns of the patient	Self-consciousness, difficulties with social interactions, depression, anxiety
Comorbidities	Overall health or previous surgeries may have implications for reconstructive options or the ability of a patient to withstand a free muscle transfer

The dominant concern in upper facial paralysis is impaired eye closure, which can predispose the eye to corneal exposure and threaten vision. In the lower face, loss of oral competence and the ability to smile are primary concerns. Beyond functional implications, altered cosmesis can be distressing for the patient. Although resulting asymmetry may be less prominent in bilateral compared with unilateral facial paralysis, unnatural resting tone and right–left discrepancies due to differential denervation between the 2 sides can be cosmetically disruptive.

Table 2
Physical examination

Affected functions	Examine all distributions of the facial nerve bilaterally, noting asymmetries between the right and left sides, and evaluating the face in both repose and animation
	• Brow ptosis (including assessment for impairment of visual field)
	• Eye
	○ Static: position of lower lid (evaluating for paralytic ectropion)
	○ Dynamic
	■ Ability to close eye in light blink
	■ Ability to close eye with maximal effort
	■ Presence of Bell phenomenon (absence places the cornea at increased risk of damage from exposure)
	○ Corneal examination to assess for damage or irritation and to determine whether the cornea is sensate
	• Mouth
	○ Static: symmetry at rest
	○ Dynamic
	■ Ability to smile and symmetry thereof
	■ Oral competence
	■ Speech intelligibility
	• Nasal airway
	○ Collapse of nasal airway with forced inspiration
Associated palsies	Especially cranial nerves III, V, VI, XI, XII

A multidisciplinary approach to the patient with facial paralysis is critical to optimize outcomes. The makeup of the medical team will vary depending on the cause of the paralysis (ie, the need for infectious disease, rheumatologic, or oncologic treatment). Ophthalmologic intervention should be sought early when there exists any concern for threatened ocular integrity. Physical therapy is essential to maximize recovery in both operative and nonoperative patients. Finally, psychological or social work support can play an important role in the comprehensive care of these patients. The psychosocial effects of facial paralysis can be significant and, especially in the congenital cause population, can have lasting implications for social function.

Conservative Management

Medical management and watchful waiting

For certain causes, such as infectious, autoimmune, and idiopathic, conservative management may be warranted before consideration of surgical treatment. When applicable, medical management should be implemented and directed by appropriate specialists, depending on diagnosis. Infectious causes (bacterial or rickettsial) may benefit from antibiosis. Patients with Bell palsy or autoimmune causes may improve after a course of steroids, as may patients with viral sources (with or without the addition of antivirals). Additionally, for all patients, physical therapy by specially trained therapists can be effective in helping patients to recover strength and relearn specific movements such as eye closure and smile.

Ocular protection

Ocular protection is imperative in all patients with upper facial paralysis. Several nonsurgical modalities (**Box 1**) are used to protect the eye. These serve both as temporizing measures for patients who recover function and as adjuncts to surgery in operative situations.

> **Box 1**
> **Nonsurgical interventions for ocular protection**
>
> Lubricating drops and ointments
>
> Eyelid taping (especially at night)
>
> Protective chambers
>
> Soft contact lenses
>
> Eye patches

Surgical Intervention

When paralysis is congenital or results from physical disruption (ie, traumatic or iatrogenic) of the facial nerve, or when medical or conservative treatment fails, surgical intervention may be warranted.

In general, surgical interventions are classified as static or dynamic. Static procedures restore resting tone to improve symmetry; cosmesis; and, sometimes, function. In the eye, these procedures facilitate closure. In the lower face, they can assist with oral competence. Dynamic procedures restore movement under emotional and/or volitional control.

Static procedures

Eye closure: procedures can target either the upper or lower eyelid (often, both are operated on simultaneously)
- Upper eyelid: to achieve adequate downward excursion of the upper lid
  ○ Gold or platinum weights[7]
  ○ Palpebral spring[8]
  ○ Lateral tarsorrhaphy (rarely used except in cases of corneal anesthesia or failure of other techniques to provide corneal protection)
- Lower lid: improve position in cases of paralytic ectropion[9]
  ○ Canthoplasty or canthopexy: useful in cases of mild-to-moderate lower lid laxity
  ○ Static tendon sling may be necessary in cases of severe lower lid laxity.

Nasal airway collapse
- Alar base fixation and periosteal anchoring
- In more severe cases, alar base elevation and support through use of a tendon or fascia sling.

Brow ptosis: when this generates cosmetic or functional concern (eg, interfering with eye opening and vision), a brow lift (any standard technique) may be considered

Smile or resting tone of lower face and oral competence (not generally recommended in the pediatric population due to success with reanimation procedures and psychosocial benefits of restoring function)
- Oral commissure suspension via dermal or tendon or fascial slings
- Face lift.

Chemodenervation
- Limited utility in bilateral compared with unilateral facial paralysis
- May be beneficial when differential denervation exists between sides, leading to gross asymmetry.

Dynamic procedures

Dynamic procedures available for a given patient depend on the state of both nerve and musculature. In acquired paralysis resulting from traumatic or iatrogenic disruption of the nerve with sparing of muscle, timely reinnervation of the impacted musculature may be an option. Neural input can be restored via nerve repair or nerve transfer.

If viable musculature is absent, as in cases of prolonged denervation or congenital agenesis, options are limited to muscle transfer (free or locoregional).

Nerve repair (primary or via interpositional graft)
- Appropriate in traumatic or iatrogenic cases of acquired facial paralysis in which viable proximal and distal facial nerve stumps can be identified and accessed for repair
- In the setting of a gap between proximal and distal nerve stumps, an interpositional nerve graft will be required for repair
- Repair should be performed within the first year of paralysis; reinnervation is time-dependent and in long-standing facial paralysis (greater than 12–24 months) outcomes are less reliable due to irreversible muscle atrophy and fibrosis.

Nerve transfer
- Appropriate in traumatic or iatrogenic cases of facial paralysis in which viable distal but not proximal facial nerve stumps are available
- Native mimetic musculature must be viable (eg, reinnervation via nerve repair; nerve transfer should be performed within 12–24 months of injury)
- Unlike cases of unilateral facial paralysis, the contralateral facial nerve is most often not a potential source of neural input Donor nerve selection will depend on functionality of other cranial nerves, as well as proximity of the donor nerve to the target facial nerve
  - CN V (specifically, nerve to masseter or deep temporal nerve)
  - CN XI
  - CN XII
- When both blink and smile are to be restored, synkinesis will result if the same donor nerve is used to power both functions
- Interposition grafting between donor and recipient nerves may be required depending on the proximity of donor and recipient nerves.

Locoregional muscle transfer
- May be appropriate options for reanimation in patients who are not good candidates for (or who wish to avoid) free muscle transfer
- Masseter flap
  - Transfer of all[10] or a portion of the masseter muscle
  - May be performed via intraoral approach
  - Generally results in acceptable static tone and imparts motion to the lower face, though the vector of pull results in an unnatural smile
- Temporalis flap: the Labbé method[11] seems to be most effective
  - Disinsertion of insertion to coronoid and rerouting to commissure or periorbital region
  - Provides support or motion to both upper and lower facial regions
  - Before proceeding, availability of neurovascular input must be ensured (may be disrupted in neurosurgical procedures)
  - Generally results in acceptable static tone
  - Results of smile reanimation vary[12]
  - May result in temporal hollowing.

Free functional muscle transfer
- Generally has the potential to produce greater excursion at the commissure than does locoregional muscle transfer, with an appropriate vector

- Options exist for both upper and lower facial movements; in bilateral paralysis (donor nerves are generally limited), lower facial reanimation is the focus; blink is rarely targeted
- Unlike unilateral facial paralysis, the contralateral facial nerve is not generally an option for neural input into the transferred muscle (via cross-facial nerve graft); donor nerve options are generally the same as those considered for nerve transfers (CN V3, XI, XII)
- Multiple muscles have been described for free transfer for facial reanimation (**Box 2**); each has advantages and disadvantages, and often selection rests on surgeon and patient preference
- Free muscle transfer can be performed in a staged fashion or bilaterally simultaneously.

APPROACH TO FREE MUSCLE TRANSFER FOR SMILE IN THE PATIENT WITH BILATERAL FACIAL NERVE PARALYSIS

Here, the authors present our approach to bilateral facial reanimation in the setting of Mobius syndrome. These patients require bilateral transfer of both nerve and muscle units due to congenital absence of the facial nerve and mimetic musculature.

Both the hypoglossal and spinal accessory nerves have been used to power free muscle transfers in these patients.[18,19] However, they each have unique disadvantages. The hypoglossal nerve is the third most commonly affected cranial nerve in Mobius syndrome. Thus, hypoglossal function is often impaired. Not only may it be an unreliable innervation source for a transferred muscle but sacrificing a branch may impair speech and swallowing.

The spinal accessory nerve is rarely affected in Mobius syndrome. However, its distance from target of reinnervation often necessitates an intervening nerve graft. This increases potential for axon loss and ultimately decreased neural input to the transferred muscle.

Our preferred donor is the nerve to masseter, almost always normal in patients with Mobius syndrome and other causes of facial paralysis. Sacrifice of this nerve produces no significant donor deficits. It has a well-defined course[20] and lies in close proximity to the recipient nerve of the muscle flap, permitting primary coaptation.

Box 2
Potential donor muscles for smile reanimation

Muscles described for use in free functional transfers

Gracilis

Pectoralis minor

Rectus abdominis

Latissimus dorsi

Extensor carpi radialis brevis

Serratus anterior

Rectus femoris

Abductor hallucis

Data from Refs.[13–17]

Outcomes studies prove it capable of generating powerful excursion of transferred musculature in smile and also improving lower lip tone to improve oral competence and speech.[21,22] Despite relative inability to achieve spontaneous smile, many patients report eventual ability to smile without clenching teeth or without significant conscious effort.[22–24]

Our preferred muscle for transfer is the partial gracilis, a reliable flap with consistent neurovascular anatomy.[25,26] Harvest leaves a relatively well-hidden scar in the upper medial thigh and minimal donor deficit.[27] Through careful dissection, flap volume is minimized to avoid excessive bulk (while maximizing excursive function).

In children, although our goal is to have bilateral muscle transfer performed before school age, we generally wait until the patient is at least 4 years old before proceeding with the first muscle transfer. This allows anatomic structures (eg, neurovascular pedicles) to be of optimal size and, more importantly, ensures adequate maturity on the part of the patient to be able to participate in postoperative rehabilitation and care of their flaps.

Although some surgeons favor simultaneous bilateral facial reanimation,[28] our preference is to perform staged operations. We reconstruct only 1 side at a time, generally waiting at least 3 months between the 2 surgeries. We do this to decrease procedure length and to minimize chances of postoperative or intraoperative positional compromise of a newly transferred flap. It also permits matching of the insertion geometry.

We use a 2-team approach. While 1 team prepares the face for inset of the muscle flap, the other is at the leg, harvesting and preparing the gracilis flap.

Facial dissection and preparation for muscle transfer
Incision (**Fig. 1**): preauricular
- Superior extent: scalp, in the region of the upper pole of the ear
- Courses inferiorly, preauricularly
- Curves postauricularly as it rounds the lobe
- Extends inferiorly, parallel to the mandibular body, placed in a neck crease; distal extent is midway along the mandibular body

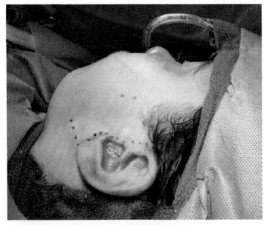

Fig. 1. A preauricular incision is designed, extending from the upper pole of the ear superiorly to below the lobule inferiorly. Inferiorly, it is placed within a neck crease, running parallel to the body of the mandible and extending to approximately its midpoint.

Dissection: mimetic musculature, useful for orientation in other forms of facial paralysis, is absent in patients with Mobius syndrome

- Plane of dissection: superficial to the parotid fascia, deep to subcutaneous fat
- Anterior limit of dissection: anterior border of the masseter
  - After facial vessels are identified (see later discussion) dissection continues to the oral commissure and upper lip
- Superior extent of dissection: body of zygoma

Vasculature: the facial artery and vein are the preferred donor vessels

- Facial vein: runs parallel to the anterior border of the masseter, coursing superiorly toward the mandibular body; transect this superiorly (distally) for coaptation to recipient vein
  - If the facial vein is absent, a large transverse facial vein is usually available for supply
- Facial artery: runs parallel to the mandibular body, anterior to the facial vein, traveling medially toward the oral commissure; transect this close to the oral commissure for coaptation

Placement of sutures for tensioning and definition of vector of smile

- As stitches are placed, the needles are maintained on the suture and tagged for further use (**Fig. 2**)
- Sutures are placed along the course of the facial artery, around the commissure, and onto the upper lip
  - If orbicularis oris is present, these sutures are placed through orbicularis fibers above and below the commissure
  - In Mobius syndrome, the orbicularis is most commonly absent
- Sequential placement
  - First stitch: at the commissure
  - Second stitch: lower lip, creating a vector such that tension generates bilabial closure
  - Third and fourth stitches: upper lip, along the course of the facial artery
- Avoid placing stitches too superficially because this can generate eversion of the upper lip with tension; placing stitches too deeply can lead to inversion
- Simultaneous traction on all sutures should generate a natural-appearing gentle nasolabial crease

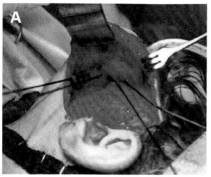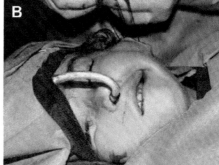

Fig. 2. Sutures are placed around the upper lip, the commissure, and the lateral lower lip to define the vector of smile (*A*). When tension is applied to all sutures simultaneously, a gentle, realistic nasolabial crease should be created (*B*).

o At the second stage, this should be planned to be made symmetric with the contralateral side.

Dissection of masseteric branch (**Fig. 3**)

- The nerve to masseter is reliably located 3 cm anterior to the tragus and 1 cm inferior to the zygomatic arch (this landmarking has proven reliable in both adults and children)[20,29]
- The nerve travels inferomedially between the intermediate and deep lobes of the masseter[30]
- Blunt spreading through the masseter, beginning at the above landmark, will generally lead to identification
- Stimulation with a nerve stimulator can assist in identification; once identified, the nerve is dissected free from surrounding tissues.

Gracilis harvest (**Fig. 4**): similar to harvest for other free functional transfers but place emphasis on minimizing the incision and the size of the flap transferred

Incision: short, 8 cm, at the anterior border of the gracilis

Dissection

- The gracilis is identified just posterior to the adductor longus
- The neurovascular pedicle is protected; it is located between the adductor magnus and adductor longus and enters the gracilis on its undersurface, approximately 6 cm distal to its origin

Length determination and debulking of the muscle

- The length of gracilis required is 2 cm greater than the distance between the oral commissure and the tragus (the extra 2 cm is for suture placement)
- The entrance of the pedicle into the muscle should be at the midpoint of the section harvested; on average, 9 to 11 cm of muscle is required, depending on patient dimensions
- Minimizing cross-section
  - o The topographic portion of the muscle that may be harvested alone depends on the course of the pedicle
  - o Typically, only the anterior 30% to 40% of the muscle is harvested (sometimes a central section must be harvested instead)

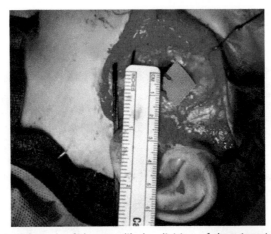

Fig. 3. The masseteric branch of the mandibular division of the trigeminal nerve is found 3 cm anterior to the tragus and 1 cm inferior to the zygomatic arch. It is identified deep within the masseter. Approximately 1 cm of length can be obtained through careful dissection.

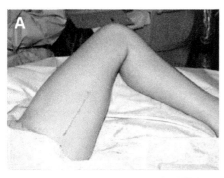
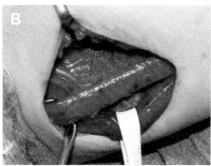
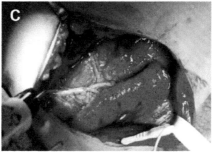

Fig. 4. The gracilis is harvested through a minimized incision in the medial thigh. This incision is centered at the expected location of the pedicle (*A*). Once dissected, the gracilis is split longitudinally such that only the anterior portion is harvested (*B*). The nerve to the gracilis is stimulated to ensure appropriate contraction of the muscle section before transfer (*C*).

   o The selected portion of muscle is stimulated before transfer to face to ensure satisfactory function.
Muscle inset
   Orientation: the distal end of the gracilis at harvest is placed at the commissure
   Muscle anchoring and neurovascular coaptation (**Fig. 5**)
   • The end of the muscle to be placed at the commissure is oversewn with mattress stitches that serve as anchor points for the previously-placed commissure or lip stitches
   • The previously-placed commissure stitches are placed through the muscle, around the mattress stitches, evenly spaced, approximately 1 cm from the muscle edge

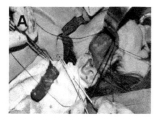
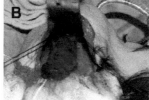
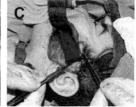

Fig. 5. The previously-placed commissure stitches are placed around the mattress stitches at the distal end of the gracilis. The mattress stitches provide strong anchor points for the commissure stitches.

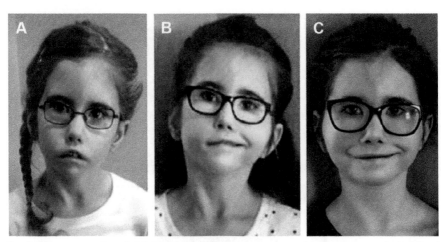

Fig. 6. The same patient (with Mobius syndrome) in attempted smile preoperatively (*A*), after first stage (*left*) gracilis transfer to masseteric nerve (*B*), and after second stage (*right*) gracilis transfer to masseteric nerve (*C*).

- Neurovascular coaptation: neurorrhaphy is performed after vascular anastomoses
- The origin of the gracilis is inset in the tragal region following neurovascular coaptation
  - Anchor securely to temporal fascia
  - Unlike cases of unilateral paralysis, there is no normal contralateral tension for reference to match the tension of muscle inset; instead, tension is set such that there is slight movement at the oral commissure
    - Some excess muscle may need to be trimmed at the tragal end of the flap

Drain placement: a Penrose drain is placed just behind the ear, away from the vessels.

Postoperative management

Muscle function is often first noted after approximately 6 to 7 weeks (**Fig. 6**)[22]

In the Mobius syndrome population, little physical therapy is generally required to train new movement

Maximal excursion usually occurs shortly after the first signs of movement, in as little as 2 weeks.

SUMMARY

Treatment of the patient with bilateral facial paralysis follows many of the same principles of management of unilateral paralysis. However, facial reanimation in this population, especially in the setting of congenital palsy, is limited to muscle transfer (generally free) without the potential for cross-facial nerve grafting. Bilateral partial gracilis transfer with innervation from the nerve to masseter produces effective results in terms of smile, oral competence, and speech.

REFERENCES

1. Gaudin RA, Jowett N, Banks CA, et al. Bilateral facial paralysis: a 13-year experience. Plast Reconstr Surg 2016;138(4):879–87.

2. Stahl N, Ferit T. Recurrent bilateral peripheral facial palsy. J Laryngol Otol 1989; 103(1):117–9.

3. Jain V, Deshmukh A, Gollomp S. Bilateral facial paralysis: Case presentation and discussion of differential diagnosis. J Gen Intern Med 2006;21(7). https://doi.org/10.1111/j.1525-1497.2006.00466.x.

4. Briegel W. Self-perception of children and adolescents with Mobius sequence. Res Dev Disabil 2012;33(1):54–9.

5. Kadakia S, Helman SN, Schwedhelm T, et al. Examining the genetics of congenital facial paralysis—a closer look at Moebius syndrome. Oral Maxillofac Surg 2015;19(2):109–16.

6. Pastuszak AL, Schuler L, Speck-Martins CE, et al. Use of misoprostol during pregnancy and Mobius' syndrome in infants. N Engl J Med 1998;338(26):1881–5.

7. Manktelow RT. Use of the gold weight for lagophthalmos. Operat Tech Plast Reconstr Surg 1999;6(3):157–8.

8. Levine RE, Shapiro JP. Reanimation of the paralyzed eyelid with the enhanced palpebral spring or the gold weight: Modern replacements for tarsorrhaphy. Facial Plast Surg 2001;16(4):325–36.

9. Pepper JP, Kim JC, Massry GG. A surgical algorithm for lower eyelid resuspension in facial nerve paralysis. Operat Tech Plast Reconstr Surg 2012;23(4):248–52.

10. Baker DC, Conley J. Regional muscle transposition for rehabilitation of the paralyzed face. Clin Plast Surg 1979;6(3):317–31. Available at: http://www.ncbi.nlm.nih.gov/pubmed/385211.

11. Labbé D, Huault M. Lengthening temporalis myoplasty and lip reanimation. Plast Reconstr Surg 2000;105(4):1289–97.

12. Bos R, Reddy SG, Mommaerts MY. Lengthening temporalis myoplasty versus free muscle transfer with the gracilis flap for long-standing facial paralysis: a systematic review of outcomes. J Craniomaxillofac Surg 2016;44(8):940–51.

13. Terzis JK. Pectoralis minor: a unique muscle for correction of facial palsy. Plast Reconstr Surg 1989;83(5):767–76.

14. Yang D, Morris SF, Tang M, et al. A modified longitudinally split segmental rectus femoris muscle flap transfer for facial reanimation: Anatomic basis and clinical applications. J Plast Reconstr Aesthet Surg 2006;59(8):807–14.

15. Dellon AL, Mackinnon SE. Segmentally innervated latissimus dorsi muscle. Microsurgical transfer for facial reanimation. J Reconstr Microsurg 1985;2(1):7–12.

16. Liu AT, Lin Q, Jiang H, et al. Facial reanimation by one-stage microneurovascular free abductor hallucis muscle transplantation: Personal experience and long-term outcomes. Plast Reconstr Surg 2012;130(2):325–35.

17. Sugg KB, Kim JC. Dynamic reconstruction of the paralyzed face, part II: Extensor digitorum brevis, serratus anterior, and anterolateral thigh. Oper Tech Otolaryngol Head Neck Surg 2012;23(4):275–81.

18. Zuker RM, Manktelow RT. A smile for the Mobius' syndrome patient. Ann Plast Surg 1989;22(3):188–94.

19. Terzis JK, Noah EM. Dynamic restoration in Mobius and Mobius-like patients. Plast Reconstr Surg 2003;111(1):40–55.

20. Borschel GH, Kawamura DH, Kasukurthi R, et al. The motor nerve to the masseter muscle: An anatomic and histomorphometric study to facilitate its use in facial reanimation. J Plast Reconstr Aesthet Surg 2012;65(3):363–6.

21. Bae YC, Zuker RM, Manktelow RT, et al. A comparison of commissure excursion following gracilis muscle transplantation for facial paralysis using a cross-face

nerve graft versus the motor nerve to the masseter nerve. Plast Reconstr Surg 2006;117(7):2407–13.

22. Zuker RM, Goldberg CS, Manktelow RT. Facial animation in children with Mobius syndrome after segmental gracilis muscle transplant. Plast Reconstr Surg 2000; 106(1):1–8.

23. Lifchez SD, Matloub HS, Gosain AK. Cortical adaptation to restoration of smiling after free muscle transfer innervated by the nerve to the masseter. Plast Reconstr Surg 2005;115(6):1472–9.

24. Marre D, Hontanilla B. Brain plasticity in Mobius syndrome after unilateral muscle transfer: case report and review of the literature. Ann Plast Surg 2012;68(1): 97–100.

25. Juricic M, Vaysse P, Guitard J, et al. Anatomic basis for use of a gracilis muscle flap. Surg Radiol Anat 1993;15(3):163–8.

26. Morris SF, Yang D. Gracilis muscle: Arterial and neural basis for subdivision. Ann Plast Surg 1999;42(6):630–3.

27. Deutinger M, Kuzbari R, Patemostro-Sluga T, et al. Donor-site morbidity of the gracilis flap. Plast Reconstr Surg 1995;95(7):1240–4.

28. Lindsay RW, Hadlock TA, Cheney ML. Bilateral simultaneous free gracilis muscle transfer: A realistic option in management of bilateral facial paralysis. Otolaryngol Head Neck Surg 2009;141(1):139–41.

29. Mundschenk MB, Sachanandani NS, Borschel GH, et al. Motor nerve to the masseter: A pediatric anatomic study and the "3:1 rule. J Plast Reconstr Aesthet Surg 2018;71(1):54–6.

30. Fisher MD, Zhang Y, Erdmann D, et al. Dissection of the masseter branch of the trigeminal nerve for facial reanimation. Plast Reconstr Surg 2013;131(5):1065–7.

Moving?

Make sure your subscription moves with you!

To notify us of your new address, find your **Clinics Account Number** (located on your mailing label above your name), and contact customer service at:

Email: journalscustomerservice-usa@elsevier.com

800-654-2452 (subscribers in the U.S. & Canada)
314-447-8871 (subscribers outside of the U.S. & Canada)

Fax number: 314-447-8029

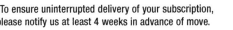

Elsevier Health Sciences Division
Subscription Customer Service
3251 Riverport Lane
Maryland Heights, MO 63043

*To ensure uninterrupted delivery of your subscription, please notify us at least 4 weeks in advance of move.